PHYSICAL PRINCIPLES OF MEDICAL IMAGING

Perry Sprawls, Jr., Ph.D., F.A.C.R.
Professor of Radiology
Emory University School of Medicine
Atlanta, Georgia

AN ASPEN PUBLICATION®
Aspen Publishers, Inc.

1987

Rockville, Maryland
Royal Tunbridge Wells

Library of Congress Cataloging-in-Publication Data

Sprawls, Perry.
Physical prinicples of medical imaging.

"An Aspen publication."
Includes bibliographies and index.
1. Diagnostic imaging. 2. Medical physics. I. Title.
[DNLM: 1. Health Physics. 2. Nuclear Magnetic Resonance.
3. Radiography. 4. Technology, Radiologic.
5. Tomography, X-Ray Computed. Ultrasonic Diagnosis.
WN 110 S767pb]
RC78.7.D53S63   1987   616.07'54   87-1223
ISBN: 0-87189-644-3

The authors have made every effort to ensure the accuracy of the information herein. However, appropriate information sources should be consulted, especially for new or unfamiliar drugs or procedures. It is the responsibility of every practitioner to evaluate the appropriateness of a particular opinion in the context of actual clinical situations and with due consideration to new developments. Authors, editors, and the publisher cannot be held responsible for any typographical or other errors found in this book.

Editorial Services: Carolyn Ormes

Library of Congress Catalog Card Number: 87-1223
ISBN: 0-87189-644-3

Printed in the United States of America

1 2 3 4 5

Contents

Preface

The effective use of any medical imaging modality and the interpretation of images requires some understanding of the physical principles of the image formation process. This is because the ability to visualize specific anatomical structures or pathologic conditions depends on the inherent characteristics of a particular modality and the set of imaging factors selected by the user. The relationship between visibility and imaging factors is rather complex and often involves compromises and trade-offs among the different aspects of image quality.

All imaging methods deposit some form of energy in the patient's body. This is not always without risk. Radiation exposure is usually a variable factor and often has an effect on image quality. An optimized image procedure is one in which these two factors, image quality and radiation exposure, are properly balanced.

This book provides the physics and scientific knowledge that will enable the physician to make appropriate technical decisions in all phases of the imaging process.

It is written primarily for physicians studying in a radiology residency program but is also a useful reference for the practicing radiologist who is faced with day-to-day decisions concerning imaging equipment, procedures, and patient safety.

This text contains much of the material from the author's previous books: *The Physical Principles of Diagnostic Radiology* and *The Physics and Instrumentation of Nuclear Medicine*. That material has been updated and supplemented, particularly in the areas of computed tomography and magnetic resonance imaging.

The selection of topics and presentation of concepts is based on the physics component of the radiology residency program at Emory University. It assumes no previous knowledge of physics but rather a sincere desire on the part of the reader to understand the physical principles of the medical imaging profession.

The specific objectives are to enhance the reader's ability to:

- understand the basic principles of image formation
- select imaging factors that are appropriate for specific clinical requirements
- optimize imaging procedures with respect to image quality and patient exposure
- communicate effectively with members of the technical staff
- make intelligent decisions when selecting equipment and imaging supplies.

Acknowledgments

The preparation of this book has been aided by the significant contributions of many individuals, whom I gratefully acknowledge.

Margaret Nix typed and edited the manuscript and coordinated its production. Dr. Jack E. Peterson has provided much valuable advice and editorial support. Jake D. Paulk, Alan Foust, and Lee Burns produced the illustrations.

My wife Charlotte has graciously provided editorial assistance. Several colleagues have reviewed specific parts of the manuscript and contributed many helpful suggestions. These include Drs. Jack E. Peterson, Robert H. Rohrer, Gary T. Barnes, R. Roger Sankey, and Robert Harbot.

I wish to express my sincere appreciation to Dr. H.S. Weens, former Chairman, Department of Radiology, for his many years of encouragement and support in the development of diagnostic radiological physics at Emory University. It was his interest and high standards in training future radiologists that has made this book possible.

The support and guidance of Dr. William J. Casarella, Chairman, Department of Radiology, has been a significant factor in the development of the educational programs and materials for the new imaging modalities.

Chapter 1

Image Characteristics and Quality

INTRODUCTION AND OVERVIEW

To the human observer, the internal structures and functions of the human body are not generally visible. However, by various technologies, images can be created through which the medical professional can look into the body to diagnose abnormal conditions and guide therapeutic procedures. The medical image is a window to the body. No image window reveals everything. Different medical-imaging methods reveal different characteristics of the human body. With each method, the range of image quality and structure visibility can be considerable, depending on characteristics of the imaging equipment, skill of the operator, and compromises with factors such as patient radiation exposure and imaging time.

Figure 1-1 is an overview of the medical imaging process. The five major components are the patient, the imaging system, the system operator, the image itself, and the observer. The objective is to make an object or condition within the patient's body visible to the observer. The visibility of specific anatomical features depends on the characteristics of the imaging system and the manner in which it is operated. Most medical imaging systems have a considerable number of variables that must be selected by the operator. They can be changeable system components, such as intensifying screens in radiography, transducers in sonography, or coils in magnetic resonance imaging (MRI). However, most variables are adjustable physical quantities associated with the imaging process such as kilovoltage in radiography, gain in sonography, and echo time (TE) in MRI. The values selected will determine the quality of the image and the visibility of specific body features.

The ability of an observer to detect signs of a pathologic process depends on a combination of three major factors: (1) image quality, (2) viewing conditions, and (3) observer performance characteristics.

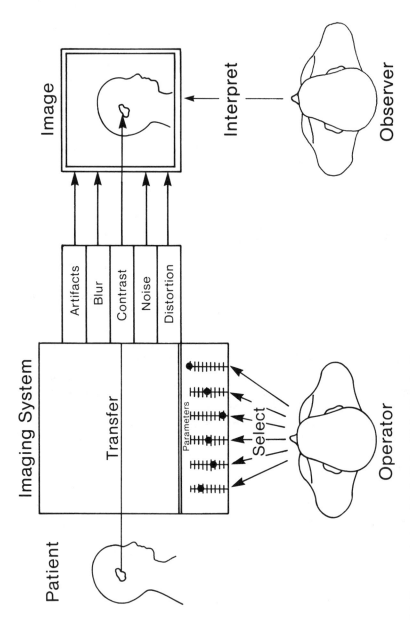

Figure 1-1 Components Associated with the Medical Imaging Process

IMAGE QUALITY

The quality of a medical image is determined by the imaging method, the characteristics of the equipment, and the imaging variables selected by the operator. Image quality is not a single factor but is a composite of at least five factors: contrast, blur, noise, artifacts, and distortion, as shown in Figure 1-1. The relationships between image quality factors and imaging system variables are discussed in detail in later chapters.

The human body contains many structures and objects that are simultaneously imaged by most imaging methods. We often consider a single object in relation to its immediate background. In fact, with most imaging procedures the visibility of an object is determined by this relationship rather than by the overall characteristics of the total image.

Consider Figure 1-2. The task of every imaging system is to translate a specific tissue characteristic into image shades of gray or color. If contrast is adequate, the object will be visible. The degree of contrast in the image depends on characteristics of both the object and the imaging system.

Image Contrast

Contrast means difference. In an image, contrast can be in the form of different shades of gray, light intensities, or colors. Contrast is the most fundamental characteristic of an image. An object within the body will be visible in an image only if it has sufficient physical contrast relative to surrounding tissue. However, image contrast much beyond that required for good object visibility generally serves no useful purpose and in many cases is undesirable.

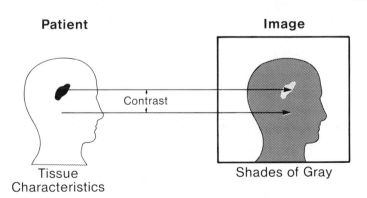

Figure 1-2 Medical Imaging Is the Process of Converting Tissue Characteristics into a Visual Image

The physical contrast of an object must represent a difference in one or more tissue characteristics. For example, in radiography, objects can be imaged relative to their surrounding tissue if there is an adequate difference in either density or atomic number and if the object is sufficiently thick.

When a value is assigned to contrast, it refers to the difference between two specific points or areas in an image. In most cases we are interested in the contrast between a specific structure or object in the image and the area around it or its background.

Contrast Sensitivity

The degree of physical object contrast required for an object to be visible in an image depends on the imaging method and the characteristics of the imaging system. The primary characteristic of an imaging system that establishes the relationship between image contrast and object contrast is its contrast sensitivity. Consider the situation shown in Figure 1-3. The circular objects are the same size but are filled with different concentrations of iodine contrast medium. That is, they have different levels of object contrast. When the imaging system has a relatively low contrast sensitivity, only objects with a high concentration of iodine (ie, high object contrast) will be visible in the image. If the imaging system has a high contrast sensitivity, the lower-contrast objects will also be visible.

We emphasize that contrast sensitivity is a characteristic of the imaging method and the variables of the particular imaging system. It is the characteristic that relates to the system's ability to translate physical object contrast into image contrast. The contrast transfer characteristic of an imaging system can be considered from two perspectives. From the perspective of adequate image contrast for object visibility, an increase in system contrast sensitivity causes lower-contrast objects to become visible. However, if we consider an object with a fixed degree of physical contrast (ie, a fixed concentration of contrast medium), then increasing contrast sensitivity will increase image contrast.

It is difficult to compare the contrast sensitivity of various imaging methods because many are based on different tissue characteristics. However, certain methods do have higher contrast sensitivity than others. For example, computed tomography (CT) generally has a higher contrast sensitivity than conventional radiography. This is demonstrated by the ability of CT to image soft tissue objects (masses) that cannot be imaged with radiography. The specific factors that determine the contrast sensitivity of each imaging method are considered in later chapters.

Consider Figure 1-4. Here is a series of objects with different degrees of physical contrast. They could be vessels filled with different concentrations of contrast medium. The highest concentration (and contrast) is at the bottom. Now imagine a curtain coming down from the top and covering some of the objects so

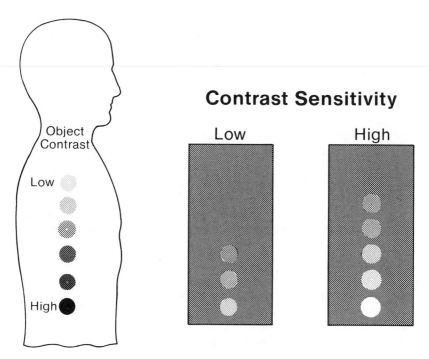

Figure 1-3 Increasing Contrast Sensitivity Increases Image Contrast and the Visibility of Objects in the Body

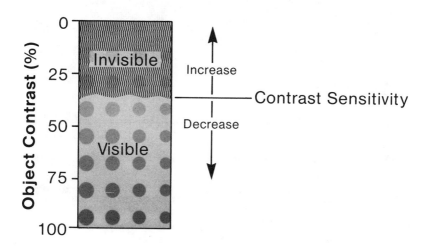

Figure 1-4 Effect of Contrast Sensitivity on Object Visibility

that they are no longer visible. Contrast sensitivity is the characteristic of the imaging system that raises and lowers the curtain. Increasing sensitivity raises the curtain and allows us to see more objects in the body. A system with low contrast sensitivity allows us to visualize only objects with relatively high inherent physical contrast.

Blur and Visibility of Detail

Structures and objects in the body vary not only in physical contrast but also in size. Objects range from large organs and bones to small structural features such as trabecula patterns and small calcifications. It is the small anatomical features that add detail to a medical image. Each imaging method has a limit as to the smallest object that can be imaged and thus on visibility of detail. Visibility of detail is limited because all imaging methods introduce blurring into the process. The primary effect of image blur is to reduce the contrast and visibility of small objects or detail.

Consider Figure 1-5, which represents the various objects in the body in terms of both physical contrast and size. As we said, the boundary between visible and invisible objects is determined by the contrast sensitivity of the imaging system. We now extend the idea of our curtain to include the effect of blur. It has little effect on the visibility of large objects but it reduces the contrast and visibility of small objects. When blur is present, and it always is, our curtain of invisibility covers small objects and image detail. Blur and visibility of detail are discussed in more depth in Chapter 18.

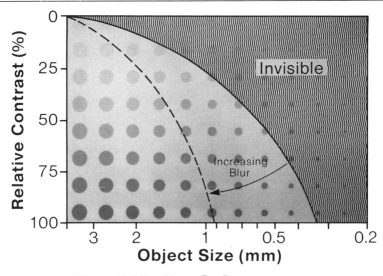

Figure 1-5 Effect of Blur on Visibility of Image Detail

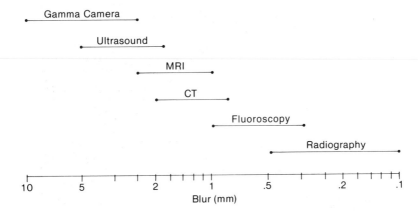

Figure 1-6 Range of Blur Values and Visibility of Detail Obtained with Various Imaging Methods

---

The amount of blur in an image can be quantified in units of length. This value represents the width of the blurred image of a small object. Figure 1-6 compares the approximate blur values for medical imaging methods. As a general rule, the smallest object or detail that can be imaged has approximately the same dimensions as those of the image blur.

Noise

Another characteristic of all medical images is image noise. Image noise, sometimes referred to as image mottle, gives an image a textured or grainy appearance. The source and amount of image noise depend on the imaging method and are discussed in more detail in Chapter 21. We now briefly consider the effect of image noise on visibility.

In Figure 1-7 we find our familiar array of body objects arranged according to physical contrast and size. We now add a third factor, noise, which will affect the boundary between visible and invisible objects. The general effect of increasing image noise is to lower the curtain and reduce object visibility. In most medical imaging situations the effect of noise is most significant on the low-contrast objects that are already close to the visibility threshold.

Artifacts

We have seen that several characteristics of an imaging method (contrast sensitivity, blur, and noise) cause certain body objects to be invisible. Another problem is that most imaging methods can create image features that do not

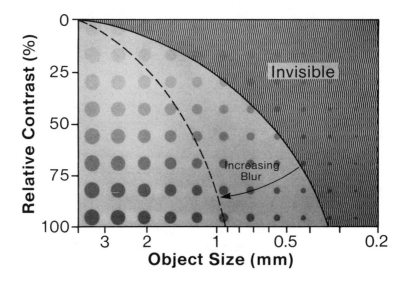

Figure 1-7 Effect of Noise on Object Visibility

represent a body structure or object. These are image artifacts. In many situations an artifact does not significantly affect object visibility and diagnostic accuracy. But artifacts can obscure a part of an image or may be interpreted as an anatomical feature. A variety of factors associated with each imaging method can cause image artifacts.

Distortion

A medical image should not only make internal body objects visible, but should give an accurate impression of their size, shape, and relative positions. An imaging procedure can, however, introduce distortion of these three factors.

Compromises

It would be logical to raise the question as to why we do not adjust each imaging procedure to yield maximum visibility. The reason is that in many cases the variables that affect image quality also affect factors such as radiation exposure to the patient and imaging time. In general, an imaging procedure should be set up to produce adequate image quality and visibility without excessive patient exposure or imaging time.

In many situations, if a variable is changed to improve one characteristic of image quality, such as noise, it often adversely affects another characteristic, such as blur and visibility of detail. Therefore an imaging procedure must be selected according to the specific requirements of the clinical examination.

TISSUE CHARACTERISTICS AND IMAGE VIEWS

A combination of two factors makes each imaging method unique. These are the tissue characteristics which are visible in the image and the viewing perspective.

The specific tissue characteristics that produce the various shades of gray and image contrast vary among the various modalities and methods.

A radiologist uses an image to search for signs of a pathologic condition or injury in the body. Signs can be observed only if the condition produces a physical change in the associated tissue. Many pathologic conditions produce a change in a physical characteristic that can be imaged by one method but not another.

Imaging methods create images that show the body from one of two perspectives, through either projection or tomographic imaging. There are advantages and disadvantages to each.

In projection imaging (radiography and fluoroscopy), images are formed by projecting an x-ray beam through the patient's body and casting shadows onto an appropriate receptor that converts the invisible x-ray image into a visible light image. The gamma camera records a projection image that represents the distribution of radioactive material in the body. The primary advantage of this type of image is that a large volume of the patient's body can be viewed with one image. A disadvantage is that structures and objects are often superimposed so that the image of one might interfere with the visibility of another. Projection imaging produces spatial distortion that is generally not a major problem in most clinical applications.

Tomographic imaging, ie, conventional tomography, computed tomography (CT), sonography, single photon emission tomography (SPECT), positron emission tomography (PET), and MRI, produces images of selected planes or slices of tissue in the patient's body. The general advantage of a tomographic image is the increased visibility of objects within the imaged plane. One factor that contributes to this is the absence of overlying objects. The major disadvantage is that only a small slice of a patient's body can be visualized with one image. Therefore, most tomographic procedures usually require many images to survey an entire organ system or body cavity.

IMAGE VIEWING CONDITIONS

Our ability to see a specific object or feature in an image depends on the conditions under which we view the image. We must deal with the effects of viewing conditions in many activities in addition to the professional interpretation of medical images. Dim candlelight enhances the pleasure of a fine dinner but often makes it difficult to read the menu. The glare of an oncoming automobile headlight reduces our ability to see objects in the road and also produces discomfort and stress. We quickly learn that there is an optimum viewing distance for television sets, newspapers, etc. A small object dropped onto the smooth surface of the dining table is easier to see than an object dropped onto a textured carpet or sandy beach. With these experiences in mind, let us consider the factors associated with image viewing conditions and how they affect our ability to visualize body structures.

Figure 1-8 shows the primary factors that affect our ability to see or detect an object in an image. We will assume a circular object located within a larger background area. The ability of an observer to detect the object depends on a combination of factors including object contrast and size, background, brightness (luminance) and structure (texture), glare produced by other light sources, distance between the image and the observer, and the time available to search for the object.

Figure 1-9 is an image of the array of objects we used to demonstrate the effects of image quality factors. We now use it to demonstrate how the factors associated with the viewing process affect our ability to see the objects. You can use this actual image to test the factors discussed below.

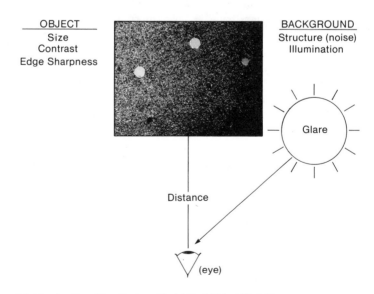

Figure 1-8 Viewing Condition Factors That Affect Object Visibility

Object Contrast

The ability to see or detect an object is heavily influenced by the contrast between the object and its background. For most viewing tasks there is not a specific threshold contrast at which the object suddenly becomes visible. Instead, the accuracy of seeing or detecting a specific object increases with contrast.

The contrast sensitivity of the human viewer changes with viewing conditions. When viewer contrast sensitivity is low, an object must have a relatively high contrast to be visible. The degree of contrast required depends on conditions that alter the contrast sensitivity of the observer: background brightness, object size, viewing distance, glare, and background structure.

Background Brightness

The human eye can function over a large range of light levels or brightness, but vision is not equally sensitive at all brightness levels. The ability to detect objects generally increases with increasing background brightness or image illumination. To be detected in areas of low brightness, an object must have a relatively high level of contrast with respect to its background. This can be demonstrated with the image in Figure 1-9. View this image with different levels of illumination. You will notice that under low illumination you cannot see all of the low-contrast objects. A higher level of object contrast is required for visibility.

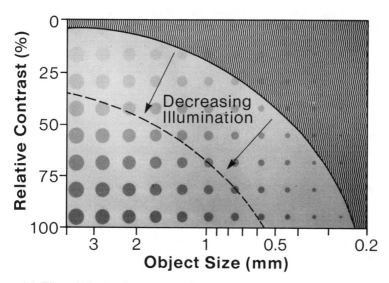

Figure 1-9 Effect of Viewing Conditions on Object Visibility

Object Size

The relationship between the degree of contrast required for detectability and for background brightness is influenced by the size of the object. Small objects require either a higher level of contrast or increased background brightness to be detected.

The detectability of an object is more closely related to the angle it forms in the visual field. The angle is the ratio of object diameter to the distance between image and observer. In principle, a small object will have the same detectability at close range as a larger object viewed at a greater distance.

Viewing Distance

The relationship between visibility and viewing distance is affected by several factors. When the viewing distance is reduced, an object creates a larger angle and is generally easier to see. However, the eye does not focus and exhibit maximum contrast sensitivity at close range. Therefore, the relationship between detectability and viewing distance generally peaks at a distance of approximately 2 ft.

Glare

Glare is produced by bright areas or light sources in the field of view and has several undesirable effects. One effect is to reduce the perceived contrast of the objects viewed. When light from the glare-producing source enters the eye, some of it is scattered over other areas within the visual field. This in turn reduces contrast sensitivity. The extent to which it is reduced depends on the brightness and size of the glare source and its proximity to the object viewed.

Background Structure

The structure or texture of an object's background has a significant effect on its visibility. A smooth background produces maximum visibility; visibility of low-contrast objects is often reduced because of the texture of surrounding tissues or image noise.

OBSERVER PERFORMANCE

In many situations, the presence of a specific object or sign is not obvious but requires establishment by a trained observer. The criteria used to establish the presence of a specific sign often vary among observers. Individual observers also use different criteria, often influenced by the clinical significance of a specific observation.

Let us assume we have a relatively large number of cases to be examined by means of a medical imaging procedure, and that a specific pathologic condition is present in some and absent in others. The ideal situation would be if the condition were diagnosed as positive when present and negative when absent. In actual practice, this is usually not achieved. A more realistic situation is represented in Figure 1-10. Here we see that a fraction of the pathological conditions were diagnosed as positive. This fraction (or percentage) represents the *sensitivity* of the specific diagnostic procedure. We also see that the condition was not always diagnosed as negative when absent. The percentage of these cases diagnosed as negative represents the *specificity* of the procedure.

The diagnoses derived from the imaging procedure divide the cases into four categories, as shown in Figure 1-11: true positives, true negatives, false positives, and false negatives. In the ideal situation, there are only true positives and true negatives. This would be a diagnostic process with 100% accuracy.

False negatives and false positives occur for a number of reasons, including inherent limitations of a specific imaging method, selection of inappropriate imaging factors, poor viewing conditions, and the performance of the observer (radiologist).

In general, if an observer is aggressive in trying to increase the number of true positives (sensitivity), the number of false negatives (decreased specificity) also increases. The relationship between sensitivity and specificity for a specific diagnostic test (including observer performance) can be described by a graph (shown in Figure 1-12) known as a receiver operating characteristic (ROC) curve.

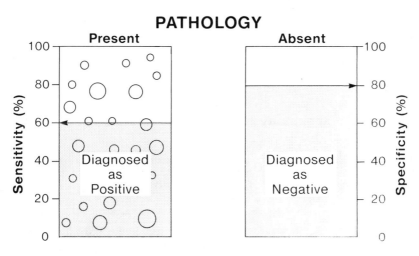

Figure 1-10 Sensitivity and Specificity

PATHOLOGY

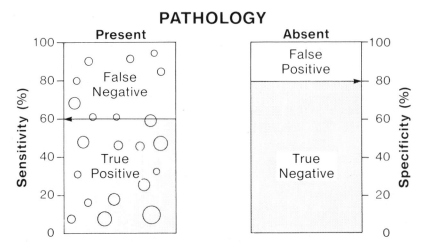

Figure 1-11 Relationship of True and False Diagnostic Decisions to Sensitivity and Specificity

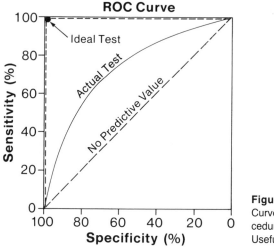

Figure 1-12 Comparison of ROC Curves for an Ideal Diagnostic Procedure with One That Produces No Useful Information

The ideal diagnostic test produces 100% sensitivity and 100% specificity as shown. If a diagnostic procedure has no predictive value, and the diagnosis is obtained by a random selection process, the relationship between sensitivity and specificity is linear as shown. The observer determines the actual operating point along this line. Since this particular diagnostic procedure is providing no useful information, an attempt to increase the sensitivity by calling a greater number of positives will produce a proportionate decrease in the specificity.

The relationship between sensitivity and specificity for most medical imaging procedures is between the ideal and no predictive value. The ROC curve shown in Figure 1-13 is typical. The characteristics of the imaging method and the quality of the resulting image determine the shape of the curve and the relationship between sensitivity and specificity for a specific pathological condition. The criteria used by the observer to make the diagnosis determine the point on the curve that produces the actual sensitivity and specificity values.

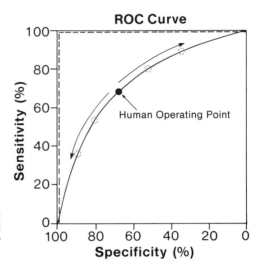

Figure 1-13 An ROC Curve for a Specific Imaging Procedure. The Actual Operating Point Is Determined by Characteristics of the Observer

Chapter 2

Energy and Radiation

INTRODUCTION AND OVERVIEW

There are two components of the physical universe: energy and matter. In most physical processes there is a constant interaction and exchange between the two; medical imaging is no exception. In all imaging methods, images are formed by the interaction of energy and human tissue (matter). A variety of energy types are used in medical imaging. This is, in part, what accounts for the difference in imaging methods. In this chapter we review some basic energy concepts and then look in detail at radiation, which is energy on the move, and the role of electrons in energy transfer.

Images of internal body structures require a transfer of energy from an energy source to the human body and then from the body to an appropriate receptor, as shown in Figure 2-1. Although the types might be different, certain characteristics apply to all energy used in imaging.

A basic requirement is that the energy must be able to penetrate the human body. Visible light is the primary type of energy used to transfer image information in everyday life. However, because it usually cannot penetrate the human body, we must use other energy types for internal body imaging.

Another characteristic of any energy used for imaging is that it must interact with internal body structures in a manner that will create image information.

A common element of all imaging methods is that a large portion of the energy used is deposited in the human tissue. It does not reside in the body as the same type of energy but is converted into other energy forms such as heat and chemical change. The possibility that the deposited energy will produce an undesirable biological effect must always be considered.

As we approach the process of medical imaging, it is helpful to recognize two broad categories of energy. One category is the group of energy forms that require a material in which to exist. The other category is energy that requires no material

17

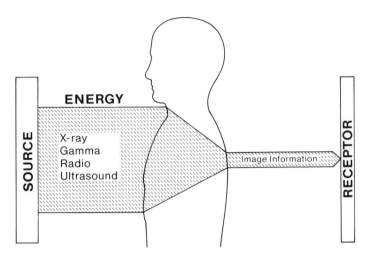

Figure 2-1 Role of Energy in Medical Imaging

object for its existence. Although the latter category does not require matter for its existence, it is always created within a material substance and is constantly moving and transferring energy from one location to another. This form of energy is radiation; all energy forms used for medical imaging, with the exception of ultrasound, are forms of radiation.

ENERGY FORMS AND CONVERSION

The significance of matter-related energy forms in medical imaging is that they supply the energy to form radiation and later recapture it when the radiation is absorbed.

A basic physical principle of the universe is that energy can be neither created nor destroyed. However, we can transform it from one form or type to another. Figure 2-2 shows some of the energy forms used in the production of an x-ray image. Various components of the imaging system convert the energy from one form to another.

RADIATION

Radiation is energy that moves through space from one object, the source, to another object where it is absorbed. Radiation sources are generally collections of matter or devices that convert other forms of energy into radiation. In some cases the energy to be converted is stored within the object. Examples are the sun and radioactive materials. In other cases the radiation source is only an energy

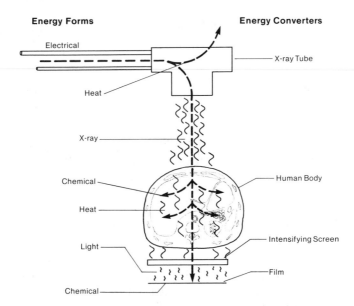

Figure 2-2 Forms of Energy Involved in the Production of an X-Ray Image

converter, and other forms of energy must be applied in order to produce radiation; light bulbs and x-ray tubes are examples.

Most forms of radiation can penetrate through a certain amount of matter. But in most situations, radiation energy is eventually absorbed by the material and converted into another energy form.

Electromagnetic Radiation

There are two general types of radiation, as shown in Figure 2-3. In one type, the energy is "packaged" in small units known as photons or quanta. A photon or quantum of energy contains no matter, only energy. Since it contains no matter, it has no mass or weight. This type of radiation is designated electromagnetic radiation. Within the electromagnetic radiation family are a number of specific radiation types that are used for different purposes. These include such familiar radiations as radio signals, light, x-radiation, and gamma radiation. The designations are determined by the amount of energy packaged in each photon.

Particle Radiation

The other general type of radiation consists of small particles of matter moving through space at a very high velocity. They carry energy because of their motion. Particle radiation comes primarily from radioactive materials, outer space, or

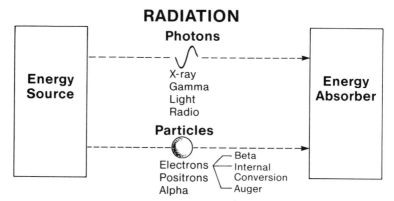

Figure 2-3 Comparison of the Two Basic Types of Radiation

machines that accelerate particles to very high velocities, such as linear accelerators, betatrons, and cyclotrons. Particle radiation differs from electromagnetic radiation in that the particles consist of matter and have mass. The type of particle radiation encountered most frequently in clinical medicine is high-velocity electron radiation. Particle radiation is generally not used as an imaging radiation because of its low tissue penetration. Also, when x-radiation interacts with matter, such as human tissue, it transfers energy to electrons, thus creating a form of electron radiation within the material. Several types of particle radiation are produced as byproducts of photon production by a number of radioactive materials used in medical imaging.

ENERGY UNITS AND RELATED QUANTITIES

There are occasions on which we must consider the quantity of energy involved in a process. Many units are used to quantify energy because of the different unit systems (metric, British, etc.) and the considerable range of unit sizes. At this time, we consider only those energy units encountered in radiological and medical imaging procedures. The primary difference among the energy units to be considered is their size, which in turn determines their specific usage. We use the basic x-ray system in Figure 2-4 to introduce the various energy units.

Joule

The joule (J) is the fundamental unit of energy in the metric International System of Units (SI*). It is the largest unit encountered in radiology. One joule is

*From the French name, Le Système International d'Unités.

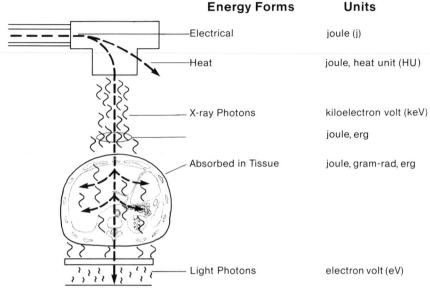

Energy Forms	Units
Electrical	joule (j)
Heat	joule, heat unit (HU)
X-ray Photons	kiloelectron volt (keV)
	joule, erg
Absorbed in Tissue	joule, gram-rad, erg
Light Photons	electron volt (eV)

Figure 2-4 Energy Units Encountered in X-Ray Imaging

equivalent to 1 watt-second. A 100-watt light bulb dissipates 100 J of energy per second. In the next chapter we consider the full range of quantities and units used specifically for radiation; several are energy-related and are defined in terms of the joule or other energy units.

In general the joule is used when relatively large quantities of energy are involved.

Heat Unit

The heat unit was developed within radiology as a convenient unit for expressing the amount of heat energy produced by an x-ray tube. One heat unit is 71% of a joule. The use of the heat unit is discussed in Chapter 9; it is gradually being replaced by the joule.

Gram-Rad

The gram-rad is another unit developed in radiology to express the total radiation energy absorbed by the body. Its usage is discussed in the following chapter. A general trend is to use the joule for this application rather than the gram-rad.

Erg

The erg is a metric energy unit but is not an SI unit. It is much smaller than the joule. Its primary use in radiology is to express the amount of radiation energy absorbed in tissue.

Electron Volt

The electron volt (eV) is the smallest energy unit. It and its multiples, kiloelectron volt (keV) and megaelectron volt (MeV), are used to express the energy of individual electrons and photons. The energy of individual light photons is in the range of a few electron volts. X-ray and gamma photons used in imaging procedures have energies ranging from approximately fifteen to several hundred kiloelectron volts.

The relationships of the three basic energy units are

$$1 \text{ joule} = 10^7 \text{ ergs}$$
$$1 \text{ joule} = 6.24 \times 10^{18} \text{ electron volts.}$$

Power

Power is the term that expresses the rate at which energy is transferred in a particular process. The watt is the unit for expressing power. One watt is equivalent to an energy transfer or conversion at the rate of 1 J/sec. As mentioned above, a 100-watt light bulb converts energy at the rate of 100 J/sec. In medical imaging, power is used to describe the capability of x-ray generators, the limitations of x-ray tubes, the output of ultrasound transducers, the rate at which energy is deposited in tissue during magnetic resonance imaging (MRI), etc.

Intensity

Intensity is the spatial concentration of power and expresses the rate at which energy passes through a unit area. It is typically expressed in watts per square meter or watts per square centimeter. Intensity is also used to express relative values of x-ray exposure rate, light brightness, radio frequency (RF) signal strength in MRI, etc.

THE QUANTUM NATURE OF RADIATION

We have seen that electromagnetic radiation is packaged as individual photons or quanta. This is sometimes referred to as the quantum nature of radiation and

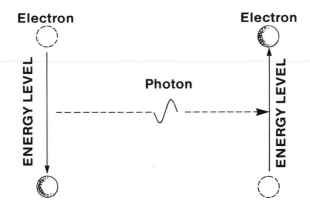

Figure 2-5 The Quantum Nature of Radiation and Matter

becomes an important concept in understanding how radiation is created and absorbed.

Figure 2-5 illustrates the basic quantum characteristics of both radiation and matter. When we consider the structure of matter in Chapter 4 we will find that electrons within atoms generally reside at specific energy levels rather than at arbitrary energy levels. Electrons can move from one energy level to another, but they must go all the way or not at all. These discrete electron energy levels give matter certain quantum characteristics. In simple terms, matter prefers to exchange energy in predefined quantities rather than in arbitrary amounts. Radiation travels through space as a shower of individual photons.

Eventually the photon is absorbed by transferring its energy back to an electron. The chance of its absorption is greatly enhanced if it encounters a material with electron energy levels close to its energy content. The important point here is that radiation photons are created and absorbed individually through energy exchanges within certain materials.

Although radiation photons are differentiated by several physical quantities, as shown in Figure 2-6, all electromagnetic radiation travels with the same velocity through space. Because light is one of the most common forms of electromagnetic radiation and its velocity is known, it is often said that electromagnetic radiations travel with the speed of light. In free space, this is a velocity of about 3×10^8 m/ sec. If we assume that the average x-ray photon travels 1 m between the time it is created and the time it is absorbed, the average lifetime of a photon would be 3.3×10^{-9} seconds. Photons cannot be stored or suspended in space. Once a photon is created and emitted by a source, it travels at this very high velocity until it interacts with and is absorbed by some material. In its very short lifetime, the photon moves a small amount of energy from the source to the absorbing material.

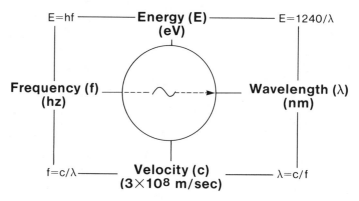

Figure 2-6 Physical Characteristics of a Photon

In Figure 2-7 the scales for the three quantities are shown in relationship to the various types of radiation. While it is possible to characterize any radiation by its photon energy, wavelength, or frequency, the common practice is to use different quantities for different types of radiations, as discussed below.

Photon Energy

Since a photon is simply a unit of energy, its most important characteristic is the quantity of energy it contains. Photon energies are usually specified in units of electron volts or appropriate multiples.

If the various types of electromagnetic radiation were ordered with respect to photon energies, as shown in Figure 2-7, the scale would show the electromagnetic spectrum. It is the energy of the individual photons that determines the type of electromagnetic radiation: light, x-ray, radio signals, etc.

An important aspect of photon energy is that it generally determines the penetrating ability of the radiation. The lower energy x-ray photons are often referred to as soft radiation, whereas those at the higher-energy end of the spectrum would be so-called hard radiation. In most situations, high-energy (hard) x-radiation is more penetrating than the softer portion of the spectrum.

If the individual units of energy, photons or particles, have energies that exceed the binding energy of electrons in the matter through which the radiation is passing, the radiation can interact, dislodge the electrons, and ionize the matter.

The minimum radiation energy that can produce ionization varies from one material to another, depending on the specific electron binding energies. Electron binding energy is discussed in more detail in Chapter 4. The ionization energies for many of the elements found in tissue range between 5 eV and 20 eV. Therefore, all radiations with energies exceeding these values are ionizing radiations.

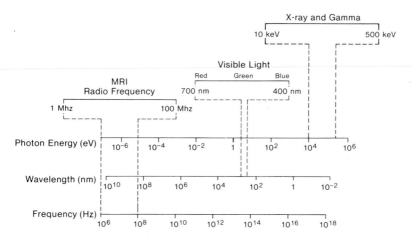

Figure 2-7 The Electromagnetic Spectrum

Photon energy quantities are generally used to describe radiation with relatively high photon energy, such as x-ray, gamma, and cosmic radiation.

Frequency

Frequency is a rate of vibration or oscillation. One of the laws of physics that applies to electromagnetic radiation is that a photon's energy (E) and frequency (f) are directly proportional, with the relationship being

$$E = hf.$$

In this relationship, h is Planck's constant, which has a value of 6.625×10^{-27} erg-second, and f is frequency in hertz (Hz, cycles per second).

Frequency is the most common quantity used to characterize radiations in the lower end, or the RF portion, of the electromagnetic spectrum and includes radiation used for radio and television broadcasts, microwave communications and cooking, and MRI. For example, in MRI, protons emit signals with a frequency of 42.58 MHz when placed in a 1-tesla magnetic field. Although, theoretically, x-radiation has an associated frequency, the concept is never used.

Wavelength

Various physical phenomena observed with electromagnetic radiation suggest that the radiation has certain wavelike properties. A characteristic of a wave is the distance between two successive peaks, which is the wavelength (λ). This is also the distance the radiation moves forward during the period of one oscillation.

Wavelength can be expressed in any unit of length. Radio and television signals have relatively long wavelengths that are usually expressed in meters. For higher energy photons, such as light and x-ray, two smaller length units are used. These are:

$$1 \text{ Ångstrom unit (Å)} = 10^{-10} \text{ m}$$
$$1 \text{ nanometer (nm)} = 10^{-9} \text{ m.}$$

The relationship between photon energy and wavelength is

$$E \text{ (keV)} = 1.24/\lambda \text{ (nm).}$$

This relationship allows the conversion of photon energy into wavelength and vice versa. In some literature, x-ray photon spectra are given in terms of wavelength rather than photon energy. This causes the spectrum curve to have an entirely different appearance. By using the relationship given above, it is possible to convert a spectrum of one kind into the other. Since energy and wavelength are inversely related, the highest energy on the spectrum corresponds to the shortest wavelength.

Wavelength is most frequently used to describe light. At one time it was used to describe x-radiation but that practice is now uncommon. Wavelength is often used to describe radio-type radiations. General terms like "shortwave" and "microwave" refer to the wavelength characteristics of the radiation.

ELECTRONS AND ENERGY

Electrons are the smallest particles found in matter. An electron has a mass of 9.1×10^{-28} g, which means it would take 10.9×10^{26} electrons to equal the weight of 1 cm^3 of water. The question might be raised as to why such a small particle can be the foundation of our modern technology. The answer is simple—numbers. Tremendous numbers of electrons are involved in most applications. For example, when a 100-watt light bulb is turned on, electrons race through the wires carrying energy to it at the rate of 5.2×10^{18} electrons per second. In addition to its mass, each electron carries a 1-unit negative electrical charge. It is the charge of an electron that enables it to interact with other electrons and particles within atoms.

Because an electron has both mass and electrical charge, it can possess energy of several types, as shown in Figure 2-8. It is the ability of an electron to take up, transport, and give up energy that makes it useful in the x-ray system.

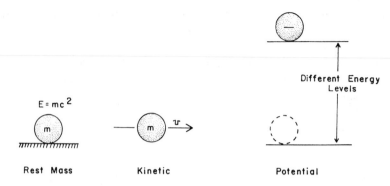

Figure 2-8 Types of Energy Associated with Electrons

Rest Mass Energy

Even when an electron is at rest and has no apparent motion, it still has energy. In fact, according to the laws of physics, an object has some energy just because of its mass. Under certain conditions, mass can be converted into energy and vice versa. Einstein's famous equation

$$E = mc^2$$

predicts the amount of energy that could be obtained if an object with a mass, m, were completely converted. In this relationship, c is the speed of light. Although it is not possible with our present technology to convert most objects into energy, certain radioactive materials emit particles, called positrons, that can annihilate electrons. When this happens, the electron's entire mass is converted into energy. According to Einstein's relationship, each electron will yield 510 keV. This energy appears as a photon. The annihilation of positrons and electrons is the basis for positron emission tomography (PET).

Kinetic Energy

Kinetic energy is associated with motion. It is the type of energy that a moving automobile or baseball has. When electrons are moving, they also have kinetic energy.

Generally, the quantity of kinetic energy an object has is related to its mass and velocity. For large objects, like baseballs and cars, the energy is proportional to the mass of the object and the square of the velocity. Doubling the velocity of such an object increases its kinetic energy by a factor of 4. In many situations, electrons travel with extremely high velocities that approach the velocity of light. At these high velocities, the simple relationship between energy and velocity given above does not hold. One of the theories of relativity states that the mass of an object, such as an electron, changes at high velocities. Therefore, the relationship between energy and velocity becomes complex. Electrons within the typical x-ray tube can have energies in excess of 100 keV and can travel with velocities of more than one-half the speed of light.

Potential Energy

Potential energy is the type of energy possessed by an object because of its location or configuration and is essentially a relative quantity. That is, an object will have more or less energy in one location or configuration than in another. Although there is generally not a position of absolute zero potential energy, certain locations are often designated as the zero-energy level for reference.

Electrons can have two forms of potential energy. One form is related to location within an electrical circuit, and the other is related to location within an atom. One important aspect of electron potential energy is that energy from some source is required to raise an electron to a higher energy level, and that an electron gives up energy when it moves to a lower potential energy position.

Energy Exchange

Because electrons are too small to see, it is sometimes difficult to visualize what is meant by the various types of electron energy. Consider the stone shown in Figure 2-9; we will use it to demonstrate the various types of energy that also apply to electrons.

Potential energy is generally a relative quantity. In this picture, the ground level is arbitrarily designated as the zero potential energy position. When the stone is raised above the ground, it is at a higher energy level. If the stone is placed in a hole below the surface, its potential energy is negative with respect to the ground level. However, its energy is still positive with respect to a position in the bottom of a deeper hole. The stone at position A has zero potential energy (relatively speaking), zero energy because it is not moving, and a rest-mass energy proportional to its mass. (The rest-mass energy of a stone is of no practical use and is not discussed further.) When the man picks up the stone and raises it to position B, he increases its potential energy with respect to position A. The energy gained by the stone comes from the man. (We show later that electrons can be raised to higher potential energy levels by devices called power supplies.) The additional potential energy possessed by the stone at B can be used for work or can be converted into other forms of energy. If the stone were connected to a simple pulley arrangement and allowed to fall back to the ground, it could perform work by raising an object fastened to the other end of the rope.

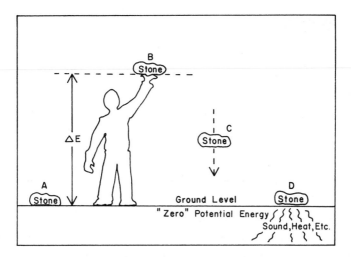

Figure 2-9 Transfer of Energy from One Form to Another

If the man releases the stone at B and allows it to fall back to the ground, its energy is converted into kinetic energy. As the stone moves downward, decreasing its potential energy, which is proportional to its distance above the ground, it constantly increases its speed and kinetic energy. Just before it hits the ground, its newly gained kinetic energy will be just equal to the potential energy supplied by the man. (Electrons undergo a similar process within x-ray tubes where they swap potential for kinetic energy.) Just as the stone reaches the surface of the ground, it will have more energy than when it was resting at position A. However, when it comes to rest on the ground at D, its energy level is the same as at A. The extra energy originally supplied by the man must be accounted for. In this situation, this energy is converted into other forms, such as sound, a small amount of heat, and mechanical energy used to alter the shape of the ground. When high-speed electrons collide with certain materials, they also lose their kinetic energy; their energy is converted into heat and x-radiation.

Energy Transfer

One of the major functions of electrons is to transport energy from one location to another. We have just seen that individual electrons can possess several forms of energy. The principle of electrical energy transportation is that electrons pick up energy in one location and then move to another where they pass the energy on to some other material. Generally the arrangement is such that the electrons then move back to the energy source and repeat the process.

SOURCE **LOAD**

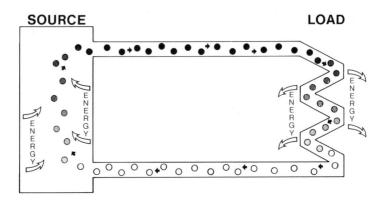

Figure 2-10 A Basic Electrical Circuit

The pathway electrons travel as they transfer energy from one point to another is a circuit. A basic electrical circuit is shown in Figure 2-10. All circuits must contain at least two components (or devices) as shown. One component, designated here as the source, can convert energy from some other form and transfer it to the electrons. Batteries are good examples of electron energy sources. The other component, designated here as a load, performs essentially the opposite function. As the electrons pass through the device they lose their energy as it is converted into some other form; a light bulb is a good example of a load in which their energy is converted into light and heat.

The energy source and load are connected with two conductors over which the electrons can freely move. The ideal conductor offers no resistance to the flow of the electrons. If the conductor offers significant resistance, the electrons lose some of their energy there. The lost energy is converted into heat. Electrical circuits neither create nor destroy electrons. The electrons are always present within the conductive materials. Energy is given to and taken from the electrons as they move around the circuit.

The energy carried by the electrons is a form of potential energy. Even though the electrons are moving through the conductors, their velocity is not sufficient to give them significant kinetic energy. When electrons are moving through free space, they can carry significant kinetic energy, but they cannot when they are moving through solid conductors. In the typical electrical circuit, one conductor has higher potential energy than the other conductor. In principle, the energy source elevates the electrons to the higher potential energy level which they maintain until they give up the energy in passing through the load device. The electrons at the lower potential level return to the energy source to repeat the process.

The connection points (terminals) between the source and load devices and the conductors are designated as either positive or negative. The electrons exit the source at the negative terminal and enter the negative terminal of the load. They then exit the positive terminal of the load device and enter the source at the positive terminal. In principle, the negative conductor contains the electrons at the high potential energy level. The positive conductor contains the electrons that have lost their energy and are returning to the source. In direct current (DC) circuits the polarities do not change. However, in alternating current (AC) circuits the polarity of the conductors is constantly alternating between negative and positive.

ELECTRICAL QUANTITIES

Each electron passing through the circuit carries a very small amount of energy. However, by collective effort, electrons can transport a tremendous amount of energy. The amount of energy transferred by an electrical circuit depends on the quantity of electrons and the energy carried by each. We now consider these specific electrical quantities and their associated units.

Current

When an electrical circuit is in operation, electrons are continuously moving or flowing through the conductor. The number of electrons that move past a given point per second is referred to as the current. Since, in the typical circuit, the number of electrons per second is quite large, a more useful unit than this number is desirable. The basic unit of current is the ampere (A). One ampere is defined as the flow of 6.25×10^{18} electrons per second. In x-ray machines, the current is typically a fraction of 1 A, and the milliampere (mA) is a more appropriate unit. As indicated in Figure 2-11, a current of 1 mA is equal to the flow of 6.25×10^{15} electrons per second past a given point. The current that flows through an x-ray tube is generally referred to as the "MA." When used to mean the *quantity,* it is written as MA. When used as the *unit,* milliampere, it is written as mA.

CURRENT

1 mA = 6.25×10^{15} electrons per second

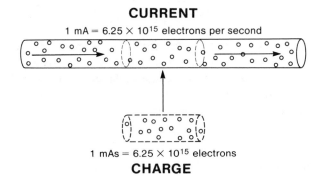

1 mAs = 6.25×10^{15} electrons

CHARGE

Figure 2-11 Electrical Current and Charge

Electron Quantity and Charge

In addition to the rate at which electrons are flowing through a circuit, ie, the current, it is often necessary to know the total quantity in a given period of time. In x-ray work the most appropriate unit for specifying electron quantity is the milliampere-second (mAs). The total quantity of electrons passing a point (MAS) is the product of the current (MA) and the time in seconds (S). Since a current of 1 mA is a flow of electrons per second, it follows that 1 mAs is a cluster of 6.25 × 10^{15} electrons, as shown in Figure 2-11.

It should be recalled that all electrons carry a negative electrical charge of the same size. In some situations the quantity of electrons might be specified in terms of the total electrical charge. If extra electrons are added to an object, it is said to have acquired a negative charge. However, if some of the free electrons are removed from an object, a positive charge is created. In either case, the total charge on the object is directly proportional to the number of electrons moved. Generally speaking, charge is a way of describing a quantity of electrons. The basic unit of charge is the coulomb (C), which is equivalent to the total charge of 6.26 × 10^{18} electrons; 1 C is equivalent to 1,000 mAs.

Voltage

We pointed out earlier that electrons could exist at different potential energy levels, because of either their different positions within the atom or their different locations within an electrical circuit. Consider the two wires or conductors shown in Figure 2-12. The electrons contained in one of the conductors are at a higher potential energy level than the electrons in the other. Generally, the electrons in the negative conductor are considered to be at the higher energy level. An electrical quantity that indicates the difference in electron potential energy between two points within a circuit is the voltage, or potential difference, suggesting a difference in potential energy. The unit used for voltage, or potential difference, is the volt. The difference in electron potential energy between two conductors is directly proportional to the voltage. Each electron will have an energy difference of 1 eV for each volt. It is the quantity of energy that an electron gains or loses, depending on direction, when it moves between two points in a circuit that are 1 V apart. In the basic x-ray machine circuit the voltage is in the order of thousands of volts (kilovolts) and is often referred to as the KV. When used to mean the *quantity,* voltage or potential, it is written KV or KV_p. When used as the *unit* it is written as kV or kVp.

Power

Power is the quantity that describes the rate at which energy is transferred. The watt is the unit of power and is equivalent to an energy transfer rate of 1 J/second.

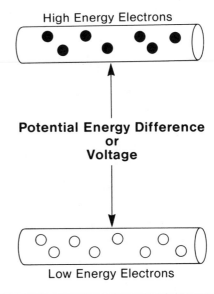

Figure 2-12 Electron Potential Energy or Voltage

High Energy Electrons

**Potential Energy Difference
or
Voltage**

Low Energy Electrons

The power in an electrical circuit is proportional to the energy carried by each electron (voltage) and the rate of electron flow (current). The specific relationship is

Power (watts) = Voltage (volts) × Current (amperes).

Total Energy

The amount of energy that an electrical circuit transfers depends on the voltage, current, and the duration (time) of the energy transfer. The fundamental unit of energy is the joule. The relationship of total transferred energy to the other electrical quantities is

Energy (joules) = Voltage (volts) × Current (amperes) × Time (seconds).

THE X-RAY CIRCUIT

The basic circuit shown in Figure 2-13 is found in all x-ray machines. The power supply that gives energy to the electrons and pumps them through the circuit is discussed in detail in Chapter 8. The voltage between the two conductors in the x-ray circuit is typically in the range of 30,000 V to 120,000 V (30 kV to 120 kV), and in radiology this kilovoltage is generally adjustable and an appropriate value can be selected by the operator of the x-ray equipment.

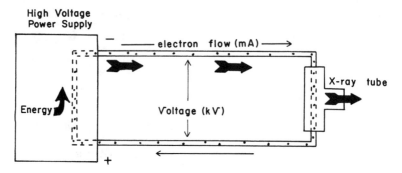

Figure 2-13 The X-Ray Circuit

In this circuit, the x-ray tube is the load. It is the place where the electrons lose their energy. The energy lost by electrons in passing through an x-ray tube is converted into heat and x-ray energy.

ALTERNATING CURRENT

In some electrical circuits, the voltage and current remain constant with respect to time, and the current always flows in the same direction. These are generally designated as direct current (DC) circuits. A battery is an example of a power supply that produces a direct current.

Some power supplies, however, produce voltages that constantly change with time. Since, in most circuits, the current is more or less proportional to the voltage, it also changes value. In most circuits of this type, the voltage periodically changes polarity and the current changes or alternates direction of flow. This is an alternating current (AC) circuit. The electricity distributed by power companies is AC. There are certain advantages to AC in that transformers can be used for stepping voltages up or down, and many motors are designed for AC operation.

If a graph of the instantaneous values of either the AC voltage or current is plotted with respect to time, it will generally be similar to the one shown in Figure 2-14. This representation of the voltage with respect to time is known as the waveform. Most AC power sources produce voltages with the sine-wave waveform, shown in Figure 2-14. This name is derived from the mathematical description of its shape.

One characteristic of an alternating voltage is its frequency. The frequency is the rate at which the voltage changes through one complete cycle. The time of one complete cycle is the period; the frequency is the reciprocal of the period. For example, the electricity distributed in the United States goes through one complete cycle in 0.0166 seconds and has a frequency of 60 cycles per second. The unit for frequency is the hertz, which is 1 cycle per second.

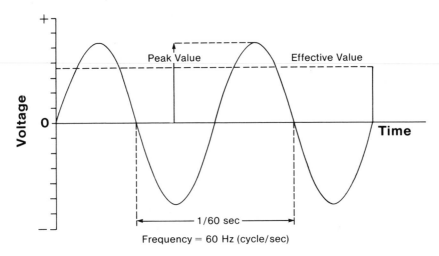

Figure 2-14 Waveform of an Alternating Voltage

During one voltage cycle, the voltage changes continuously. At two times during the period it reaches a peak, but remains there for a very short time. This means that for most of the period the circuit voltage is less than the peak value. For the purpose of energy and power calculations, an effective voltage value, rather than the peak value, should be used. For the sine-wave voltage, the effective value is 70.7% (0.707) of the peak voltage. This is the waveform factor, and its value depends on the shape of the voltage waveform.

Chapter 3

Radiation Quantities and Units

INTRODUCTION AND OVERVIEW

There are many different quantities and units used to quantify radiation, because there are a number of different aspects of an x-ray beam or gamma radiation that can be used to express the amount of radiation. The selection of the most appropriate quantity depends on the specific application. The primary objective of this chapter is to help the reader develop a conceptual understanding of the various radiation quantities and units and gain sufficient factual knowledge to support their usage.

UNIT SYSTEMS

A complicating factor is that American society is undergoing a slow change in the units used to express a variety of physical quantities. In everyday life we see this as a change from the conventional British unit system (feet, pounds, miles) to the metric system (meters, kilograms, kilometers). In radiology we are experiencing a change not only to the general metric units but also to the proposed adoption of a set of fundamental metric units known as the International System of Units (SI units). The adoption of SI radiation units is progressing rather slowly because there is nothing wrong with our conventional units, and SI units are somewhat awkward for a number of common applications. Throughout this text we use the units believed the most useful to the reader. In this chapter both unit systems are discussed and compared.

Table 3-1 is a listing of most of the physical quantities and units encountered in radiology. It is a useful reference especially for the conversion of one system of units to another.

Table 3-1 Radiation Units and Conversion Factors

Quantity	Conventional Unit	SI Unit	Conversions
Exposure	roentgen (R)	coulomb/kg of air (C/kg)	1 C/kg = 3876 R
			1 R = 258 μC/kg
Dose	rad	gray (Gy)	1 Gy = 100 rad
Dose equivalent	rem	sievert (Sv)	1 Sv = 100 rem
Activity	curie (Ci)	becquerel (Bq)	1 mCi = 37 MBq

QUANTITIES

Radiation quantities used to describe a beam of x-radiation fall into two general categories as shown in Figure 3-1. One category comprises the quantities that express the total amount of radiation, and the other comprises the quantities that express radiation concentration at a specific point. We need to develop this distinction before considering specific quantities.

A characteristic of an x-ray beam or any other type of radiation emitted from a relatively small source is that it is constantly spreading out or diverging as it moves away from the source, as shown in Figure 3-2. At any point along the beam, the width of the area covered is proportional to the distance from the source. At a

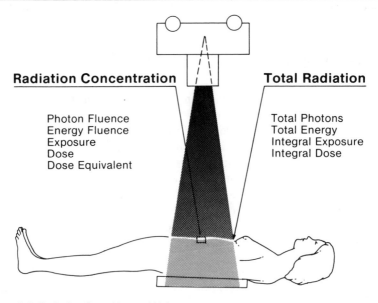

Radiation Concentration

Photon Fluence
Energy Fluence
Exposure
Dose
Dose Equivalent

Total Radiation

Total Photons
Total Energy
Integral Exposure
Integral Dose

Figure 3-1 Radiation Quantities and Units

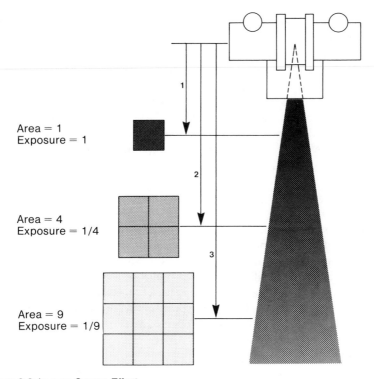

Figure 3-2 Inverse-Square Effect

distance of 1 m, the cross-sectional beam area is one unit wide and progresses to a width of two units at a distance of 2 m. At 3 m, the area is three units wide. Therefore, the area covered by our x-ray beam is increasing in proportion to the square of the distance from the source.

First, let us consider the amount of radiation passing through the three areas. We are assuming that none of the radiation is absorbed or removed from the beam before it reaches the third area. All radiation that passes through the first area will also pass through the second and third areas. In other words, the total amount of radiation is the same through all areas and does not change with distance from the source.

Now let us consider the concentration of radiation through the three areas. In the first area, all radiation is concentrated in a one-unit area. At a distance of 2 m from the source the radiation is spread over a four-unit square area, and continues to spread to cover a nine-unit square area at a distance of 3 m. If the same total amount of radiation is being distributed over larger areas it is obviously becoming less concentrated.

What we have observed here is the fact that as radiation moves away from its source, the total amount of radiation does not change but its concentration decreases. At any given distance the concentration is inversely proportional to the area covered by the beam, and the area covered by the beam is proportional to the square of the distance from the source. We can conclude that the concentration of radiation is inversely related to the square of the distance from the source. This is commonly known as the inverse-square law.

We now introduce some quantities and the associated units that can be used to express both the concentration and total amount of radiation.

PHOTONS

Since an x-ray beam and gamma radiation are showers of individual photons, the number of photons could, in principle, be used to express the amount of radiation. In practice, the number of photons is not commonly used, but it is a useful concept in understanding the nature of radiation and distinguishing between concentration and total radiation. Let us go back to the situation shown in Figure 3-1 and examine the different ways the concentration of radiation delivered to a small area on a patient's body could be expressed.

Photon Concentration (Fluence)

If we draw a 1-cm^2 area on the surface of the patient and then count the number of photons passing through the area during a radiographic procedure, we will have an indication of the concentration of radiation delivered to the patient. During a single abdominal radiographic exposure we would find that close to 10^{10} photons would have passed through our square centimeter. The more formal term for photon concentration is *photon fluence*.

Total Photons

If we count the number of photons entering the total exposed area, we will have an indication of the total amount of radiation energy delivered to the patient. This quantity depends on the size of the exposed area and the radiation concentration. If the radiation is uniformly distributed over the exposed area, the total number of photons entering the patient can be found by multiplying the concentration (fluence) by the exposed area. Changing the size of the exposed area does not affect the concentration entering at the center of the beam. However, reducing the exposed area does reduce the total number of photons and radiation entering the patient.

EXPOSURE

Concept

Exposure is the quantity most commonly used to express the amount of radiation delivered to a point. The conventional unit for exposure is the roentgen (R), and the SI unit is the coulomb per kilogram of air (C/kg):

$$1 \text{ R} = 2.58 \times 10^{-4} \text{ C/kg}$$
$$1 \text{ C/kg} = 3876 \text{ R}.$$

The reason exposure is such a widely used radiation quantity is that it can be readily measured. All forms of radiation measurement are based on an effect produced when the radiation interacts with a material. The specific effect used to measure exposure is the ionization in air produced by the radiation.

Exposure is generally measured by placing a small volume of air at the point of measurement and then measuring the amount of ionization produced within the air. The enclosure for the air volume is known as an ionization chamber. The use of ionization chambers and other radiation measuring devices is discussed in Chapter 34. The concept of exposure and its units can be developed from Figure 3-3. When a small volume of air is exposed to ionizing radiation (x-ray, gamma, etc.), some of the photons will interact with the atomic shell electrons. The interaction separates the electrons from the atom, producing an ion pair. When the negatively charged electron is removed, the atom becomes a positive ion. Within a specific mass of air the quantity of ionizations produced is determined by two factors: the concentration of radiation photons and the energy of the individual photons.

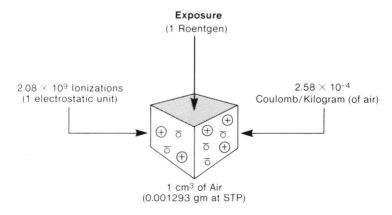

Figure 3-3 Exposure

An exposure of 1 roentgen produces 2.08×10^9 ion pairs per cm^3 of air at standard temperature and pressure (STP); 1 cm^3 of air at STP has a mass of 0.001293 g. The official definition of the roentgen is the amount of exposure that will produce 2.58×10^{-4} C (of ionization) per kg of air. A coulomb is a unit of electrical charge. Since ionization produces charged particles (ions), the amount of ionization produced can be expressed in coulombs. One coulomb of charge is produced by 6.24×10^{18} ionizations.

Exposure is a quantity of radiation concentration. For a specific photon energy, exposure is proportional to photon concentration or fluence. The relationship between exposure and photon concentration is shown in Figure 3-4; the relationship changes with photon energy because both the number of photons that will interact and the number of ionizations produced by each interacting photon is dependent on photon energy. If we assume a photon energy of 60 keV, a 1-R exposure is equivalent to a concentration of approximately 3×10^{10} photons per cm^2.

Surface Integral Exposure

Since exposure expressed in roentgens or coulombs per kilogram is a concentration, it does not express the total amount of radiation delivered to a body. The total radiation delivered, or surface integral exposure (SIE), is determined by the exposure and the dimensions of the exposed area.

The surface integral exposure is expressed in the conventional units of roentgens-square centimeters (R-cm^2). If the radiation exposure is uniform over the entire area, the SIE is the product of the exposure in roentgens and the exposure area in square centimeters. If the exposure is not the same at all points in the

Photon Fluence   Exposure   Energy Fluence
$(3.1 \times 10^{10}$ photons/cm^2) = (1 Roentgen) = (3000 ergs/cm^2)

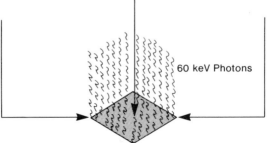

Figure 3-4 Relationship Between Exposure and Photon Concentration

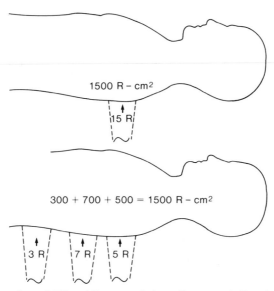

Figure 3-5 Comparison of SIE and Exposure during a Fluoroscopic Examination

exposed area, the SIE can be found by adding the exposure values for each square centimeter of exposed surface. Mathematically, this is the process of integrating the exposure over the surface area. The SIE can be measured during x-ray examinations by placing a special type of ionization chamber in the x-ray beam. The significance of SIE is that it describes total radiation imparted to a patient, whereas exposure indicates only the concentration of radiation at a specified point.

The typical fluoroscopy examination provides an excellent opportunity to compare exposure (concentration) and SIE (total radiation). In Figure 3-5 two cases are compared. In both instances the beam area was 10 cm × 10 cm (100 cm²); the total exposure time was 5 minutes at an exposure rate of 3 R/min. In both instances the SIE is 1,500 R-cm². However, the exposure depends on how the x-ray beam was moved during the examination. In the first example the beam was not moved and the resulting exposure was 15 R. In the second example, the beam was moved to different locations so that the exposure was distributed over more surface area and the concentration became less.

Another important example is illustrated in Figure 3-6. Here the same exposure (100 mR) is delivered to both patients. However, there is a difference in the exposed area: the patient on the right received 10 times as much radiation as the patient on the left.

The important point to remember is that exposure (roentgens) alone does not express the total radiation delivered to a body. The total exposed area must also be considered.

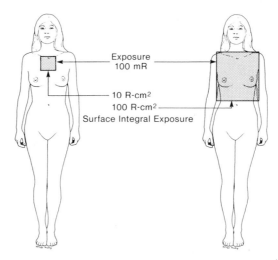

Figure 3-6 Comparison of SIE Values for a Radiographic Examination

ENERGY

An x-ray beam and other forms of radiation deliver energy to the body. In principle, the amount of radiation delivered could be expressed in units of energy (joules, ergs, kiloelectron volts, etc.). The energy content of an x-ray beam is rather difficult to measure and for that reason is not widely used in the clinical setting. However, considering the energy delivered by an x-ray beam is helpful in understanding other radiation quantities.

Energy Fluence

Energy fluence (concentration) is the amount of radiation energy delivered to a unit area. The units for expressing radiation energy concentration are either the millijoule (mJ) per square centimeter or erg per square centimeter. For a specific photon energy, fluence is proportional to exposure. The relationship between energy fluence and exposure is shown in Figure 3-4. The relationship changes with photon energy because of the change in photon interaction rates. However, if we assume a photon energy of 60 keV, the energy fluence for a 1-R exposure is approximately 0.3 mJ/cm^2.

The energy delivered by an x-ray beam can be put into perspective by comparing it to the energy delivered by sunlight (see Figure 3-7). For the x-ray exposure we will use the fluoroscopic factors of 5 minutes at the rate of 3 R/min. This 15-R exposure delivers x-ray energy to the patient with a concentration (fluence) of 4.5 mJ/cm^2 if we assume an effective photon energy of 60 keV.

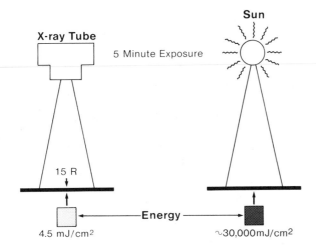

Figure 3-7 Comparison of Energy Delivered by an X-Ray Beam and Sunlight

The energy delivered by the sun depends on many factors including geographic location, season, time of day, and atmospheric conditions; a typical midday summer exposure on a clear day in Atlanta produces approximately 100 mJ/sec/cm^2. In 5 minutes a person would be exposed to an energy fluence of 30,000 mJ/cm^2. We see from this example that the energy content of an x-ray beam is relatively small in comparison to sunlight. However, x-ray and gamma radiation will generally produce a greater biological effect per unit of energy than sunlight because of two significant differences: x- and gamma radiation penetrate and deposit energy within the internal tissue, and the high energy content of the individual photons produces a greater concentration of energy at the points where they are absorbed within individual atoms.

Total Energy

The total energy imparted to a body by an x-ray beam is determined by the energy fluence (concentration) and the size of the exposed area. If the radiation is uniformly distributed over the area, the total energy delivered is the product of the fluence and the surface area.

ABSORBED DOSE

Concept

A human body absorbs most of the radiation energy delivered to it. The portion of an x-ray beam that is absorbed depends on the penetrating ability of the radiation and the size and density of the body section exposed. In most clinical situations more than 90% is absorbed. In nuclear imaging procedures, a large percentage of the energy emitted by radionuclides is absorbed in the body. Two aspects of the absorbed radiation energy must be considered: the amount (concentration) absorbed at various locations throughout the body and the total amount absorbed.

Absorbed dose is the quantity that expresses the concentration of radiation energy absorbed at a specific point within the body tissue. Since an x-ray beam is attenuated by absorption as it passes through the body, all tissues within the beam will not absorb the same dose. The absorbed dose will be much greater for the tissues near the entrance surface than for those deeper within the body. Absorbed dose is defined as the quantity of radiation energy absorbed per unit mass of tissue.

Units

The conventional unit for absorbed dose is the rad, which is equivalent to 100 ergs of absorbed energy per g of tissue. The SI unit is the gray (Gy), which is equivalent to the absorption of 1 J of radiation energy per kg of tissue. The relationship between the two units is

$$1 \text{ rad } = \ 100 \text{ erg/g } = \ 0.01 \text{ J/kg } = \ 0.01 \text{ Gy}$$
$$1 \text{ Gy } = \ 100 \text{ rad.}$$

For a specific type of tissue and photon energy spectrum, the absorbed dose is proportional to the exposure delivered to the tissue. The ratio, f, between dose (rads) and exposure (roentgens) is shown in Figure 3-8 for soft tissue and bone over the photon energy range normally encountered in diagnostic procedures. The absorbed dose in soft tissue is slightly less than 1 rad/R of exposure throughout the photon energy range. The relationship for bone undergoes a considerable variation with photon energy. For a typical diagnostic x-ray spectrum, a bone exposure of 1 R will produce an absorbed dose of approximately 3 rad.

Integral Dose

Integral dose is the total amount of energy absorbed in the body. It is determined not only by the absorbed dose values but also by the total mass of tissue exposed.

The conventional unit for integral dose is the gram-rad, which is equivalent to 100 ergs of absorbed energy. The concept behind the use of this unit is that if we add the absorbed doses (rads) for each gram of tissue in the body, we will have an indication of total absorbed energy. Since integral dose is a quantity of energy, the SI unit used is the joule. The relationship between the two units is

$$1 \text{ J } = \ 1{,}000 \text{ gram-rad.}$$

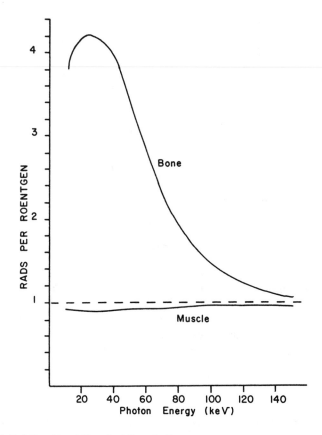

Figure 3-8 Relationship of Absorbed Dose to Exposure

Integral dose (total absorbed radiation energy) is probably the radiation quantity that most closely correlates with potential radiation damage during a diagnostic procedure. This is because it reflects not only the concentration of the radiation absorbed in the tissue but also the amount of tissue affected by the radiation.

There is no practical method for measuring integral dose in the human body. However, since most of the radiation energy delivered to a body is absorbed, the integral dose can be estimated to within a few percent from the total energy delivered to the body.

Computed tomography can be used to demonstrate integral dose, as illustrated in Figure 3-9. We begin with a one-slice examination and assume that the average dose to the tissue in the slice is 5 rad. If there are 400 g of tissue in the slice, the integral dose will be 2,000 gram-rad. If we now perform an examination of 10 slices, but all other factors remain the same, the dose (energy concentration) in

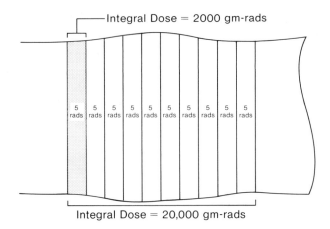

Figure 3-9 Integral Dose in Computed Tomography

each slice will remain the same. However, the integral dose (total energy) increases in proportion to the number of slices and is now 20,000 gram-rad. In this example we made the simplifying assumption that no radiation is scattered from one slice to another. In reality, some radiation is exchanged between contiguous slices but that does not affect the concept presented.

BIOLOGICAL IMPACT

It is sometimes desirable to express the actual or relative biological impact of radiation. It is necessary to develop a distinction between the biological impact and the physical quantity of radiation because all types of radiation do not have the same potential for producing biological change. For example, one rad of one type of radiation might produce significantly more radiation damage than one rad of another type. In other words, the biological impact is determined by both the quantity of radiation and its ability to produce biological effects. Two radiation quantities are associated with biological impact.

Dose Equivalent

Dose equivalent (H) is the quantity commonly used to express the biological impact of radiation on persons receiving occupational or environmental exposures. Personnel exposure in a clinical facility is often determined and recorded as a dose equivalent.

Dose equivalent is proportional to the absorbed dose (D), the quality factor (Q), and other modifying factors (N) of the specific type of radiation. Most radiations encountered in diagnostic procedures (x-ray, gamma, and beta) have quality and modifying factor values of 1. Therefore, the dose equivalent is numerically equal to the absorbed dose. Some radiation types consisting of large (relative to electrons) particles have quality factor values greater than 1. For example, alpha particles have a quality factor value of approximately 20.

The conventional unit for dose equivalent is the rem, and the SI unit is the sievert (Sv). When the quality factor is 1, the different relationships between dose equivalent (H) and absorbed dose (D) are

$$H(rem) = D(rad)$$

$$H(Sv) = D(Gy).$$

Dose equivalent values can be converted from one system of units to the other by:

$$1 \; Sv = 100 \; rem.$$

Figure 3-10 is a summary of the general relationship among the three quantities: exposure, absorbed dose, and dose equivalent. Although each expresses a different aspect of radiation, they all express radiation concentration. For the types of radiation used in diagnostic procedures, the factors that relate the three quantities have values of approximately 1 in soft tissue. Therefore, an exposure of 1 R produces an absorbed dose of approximately 1 rad, which, in turn, produces a dose equivalent of 1 rem.

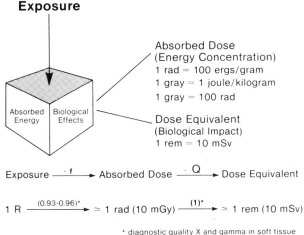

Figure 3-10 Relationship of Exposure, Absorbed Dose, and Dose Equivalent

Relative Biological Effectiveness

When specific radiation effects rather than general risk are being considered, the relative biological effectiveness (RBE) of the radiation must be taken into account. The value of the RBE depends on characteristics of the radiation and the specific biological effects being considered. This radiation characteristic is generally not used in association with diagnostic procedures. Additional discussions of the concept can be found in radiation biology texts.

LIGHT

The basic light quantities and units encountered in radiology can be conveniently divided into two categories: those that express the amount of light emitted by a source and those that describe the amount of light falling on a surface, such as a piece of film. The relationships of several light quantities and units are shown in Figure 3-11.

Luminance

Luminance is the light quantity generally referred to as brightness. It describes the amount of light being emitted from the surface of the light source. The basic

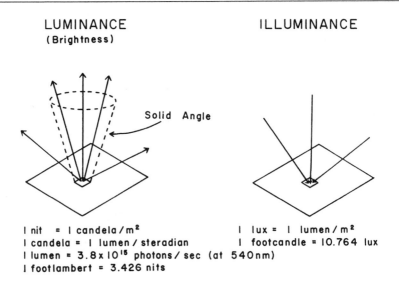

LUMINANCE (Brightness)   ILLUMINANCE

Solid Angle

I nit   = I candela / m²   I lux = I lumen / m²
I candela = I lumen / steradian   I footcandle = 10.764 lux
I lumen = 3.8 x 10¹⁵ photons / sec (at 540nm)
I footlambert = 3.426 nits

Figure 3-11 Light Quantities and Units Encountered in Radiology

unit of luminance (brightness) is the nit, which is equivalent to 1 candela per m² of source area.

The concept of luminance is somewhat easier to understand if it is related to the number of light photons involved. The quantity for specifying an amount of light is the lumen. One lumen of light with wavelengths encountered in x-ray imaging systems (540 nm) is equivalent to 3.8×10^{15} photons per second. Another factor that determines luminance is the concentration of light in a given direction. This can be described in terms of a cone or solid angle that is measured in units of steradians (sr).

If a light source produces an intensity of 1 cd/m² of surface area, it has a luminance of 1 nit. Perhaps it is more realistic to consider the quantity of light that would be emitted from a 1-mm² area of a source, such as the output screen of an image intensifier. One millimeter square is 10^{-6} m². If the intensifier has a luminance (brightness) of 1 nit, the intensity from an area of 1 mm² would be 10^{-6} lumen in a 1-unit solid angle. This would be equivalent to 3.8×10^{9} photons per second, leaving the 1-mm² area through a cone (solid angle) of 1 sr.

Another unit used for specifying luminance is the foot-lambert, which is equivalent to 3.426 nits.

Illuminance

Illuminance is a specification of the quantity of light falling on or illuminating a surface. The basic unit is the lux. A surface has an illuminance of 1 lux when it receives 1 lumen/m² of surface area. Consider a small area on a piece of film that is 1 mm². For light with a wavelength of 540 nm, there are 3.8×10^{15} photons per second per lumen. An illuminance to the film of 1 lux would be equivalent to 3.8×10^{9} photons per sec to a 1-mm² area. The total light exposure to a film is found by multiplying the illuminance, in lux, by the exposure time, in seconds, and is expressed in units of lux-seconds.

Another unit used in some literature for specifying illuminance is the foot-candle, which is equivalent to 10.764 lux.

RADIO FREQUENCY RADIATION

Radio frequency (RF) radiation is used in magnetic resonance imaging (MRI). During an imaging procedure, pulses of RF energy are applied to the patient's body where most of it is absorbed. Conventional energy units are used to express the amount of RF energy imparted to the body.

Power is the rate at which energy is transferred. The unit for power is the watt, which is equivalent to an energy transfer at the rate of 1 joule/second. During the acquisition phase of MRI, the system transfers energy to the patient's body at some specific power level. The actual power (watts) used depends on many factors associated with the examination.

From the standpoint of effect on the patient's body a more significant quantity is the concentration of power in the tissue. This is expressed in the units of watts per kilogram of tissue and is designated the specific absorption rate (SAR). Since RF energy is not uniformly distributed within the body, two quantities must be considered: the SAR in a specific location and the average SAR within the total body. The RF energy absorbed by the tissue is converted into heat. Therefore, the power concentration is an indication of the rate at which heat is produced within specific tissue.

Chapter 4

Characteristics and Structure of Matter

INTRODUCTION AND OVERVIEW

Radiation is created and then later absorbed within some material substance or matter. Certain materials are more suitable than others as both radiation sources and absorbers. In this chapter we consider some basic physical characteristics of matter that determine how the materials interact with radiation. Radiation interactions, both formation and absorption, occur within individual atoms. We therefore begin with a brief review of atomic structure with an emphasis on atomic characteristics that affect interactions. We then discuss the collective properties of atoms within a material.

Atoms consist of two major regions: the nucleus and the electron shells. Each region has a role in radiation interactions. The nucleus is the source of energy for the radiations used in nuclear medicine procedures. Although the nucleus is not the source of x-ray energy, it is involved in the production of x-ray photons. In most instances radiation is absorbed by interacting with the electrons located in the shells surrounding the nucleus. Electrons also produce one form of x-radiation.

NUCLEAR STRUCTURE

The conventional model of an atom consists of a nucleus containing neutrons and protons surrounded by electrons located in specific orbits or shells, as shown in Figure 4-1. The nucleus is shown as a ball or cluster of particles at the center of the atom. The nucleus is quite small in comparison to the total dimensions of the atom. However, most of the mass of the atom is contained within the nucleus. The components of the atom in Figure 4-1 are not drawn to scale. Actually, the electrons in the K, L, and M shells are much smaller than the protons and neutrons that make up the nucleus, and the electrons are located at a much greater distance from the nucleus than shown.

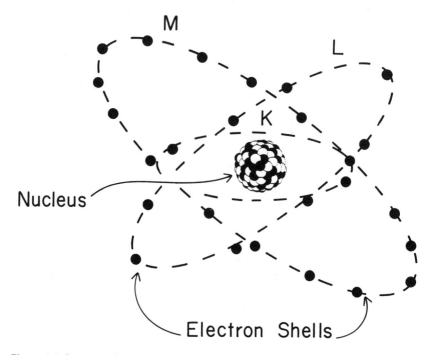

Figure 4-1 Structure of an Atom

Composition

All nuclei are composed of two basic particles, neutrons and protons. Neutrons and protons are almost the same size but differ in their electrical charge. Neutrons have no electrical charge and contribute only mass to the nucleus. Each proton has a positive charge equal in strength to the negative charge carried by an electron.

Most physical and chemical characteristics of a substance relate to the nuclei's neutron-proton composition. The number of protons in a nucleus is the atomic number (Z) and establishes the chemical identity of the atom. Each atomic number corresponds to a different chemical element; there are now approximately 106 known chemical elements that correspond to nuclei containing from 1 to 106 protons.

Because of their very small size it is not convenient to express the mass of nuclei and atomic particles in the conventional unit of kilograms. A more appropriate unit is the atomic mass unit (amu), the reference for which is a carbon atom with a mass number of 12, which is assigned a mass of 12.000 amu. The relationship between the atomic mass unit and kilogram is

$$1 \text{ amu} = 1.66 \times 10^{-27} \text{ kg}.$$

The difference in mass between a neutron and proton is quite small: approximately 0.1%. The larger difference is between the mass of these two particles and the mass of an electron. More than 1,800 electrons are required to equal the mass of a proton or neutron.

The total number of particles (neutrons and protons) in a nucleus is the mass number (A). Since neutrons and protons have approximately the same mass, the total mass or weight of a nucleus is, within certain limits, proportional to the mass number. However, the nuclear mass is not precisely proportional to the mass number because neutrons and protons do not have the same mass, and some of the mass is converted into energy when the nucleus is formed. The relationship between mass and energy is considered in more detail later.

There is a standard method for labeling different nuclear compositions: The mass number is designated by either a superscript preceding the chemical symbol, such as ^{14}C or ^{131}I, or by a number following the symbol, such as C-14, I-131, etc. The atomic number is added as a subscript preceding the chemical symbol. Adding the atomic number to the symbol is somewhat redundant since only one atomic number is associated with each chemical symbol or element.

With the exception of ordinary hydrogen, all nuclei contain neutrons and protons. The lighter elements (with low atomic and mass numbers) contain almost equal numbers of neutrons and protons. As the size of the nucleus is increased, the ratio of neutrons to protons increases to a maximum of about 1.3 neutrons per proton for materials with very high atomic numbers. The number of neutrons in a specific nucleus can be obtained by subtracting the atomic number from the mass number. One chemical element may have nuclei containing different numbers of neutrons. This variation in neutron composition usually determines if a nucleus is radioactive.

Nuclides

As stated previously, there are 106 different atomic numbers or elements. Since one element can have several different neutron numbers, there are obviously more than 106 different nuclear compositions. Actually, at least 1,300 different neutron-proton combinations are now known. The term *element* refers to the classification of a substance according to its atomic number, and the term *nuclide* refers to its classification by both atomic number and number of neutrons. In other words, whereas there are at least 106 different elements, there are about 1,300 different nuclides known.

The structural relationship of various nuclides is often shown on a grid generally referred to as a nuclide chart, as shown in Figure 4-2. The scale in one direction represents the number of protons (atomic number), and the scale in the other direction represents the number of neutrons. Each square in the grid represents a specific nuclear composition or nuclide. Not all areas in the chart are occupied. Many neutron-proton combinations represent unstable combinations and do not

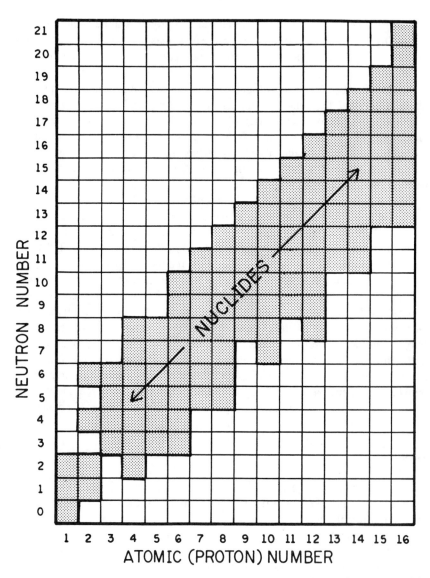

Figure 4-2 Chart of Nuclides Arranged According to the Neutron-Proton Composition of the Nucleus

exist as nuclei. The nuclides that do exist are located in a relatively narrow band that runs diagonally up through the chart.

The charts in this text show only the first 16 elements because our immediate interest is in the characteristics of the chart, and not the details of all elements.

Charts are published that show all known nuclides. Certain relationships between specific nuclides now need to be considered.

Isotopes

The nuclides of an element may contain different numbers of neutrons. Nuclides that belong to the same chemical element (and have the same atomic number) but have different numbers of neutrons are known as isotopes. It should be emphasized that the term *isotope* describes a relationship between or among nuclides rather than a specific characteristic of a given nuclide. An analogy is that persons who have the same grandparents but not the same parents are known as cousins. The isotopes of each element are located in the same vertical column of the nuclide chart as shown in Figure 4-3.

There seems to be a general misconception that the term *isotope* means radioactive. This is obviously incorrect, since every nuclide is an isotope of some other nuclide. Most elements have several isotopes. In most cases some of the isotopes of a given element are stable (not radioactive), and some are radioactive. For example, iodine has 23 known isotopes with mass numbers ranging from 117 to 139. Two of these, I-127 and I-131, are shown in Figure 4-4. The relationship between the two nuclides is that they are isotopes. I-131 is an isotope of I-127, and I-127 is also an isotope of I-131. For most elements the most common or most abundant form is the stable isotope. The radioactive forms are therefore isotopes of the more common forms, explaining the strong association isotopes have developed with radioactivity.

Isobars

Nuclides having the same mass number (total number of neutrons and protons) but different atomic numbers are known as isobars, as shown in Figure 4-5. I-131 and Xe-131 are isobars of each other. A pair of isobars cannot belong to the same chemical element. The relationship among isobars in the nuclide chart is illustrated in Figure 4-3, showing aluminum-29, silicon-29, phosphorus-29, and sulfur-29.

Our major interest in isobars is that in most radioactive transformations one nuclide will be transformed into an isobar of itself. For example, the I-131 shown in Figure 4-5 is radioactive and is converted into Xe-131 when it undergoes its normal radioactive transformation.

Isomers

Nuclei can have the same neutron-proton composition but not be identical; one nucleus can contain more energy than the other. Two nuclei that have the same

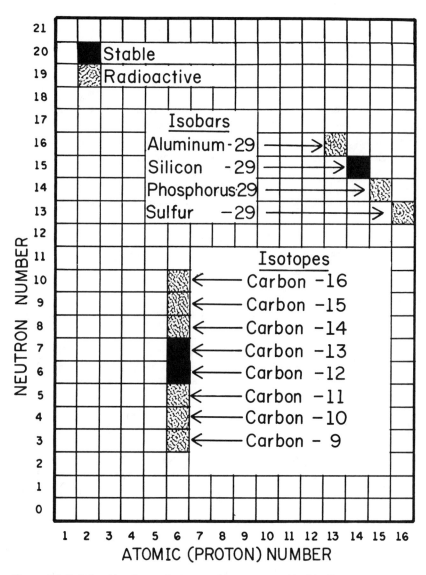

Figure 4-3 Relationships Among Isobars and Isotopes on a Nuclide Chart

composition but varying energy are known as isomers. An example of a pair of isomers is shown in Figure 4-6. Technetium-99 can exist in two energy states; the higher of the two is a temporary state generally referred to as a metastable state. The symbol for a nuclide in the metastable state is obtained by adding the letter m

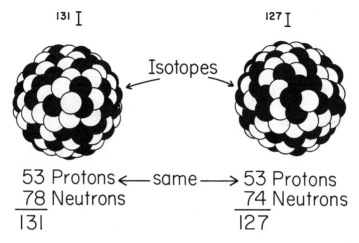

Figure 4-4 Comparison of Two Isotopes

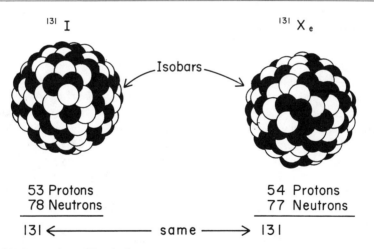

Figure 4-5 Comparison of Two Isobars

to the mass number (Tc-99m). A nucleus in the metastable state will eventually give off its excess energy and change to the other isomer. Such isomeric transitions have an important role in nuclear medicine and are discussed in detail later.

Isotones

Nuclides that have the same number of neutrons are known as isotones. This relationship, mentioned here for the sake of completeness, is not normally encountered in nuclear medicine.

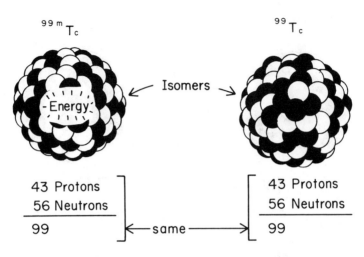

Figure 4-6 Comparison of Two Isomers

NUCLEAR STABILITY

The ability of a nucleus to emit radiation energy is related to its level of stability. Figure 4-7 illustrates three levels of nuclear stability. A *stable* nucleus will not undergo internal changes on its own. This is the condition of all non-radioactive material. The *radioactive* nuclei are stable enough to remain unchanged for a period of time, but will spontaneously undergo a transformation in which they will emit a burst of energy and become more stable; the second state is either a more stable radioactive state or a completely stable state. Many hypothetical nuclear compositions (neutron-proton mixtures) are completely *unstable* and cannot exist as intact nuclei. As stated previously, only about 1,300 different neutron-proton combinations, found among the stable and radioactive nuclides, will stick together as a nucleus.

Nuclear stability is determined by the balance of forces within the nucleus. There are forces that cause the nuclear particles (protons and neutrons) to be both attracted to and repelled from each other. Since each proton carries a positive electrical charge, protons repel each other. A short-range attraction force between all particles is also present within nuclei.

The most significant factor that determines the balance between the internal forces and therefore the nuclear stability is the ratio of the number of neutrons to the number of protons. For the smaller nuclei, a neutron-proton ratio of 1 to 1 produces maximum stability. The ratio for stability gradually increases with increasing atomic number up to a value of approximately 1.3 to 1.0 for the highest atomic numbers.

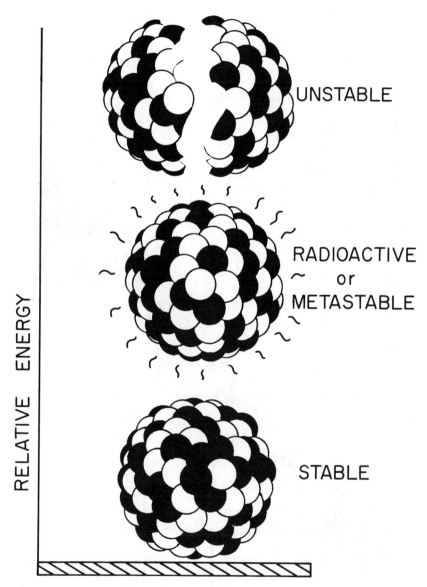

Figure 4-7 The Three Levels of Nuclear Stability.

If the neutron-proton ratio is slightly above or below the ratio for stability, the nucleus will generally be radioactive. Ratios considerably different from those required for stability are not found in nuclei because they represent completely unstable compositions. In an unstable composition, the repelling forces override the forces of attraction between the nuclear particles.

The relationship between nuclear stability and neutron-proton ratio is illustrated in Figure 4-8. The stable nuclides, those with a neutron-proton ratio of approx-

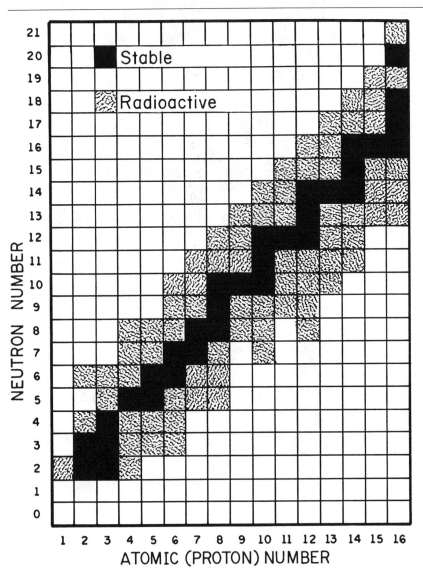

Figure 4-8 Nuclide Chart Showing the Relationship of Unstable Radioactive and Stable Nuclear Structures

imately 1 to 1, are located in a narrow band running diagonally through the nuclide chart. The radioactive nuclides are located on either side of the stable band. All other areas on the nuclide chart represent neutron-proton mixtures that cannot exist as a nuclei.

NUCLEAR ENERGY

Whenever a nucleus changes to a more stable form, it must emit energy. Several types of nuclear changes can result in the release of energy. Under certain conditions a nucleus can fission or break apart into more stable components. This process takes place in nuclear reactors where the energy released is often used to generate electrical energy. The fusion of two small nuclei to form a larger nucleus is the process that creates energy within the sun and the hydrogen bomb. In nuclear medicine, radiation energy is created when nuclei undergo spontaneous radioactive transitions to create more stable nuclear structures.

The energy emitted during nuclear transitions is created by converting a small fraction of the nuclear mass into energy. When such a conversion takes place, the relationship between the amount of energy (E) and the amount of mass (m) involved is given by Einstein's equation:

$$E = mc^2,$$

where c is the velocity of light. A significant aspect of this relationship is that a tremendous amount of energy can be created from a relatively small mass. The mass of 1 g, completely converted, would produce 25,000,000 kilowatt-hours.

In clinical applications we are interested in the amount of energy released by an individual atom. This is expressed in the unit of kiloelectron volts (keV), a relatively small unit of energy. The relationship between some other energy units and the keV are:

$$1 \text{ erg} = 6.24 \times 10^8 \text{ keV}$$
$$1 \text{ j} = 10^7 \text{ erg} = 6.24 \times 10^{15} \text{ keV}.$$

The energy released in the radioactive transitions used in nuclear medicine is typically in the range of 100 keV to 500 keV. This corresponds to a nuclear mass change of 0.0001 amu to 0.0005 amu. The amount of nuclear mass used to produce the radiation energy is relatively small.

The energy equivalent of one electron mass is 511 keV. This value is often referred to as the rest-mass energy of an electron. In some situations in nuclear medicine procedures, the masses of individual electrons are completely converted into energy. The result is a photon with the characteristic energy of 511 keV.

ELECTRONS

Electrons are located in orbits or shells in the space surrounding a nucleus and have several important roles in image formation. In certain types of radioactive transitions, the orbital electrons become involved in the actual emission of energy from the atom. When radiation interacts with materials, such as human tissue, the interaction is usually with the electrons rather than the nuclei of the atoms.

Number

The number of electrons contained in a normal atom is equal to the number of protons in the nucleus. This number is the atomic number (Z) of the particular chemical element. Each electron has a negative electrical charge equivalent in strength to the positive charge of a proton. Under normal conditions, when the number of electrons and protons in an atom is the same, the positive and negative charges balance so that the atom has no net charge. However, if an electron is removed from an atom, the atom is said to be ionized and will have a positive charge.

Energy Levels

Electrons are located in discrete shells surrounding the nucleus, identified by letters of the alphabet beginning with K for the shell closest to the nucleus as shown in Figure 4-1. Each shell has a limited electron capacity. The maximum capacity of the K shell in any atom is 2 electrons; the L shell, 8 electrons; the M shell, 18 electrons; etc. The electron shells are generally filled beginning with the K shell and extending out until the total number of electrons have been placed.

Electrons are bound to the positive nucleus of an atom by their negative electrical charge. The strength of this binding can be expressed in terms of energy. This binding energy of an electron is equal to the amount of energy that would be required to remove the electron from the atom. Binding energy is a form of electron potential energy. As with any form of potential energy, some point must be designated the zero energy level. In the case of electrons, a location outside the atom where the electron is no longer under the influence of the nucleus is designated the zero point. Consider a golf ball resting on the ground. For the golf ball, the ground level would be the zero energy level. When an electron enters an atom, it drops to a lower energy level, just as the golf ball does when it rolls into a hole. Electrons within atoms are generally considered to have negative energy, since energy from some source must be added to raise them to the zero level. Likewise, the golf ball in the hole has negative energy with respect to the surface of the ground. It takes energy from some source to lift it back to zero level.

The concept of electron energy levels can be illustrated by using an energy level diagram of the type shown in Figure 4-9. It should be noticed that this diagram represents the electrons as being down in a hole. The electrons near the bottom are the lowest energy level and would have the greatest binding energy.

As discussed previously, the electrons are arranged within the atoms in definite layers, or shells. Each shell is a different energy level. The K shell, which is closest to the nucleus, is at the lowest energy level. The diagram in Figure 4-9 is for tungsten, which has an atomic number of 74. Only the K, L, and M electron levels are shown. Additional electrons are located in the N and O shells. These shells would be located above the M shell and slightly below the zero level. It should be noticed that there is a significant energy difference between the various shells. All of the shells, except K, are subdivided into additional energy levels. For example, the L shell is divided into three levels designated LI, LII, and LIII.

The roles of electrons in radiation events usually involve one of two basic principles: (1) Energy from some source is required to move an electron to a higher shell (such as K to L) or out of the atom; (2) If an electron moves to a lower shell (ie, L to K), energy must be given up by the electron and usually appears as some type of radiation. The amount of energy involved depends on the difference in the energy levels between which the electrons move.

The binding energy for electrons in a specific shell, such as K, is related to atomic number as indicated in Figure 4-10. It should be noticed that only the K shell electrons for the higher atomic number elements have binding energies in the same range as the energies of diagnostic gamma and x-ray photons. This is significant in several types of interactions discussed later. The binding energy of the L-shell electrons is always much less than for the K, but it also increases with atomic number. For most substances, the binding energy of the outermost electrons is in the range of 5 eV to 20 eV. Obviously, these are the electrons that are the easiest to remove from an atom.

The removal of an electron from an atom is called ionization. Since x-ray and gamma photons have sufficient energy to remove electrons from atoms, they can be considered ionizing radiation. Visible light, which has photon energies below the minimum binding energy in most atoms, cannot produce ionization.

Concentration

Photons are absorbed when they collide with electrons. As a photon passes through matter, its chances of being absorbed generally depend on the concentration of available electrons within the material. The concentration, or number of electrons per cubic centimeter, is given by

$$\text{Electrons per cc} = \rho N(Z/A).$$

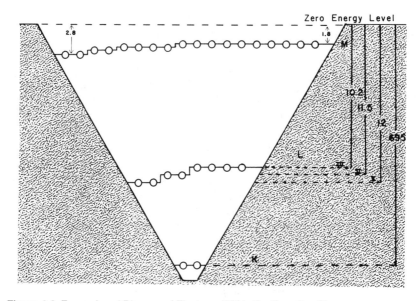

Figure 4-9 Energy Level Diagram of Electrons Within the Tungsten Atom

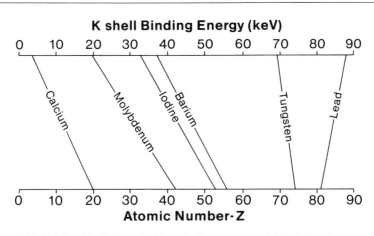

Figure 4-10 Relationship Between K-Shell Binding Energy and Atomic Number

This relationship is the number of atoms per cubic centimeter multiplied by the atomic number, which is the number of electrons per atom. Several comments concerning this relationship are in order. Avogadro's number, N, always has the same value and obviously does not change from element to element. Z and A have unique values for each chemical element. It should be noticed, however, that the number of electrons per cubic centimeter depends only on the ratio of Z to A. The elements with lower atomic numbers have approximately one neutron for each proton in the nucleus. The value of Z/A is approximately 0.5. As the atomic number and atomic weight increase, the ratio of neutrons within the nucleus also increases. This produces a decrease in the Z/A ratio, but this change is relatively small. Lead, which has an atomic number of 82 and an atomic weight of 207, has a Z/A ratio of 0.4. For most material encountered in x-ray applications, the Z/A ratio varies by less that 20%. The single exception to this is hydrogen. Normal hydrogen contains no neutrons and has a nucleus that consists of a single proton. The Z/A ratio, therefore, has a value of 1.

Since Avogadro's number is constant, and the Z/A ratio is essentially constant, the only factor that can significantly alter the electron concentration is the density of the material. Most materials, especially pure elements, have more or less unique density values. In compounds and mixtures, the density depends on the relative concentration of the various elements.

The fact that electron concentration does not significantly change with atomic number might suggest that atomic number has little to do with electron–x-ray interactions. This is, however, not the case. As x-ray photons pass through matter, the chance of interaction depends not only on electron concentration, but also on how firmly the electrons are bound within the atomic structure. Certain types of interactions occur only with firmly bound electrons. Since the binding energy of electrons increases with atomic number, the concentration of highly bound electrons increases significantly with increased atomic number.

Atomic number is essentially a characteristic of the atom and has a value that is unique to each chemical element. Many materials, such as human tissue, are not a single chemical element, but a conglomerate of compounds and mixtures. With respect to x-ray interactions, it is possible to define an effective atomic number, Z_{eff}, for compounds and mixtures. The effective atomic number is given by

$$Z_{eff} = {}^{2.94}\sqrt{f_1 Z_1^{2.94} + f_2 Z_2^{2.94} + f_3 Z_3^{2.94} + - -}.$$

In this relationship, f is the fraction of the total number of electrons associated with each element. The exponent, 2.94, is derived from the relationship between x-ray interactions and atomic number, which is discussed later.

Water, which is a major component of the human body, can be used to demonstrate the concept of effective atomic number. The water molecule contains two hydrogen atoms, which have one electron each, and one oxygen atom with eight electrons. The electron fractions, f, are therefore 0.2 for hydrogen and 0.8 for oxygen. Substitution of these values in the above relationship gives an effective atomic number for water of

$$Z = {}^{2.94}\sqrt{0.2 \cdot 1^{2.94} + 0.8 \cdot 8^{2.94}}$$

$$= 7.42.$$

In many x-ray systems, a variety of materials are involved in x-ray interactions. Many of these materials are listed in Table 4-1, along with their principal physical characteristics and relationship to the x-ray system.

Table 4-1 Physical Characteristics of Materials Involved in Photon Interactions

Material	Atomic number[a] (Z)	K electron binding energy (keV)	Density (g/cc)	Application
Beryllium	4.0		1.85	Low absorbing tube window
Fat	5.92		0.91	Body tissue
Water	7.42		1.0	Tissue "equivalent"
Muscle	7.46		1.0	Body tissue
Air	7.64		0.00129	
Aluminum	13.0		2.7	X-ray filter and penetration reference
Bone (femur)	14.0		1.87	Body tissue
Calcium	20.0		1.55	Body deposits
Copper	29.0	8.9	8.94	X-ray filter
Molybdenum	42.0	20.0	10.22	X-ray source
Silver	47.0	25.5	10.5	Absorber in film
Iodine	53.0	33.2	4.94	Contrast medium and receptor absorber
Xenon	54.0	34.5	0.0059	Receptor absorber
Barium	56.0	37.4	3.5	Contrast medium and receptor absorber
Lanthanun	56.0	38.9	6.15	Receptor absorber
Gadolinium	64.0	50.2	7.95	Receptor absorber
Tungsten	74.0	69.5	19.3	X-ray source
Lead	82.0	88.0	11.34	X-ray absorber for shielding

[a]Effective Z of tissues from Spiers (1946).

Source: Spiers FW: Effective atomic number and energy absorption in tissues. *Br J Radiol* 1946;19:218.

Chapter 5

Radioactive Transitions

INTRODUCTION AND OVERVIEW

In the previous chapter we showed that certain nuclei are not completely stable and eventually undergo an internal change that will produce a more stable nuclear structure. This spontaneous change is a radioactive transition. In some older literature this event is called a nuclear disintegration. The terminology is misleading because the nucleus does not disintegrate; it simply undergoes a slight change. This event is illustrated in Figure 5-1. The original nucleus is designated the parent, and the nucleus after the transition is designated the daughter. In radioactive transitions, energy is emitted as radiation. The types of radiation encountered in nuclear medicine are shown in Figure 5-1. The radiation is in the form of either energetic particles or photons.

Most radionuclides emit a combination of radiations; the types depend on the physical characteristics of the nucleus and are considered in more detail later. The daughter nucleus can be either stable or a radioactive or metastable nucleus that will undergo another transition in the future.

In most in-vivo nuclear medicine procedures it is desirable to use a radionuclide that emits photons in the range of 100 to 500 keV. The penetrating ability of photons is related to their energy. Many photons in this energy range can emanate from the body, but not penetrate through the detector and be lost. Particle radiation is not useful in most diagnostic procedures. In fact, it is usually undesirable because it deposits its energy in the body close to the site of origin and can contribute significantly to patient dose without contributing to diagnostic information. With many radionuclides, particle radiation is a byproduct of the transition required for desirable photon emissions.

It is often useful to construct a diagram to show changes in the nucleus and the radiation emitted during a radioactive transition. A transition diagram, sometimes referred to as a decay scheme, is shown in Figure 5-2. Two types of changes occur

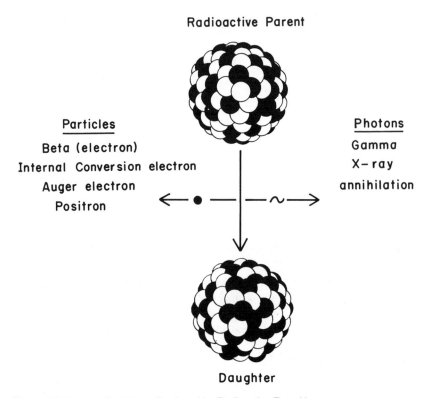

Figure 5-1 Various Radiations Produced by Radioactive Transitions

within a nucleus: loss of energy and, possibly, a change in atomic number in an isobaric transition. In the transition diagram, relative nuclear energy is represented by vertical distance and relative atomic number by horizontal distance. The actual scales are not usually shown as they are in Figure 5-2. The position of the nucleus before and after the transition is represented by horizontal lines in the diagram. In Figure 5-2 the image of a nucleus is resting on these lines. This is not generally found in the conventional diagram but is here to help us follow the transition. The steps in the transition are represented by lines running downward. The transition always moves downward because the nucleus is decreasing its energy by emitting radiation. If the atomic number changes (isobaric transition), the transition line will slant to the right or left.

The vertical distance between the parent and daughter positions represents the total transition energy. This value is always specific for the transition associated with each radioactive nuclide. But all nuclei of the same nuclide do not necessarily go from the parent to daughter state in the same way. The significance of this is discussed in detail later.

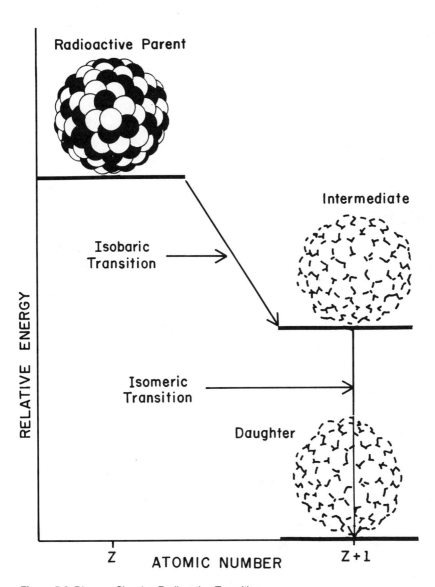

Figure 5-2 Diagram Showing Radioactive Transition

ISOBARIC TRANSITIONS

Most radioactive transitions have several steps. For most radionuclides, the first step is an isobaric transition usually followed by an isomeric transition and interactions with orbiting electrons. The three types of isobaric transitions of interest to us are (1) beta emission, (2) positron emission, and (3) electron capture.

In nuclear stability, the neutron-proton ratio (N/P) is crucial. If it is too low or too high, the nucleus will eventually rearrange itself into a more stable configuration. Beta radiation, which is the emission of energetic electrons, results when an N/P ratio is too high for stability; positron emission or electron capture occurs when it is too low for stability. These two conditions are represented by specific areas of the nuclide chart shown in Figure 5-3. Beta emitters are above the stable nuclides, and positron emitters and electron capture nuclides are below.

Beta Emission

A beta transition is illustrated in Figure 5-4. We should recall that the nuclear N/P is too high for stability. During the transition, this condition is relieved by the conversion of an internal neutron into a proton, accompanied by the emission, from the nucleus, of an electron. The electron, or beta particle, has two functions in this transition.

One function is to carry away from the nucleus a one-unit negative charge so that a neutron (no charge) can be converted into a proton with a one-unit positive charge. A fundamental principle of physics is that electrical charge cannot be created or destroyed. The only way to change the charge on an object, such as a nucleus, is to transfer electrons to or from the object. The emission of a beta particle causes the number of protons, and therefore the atomic number, of the nucleus to increase by one unit. Since the mass number, or total number of neutrons and protons, is not changed, the transition is isobaric.

The second function of the electron is to carry off a portion of the energy given up by the nucleus. The energy is carried as kinetic energy by the electron. But the energy carried by a beta particle is usually less than the total transition energy given up by the nucleus. The remaining portion is removed from the nucleus by the emission of a very small particle known as a neutrino. In each transition, the sum of the beta and neutrino energy is equal to the transition energy for the nuclide. Unlike the beta particle, the neutrino is very penetrating and carries the energy out of the patient's body.

A typical energy spectrum for a beta-emitting nuclide is shown in Figure 5-5. The maximum energy corresponds to the transition energy. This is the energy a beta particle would have in the few instances no neutrino is emitted. The average energy value indicates the radiation dose or energy deposited in the body by the beta radiation. The shape of the beta energy spectrum varies from nuclide to nuclide. The relationship between average energy and transition energy depends on the value of the transition energy and the atomic number of the nuclide. For

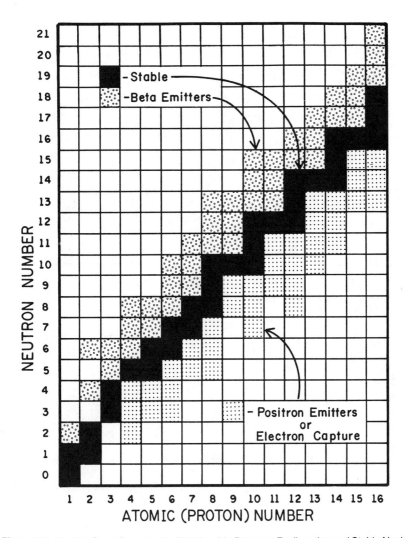

Figure 5-3 Nuclide Chart Showing the Relationship Between Radioactive and Stable Nuclear Structures

most radionuclides encountered in nuclear medicine, the average beta energy is usually between 25% and 30% of the maximum energy.

Positron Emission

Two types of transitions can occur when the nuclear N/P is too low for stability. One is positron emission. A positron is a small particle that has essentially the

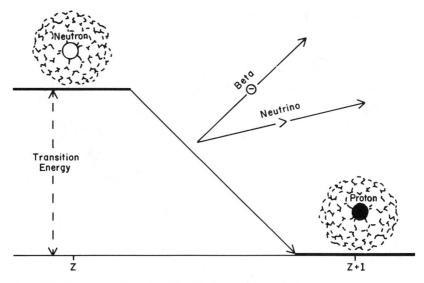

Figure 5-4 Diagram of a Transition That Produces Beta Radiation

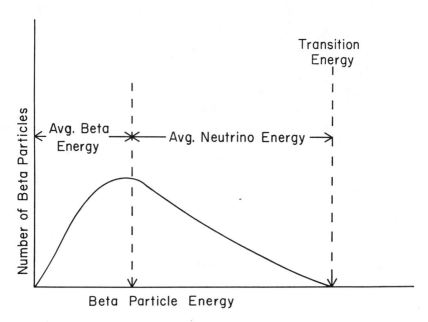

Figure 5-5 Spectrum of Beta Radiation Energy

same mass as an electron but has a positive rather than negative electrical charge. The nuclear transition resulting in the emission of a positron is illustrated in Figure 5-6. The transition energy is shared between the positron and a neutrino.

In this transition a proton is converted into a neutron as the positron particle is formed. Since a neutron is heavier than a proton, energy is required for this conversion. The energy equivalent to the mass difference between a neutron and a proton plus the energy equivalent of the positron mass is approximately 1.8 MeV. This means that the total transition energy must be at least 1.8 MeV for positron emission to occur.

The positron is the antiparticle of an electron and will enter an annihilation reaction when the two particles meet. Since electrons are normally abundant in material, positrons are annihilated soon after their emission. Positron emitters are useful in nuclear medicine because of the radiation produced when the positron is annihilated. The total masses of the positron and the electron are converted into energy according to the relationship

$$E = mc^2.$$

The energy produced is 1.022 MeV emitted as a pair of photons, each with an energy of 511 keV. Therefore, the radiation from a positron-emitting material is photons with a characteristic energy of 511 keV. The pair of photons leave the site traveling in opposite directions. This is useful in imaging, because it allows the annihilation site to be precisely determined.

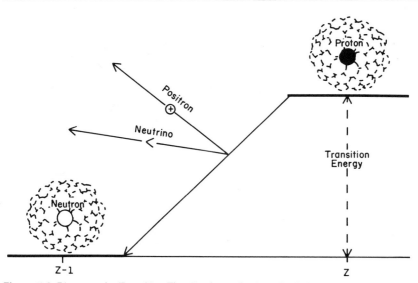

Figure 5-6 Diagram of a Transition That Produces Positron Radiation

Electron Capture

A nucleus can also relieve a low neutron-proton ratio by capturing and absorbing an electron from a shell. Since most electrons are captured from the K shell, this process is sometimes referred to as K-capture. Capture from the L and M shells is possible under some conditions, but does not occur so frequently as from the K shell. The electron capture process is illustrated in Figure 5-7. When the negative electron enters the nucleus, the positive charge of one proton is canceled and the proton is converted into a neutron. This results in the reduction of the atomic number by one unit. Since the mass number does not change, electron capture is an isobaric transition. Electron capture often competes with positron emission; if a nuclide is a positron emitter, some nuclei will emit positrons and some will capture electrons. The ratio between the two processes is specific for each nuclide.

In an electron capture transition, radiation is not emitted directly from the nucleus but results from changes within the electron shells. Electron capture creates a vacancy in one shell, which is quickly filled by an electron from a higher energy location. As the electron moves down to the K shell, it gives off an amount of energy equivalent to the difference in the binding energy of the two levels. This energy is emitted from the atom in either characteristic x-ray photons or Auger electrons. Auger electrons are produced when the energy given up by the electron

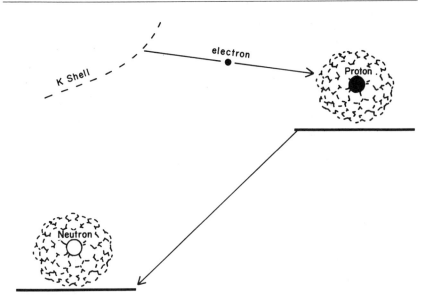

Figure 5-7 Diagram of a Transition That Produces Electron Capture

filling the K-shell vacancy is transferred to another electron, knocking it out of its shell. Most Auger electrons have relatively low energies.

Many radionuclides that undergo electron capture are used in nuclear medicine because the energy of characteristic x-ray photons is ideal for in-vivo studies.

ISOMERIC TRANSITIONS

After a radioactive nucleus undergoes an isobaric transition (beta emission, positron emission, or electron capture), it usually contains too much energy to be in its final stable or daughter state. Nuclei in these intermediate and final states are isomers, since they have the same atomic and mass numbers. Nuclei in the intermediate state will undergo an isomeric transition by emitting energy and dropping to the ground state.

Gamma Emission

In most isomeric transitions, a nucleus will emit its excess energy in the form of a gamma photon. A gamma photon is a small unit of energy that travels with the speed of light and has no mass; its most significant characteristic is its energy. The photon energies useful for diagnostic procedures are generally in the range of 100 keV to 500 keV.

The energy of a gamma photon is determined by the difference in energy between the intermediate and final states of the nucleus undergoing isomeric transition. This difference is the same for all nuclei of a specific nuclide. However, many nuclides have more than one intermediate state or energy level. When this is the case, a radionuclide might emit gamma photons with several different energies. This is illustrated in Figure 5-8.

The nuclide used in this illustration has two intermediate states or energy levels. One has an energy 500 keV above the daughter level, and the other is 300 keV higher than the first. When there are several different intermediate energy levels, it is common for some nuclei to go to one level and other nuclei to go to another level during isobaric transition. This is usually indicated on the transition diagram by showing the percentage of nuclei that go to each energy level. In the illustration considered, 80% of the nuclei go directly to intermediate energy level number 1, and 20% go directly to level number 2. The gamma photons are emitted when the nuclei move from these intermediate energy levels down to the daughter nuclide level.

Nuclei that have gone to a specific intermediate energy level might then go directly to the daughter level or to a lower intermediate level. With this in mind we can predict the gamma photon energy spectrum produced by our example nuclide. The spectrum will consist of three discrete energies as shown in Figure 5-8. Sixty percent of the parent nuclei will go to intermediate energy level number 1 and then directly to the daughter level 800 keV below. Therefore, 60% of the transitions will give rise to an 800-keV photon. Twenty percent of the nuclei that go to energy level 1 will then go to intermediate level number 2 by emitting a 300-keV photon. Forty percent of the nuclei will go through intermediate energy level number 2, either directly from the parent or from intermediate level number 1. When these nuclei drop to the daughter energy level, a 500-keV gamma photon will be emitted. It is the combination of different energy levels and different transition routes that gives rise to the different energies in the typical gamma spectrum. For most radionuclides, one or two gamma energies will account for the vast majority of transitions.

For most nuclides, the time spent by the nucleus in the intermediate state is extremely short and the isomeric transition appears to coincide with the isobaric transition. In some nuclides, however, the nuclei remain in the intermediate state for a longer time. In this case, the intermediate state is referred to as a metastable state. Metastable states are of particular interest in nuclear medicine because they make possible the separation of electron and photon radiation. In a diagnostic procedure it is undesirable to have electron radiation in the body because it contributes to radiation dosage but not to image formation. By using a nuclide that has already undergone an isobaric (electron-emitting) transition and is in a metastable state, it is possible to have a radioactive material that emits only gamma radiation.

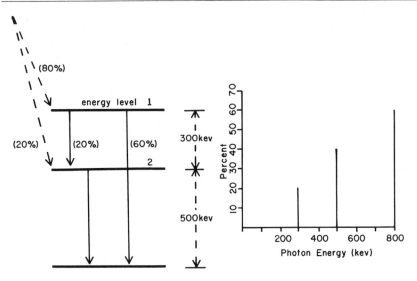

Figure 5-8 Relationship of Nuclear Energy Levels to the Energy Spectrum of Gamma Photons

Technetium-99m is a nuclide used in the metastable state. The parent nuclide is molybdenum, which undergoes an isobaric transition to technetium-99 in the metastable state. The technetium-99m will later undergo an isomeric transition to technetium-99.

Internal Conversion

Under some conditions, the energy from an isomeric transition can be transferred to an electron within the atom. This energy supplies the binding energy and expels the electron from the atom. This process is known as internal conversion (IC) and is an alternative to gamma emission. In many nuclides, isomeric transitions produce gamma photons and IC electrons. When an electron is removed from the atom by internal conversion, a vacancy is created. When the vacancy is filled by an electron from a higher energy level, energy must be emitted from the atom as a characteristic x-ray photon or an Auger electron.

The various isobaric and isomeric transitions give rise to a combination of both photon and particulate radiations. The radiations encountered in clinical procedures are summarized in Figure 5-9. Nuclei with a high N/P generally produce beta radiation; those with a low N/P produce either positrons or electron capture. All transitions are usually followed by either gamma or internal conversion

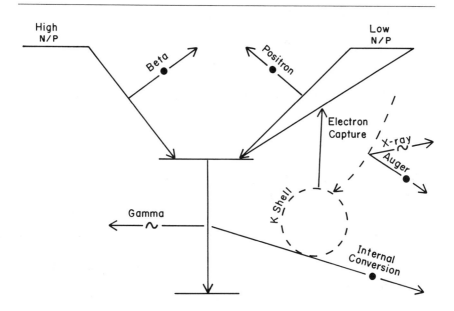

Figure 5-9 Composite Diagram Showing the Various Nuclear Transitions That Produce Radiation

electron emission. Internal conversion and electron capture lead to x-ray or Auger electron emission.

ALPHA EMISSION

Some radioactive materials emit alpha particles during their transformation. An alpha particle consists of two neutrons and two protons. Because of their size and electrical charge, alpha particles are not good penetrators and deposit their energy very close to their origin. Because of this, and the fact that alpha particles generally have more energy than other radiation forms, significant tissue doses can result from an alpha emitter within the body. Alpha emitters are generally not used in clinical medicine. An exception is radium, which is often used in therapeutic procedures. In these procedures the radium is contained in sealed metal capsules which absorb alpha radiation and let gamma radiation through to the tissue.

The transitions and principal radiations emitted by many nuclides used in clinical medicine are shown in Table 5-1.

Table 5-1 Radionuclides Used in Nuclear Medicine

Element	A	Z	$T_{1/2}$	Transition	Radiation	Yield	Energy (keV)
Hydrogen	3	1	12.3 yr	Beta	Beta	1.0	57
Carbon	11	6	20.3 min	Positron	Positron	1.0	394
					Annihilation	2.0	511
Nitrogen	13	7	10 min	Positron	Positron	1.0	488
					Annihilation	2.0	511
Carbon	14	6	5730 yr	Beta	Beta	1.0	49
Oxygen	15	8	2 min	Positron	Positron	1.0	721
					Annihilation	2.0	511
Fluorine	18	9	109 min	Positron EC (3%)	Positron	0.97	250
					Annihilation	1.94	511
Chromium	51	24	27.7 d	EC	Gamma	0.10	320
Cobalt	57	27	270 d	EC	Gamma	0.86	122
					Gamma	0.10	136
Iron	59	26	45 d	Beta	Beta	0.52	150
					Beta	0.46	81
					Gamma	0.55	1099
					Gamma	0.44	1292
Gallium	67	31	78.1 hr	EC	Gamma	0.38	93
					Gamma	0.24	185
					Gamma	0.16	300
					IC Electron	0.28	84
Zinc	69m	30	13.8 hr	Isomeric	Gamma	0.95	440

Table 5-1 continued

Element	A	Z	T$_{1/2}$	Transition	Radiation	Yield	Energy (keV)
Selenium	75	34	120 d	EC	Gamma	0.16	121
					Gamma	0.54	136
					Gamma	0.57	265
					Gamma	0.24	280
					Gamma	0.12	400
Strontium	85	38	65.1 d	EC	Gamma	0.99	514
Strontium	87m	38	2.8 hr	EC and isomeric	Gamma	0.83	388
					IC electron	0.14	372
Technetium	99m	43	6.0 hr	Isomeric	IC electron	0.09	119
					Gamma	0.88	141
Indium	111	49	2.8 d	EC	Gamma	0.90	172
					Gamma	0.94	247
Iodine	123	53	13 hr	EC	IC electron	0.13	127
					Gamma	0.84	159
					X-Ray	0.71	27
Iodine	125	53	60.2 d	EC	X-Ray	1.15	27
Iodine	131	53	8.0 d	Beta	Beta	0.90	192
					Gamma	0.82	364
					Gamma	0.07	637
Xenon	133	54	5.31 d	Beta	Beta	0.98	101
					IC electron	0.53	45
					Gamma	0.36	81
Ytterbium	169	70	32 d	EC	IC electron	0.47	108
					IC electron	0.15	196
					Gamma	0.45	63
					Gamma	0.11	130
					Gamma	0.17	177
					Gamma	0.26	198
					X-Ray	0.78	51
Mercury	197	80	65 hr	EC	IC electron	0.56	64
					IC electron	0.19	75
					Gamma	0.25	77
					X-Ray	0.36	69
Gold	198	79	2.69 d	Beta	Beta	0.99	316
					Gamma	0.96	412

EC, electron capture; IC, internal conversion.

PRODUCTION OF RADIONUCLIDES

Some radionuclides occur in nature but are generally not suitable for clinical studies. Most are made by bombarding a nucleus with a particle such as a neutron or a proton. Beta emitters are created by neutron bombardment, and positron emitters and nuclides that undergo electron capture are created by bombardment with positive particles such as protons. Neutrons can be obtained from nuclear reactors or accelerators. Positive particles are obtained from accelerators, usually cyclotrons.

Chapter 6

Radioactivity

INTRODUCTION AND OVERVIEW

One of the most important quantities associated with a sample or collection of radioactive material is its activity. Activity is the rate at which the nuclei within the sample undergo transitions and can be expressed in terms of the number of transitions per second (tps). Two units are used: the becquerel (Bq), equivalent to 1 tps, and the curie (Ci), equivalent to 3.7×10^{10} tps. The becquerel is an SI unit. The curie was first introduced as the activity of 1 g of radium. However, it was later discovered that the activity of 1 g of radium is not exactly 1 Ci, although the number of transitions per second per curie remains the same. Some useful conversions are

$$1 \text{ Ci} = 3.7 \times 10^{10} \text{ Bq}$$
$$1 \text{ mCi} = 37 \text{ MBq}$$
$$1 \text{ MBq} = 27 \text{ } \mu\text{Ci}.$$

The activity of a sample is related to two quantities used in clinical nuclear medicine. These are illustrated in Figure 6-1 and are (1) the number of radioactive (untransformed) nuclei in the sample and (2) the elapsed time. Both relationships involve the lifetime of the radioactive material. The lifetime is the time between the formation of a radioactive nucleus and its radioactive transition.

RADIOACTIVE LIFETIME

A fundamental characteristic of radioactivity is that all nuclei, even of the same radioactive nuclide, do not have the same lifetime. This is illustrated in Figure 6-2. There is no way to determine or predict the lifetime of a nucleus. However, we can determine the average lifetime of the nuclei of a specific radioactive nuclide. The average lifetime is a unique characteristic of each specific nuclide.

83

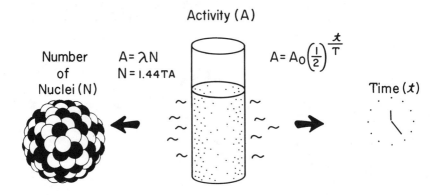

Figure 6-1 Relationship of Activity to Number of Nuclei and Elapsed Time

Formation

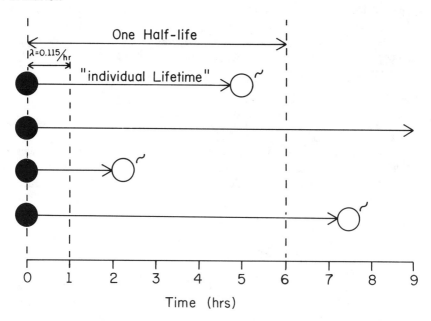

Figure 6-2 Variation in Lifetimes of Radioactive Nuclei

Half-Life

It is generally more useful to express the lifetime of a radioactive material in terms of the half-life, $T_{1/2}$, rather than the average life, T_a. The half-life is the time required for one-half of the nuclei to undergo transitions. The half-life is shorter than the average life. The specific relationship is

$$T_{1/2} = 0.693\, T_a$$
or
$$T_a = 1.44\, T_{1/2}.$$

Since half-life is proportional to the average life, the value is specific for each radionuclide. The half-lives for many nuclides of interest are given in Table 5-1 of Chapter 5.

Transformation Constant (Decay Constant)

Another way to express the lifetime characteristic of a radioactive substance is by means of the transformation constant, λ, often referred to as the *decay constant*. The transformation constant actually expresses the probability that a nucleus will undergo a transition in a stated period of time. In the example in Figure 6-2, the value of the transformation constant is 0.115 per hour. This means that a nucleus has a probability of 0.115 or an 11.5% chance of undergoing a transition in 1 hour. The value of the transformation constant is inversely related to lifetime. The probability of undergoing a transition in 1 hour is obviously much less for a radionuclide with a long lifetime (half-life). The actual relationship between the transformation constant and lifetime is:

$$T_{1/2} = \frac{0.693}{\lambda}.$$

The number, 0.693, is the natural logarithm of the number two, and frequently appears in relationships involving half-life. The transformation constant λ is the reciprocal of the average life, T_a:

$$\lambda = \frac{1}{T_a}.$$

We can summarize the lifetime characteristics of a radioactive substance: The lifetimes of nuclei within a sample vary tremendously. For a specific radioactive substance or nuclide, however, a characteristic lifetime can be expressed in terms of half-life, average life, or the transformation constant. If the value for one term is known, the others can be derived using the simple relationships above.

Quantity of Radioactive Material

Although activity does not express the amount of radioactive material present, it is proportional to the amount present at a specific time. The amount can be expressed by quantities such as mass, volume, or number of nuclei. We now consider the relationship of activity and the number of nuclei, N, in a specific sample.

We have just seen that transitions are spread over a longer time for some nuclides than for others. In other words, for a given number of radioactive nuclei, the rate of transition (activity) is inversely related to the lifetime of the nuclide. The transformation constant, λ, can be used to relate the activity to the number of nuclei in a sample. When applied to a large number of nuclei, the value of the transformation constant represents the fraction or percentage of the nuclei that will undergo a transition during one unit of time. Suppose we have a sample containing one million radioactive nuclei and the transformation constant has a value of 0.001 per second.

$$
\begin{aligned}
\text{Activity} &= \lambda \times N \\
&= (0.001/s)(1,000,000) \\
&= 1,000 \text{ transitions/second.}
\end{aligned}
$$

We should emphasize the difference between activity and amount of radioactive material, or number of nuclei. Both quantities are important when using radio-nuclides for clinical purposes. The amount of radioactive material is the quantity of radioactive nuclei or atoms in a sample, whereas the activity is the rate at which they are undergoing transitions and emitting radiation. Although activity is proportional to the number of nuclei, the proportion varies from one nuclide to another depending on its lifetime. From the relationships above, it can be seen that for a given quantity of radioactive material, activity is inversely related to half-life:

$$
\text{Activity} = .693 \times \frac{N}{T_{1/2}}
$$

$$
\text{Number of nuclei} = 1.44 \times \text{Activity} \times T_{1/2}.
$$

A relatively small amount of radioactive material can have the same activity as a larger amount if the smaller quantity has a shorter lifetime (half-life).

Cumulated Activity

The quantity of radioactive nuclei that undergo transitions in a period of time is usually designated the cumulated activity, Ã, and is expressed in the units of microcurie-hours. 1 μCi-hr is equivalent to 133 million (13.3×10^7) transitions. The relationship between cumulated activity, Ã, and the initial activity of a collection of radioactive material, A, is

$$\tilde{A} \ (\mu Ci\text{-}hr) = 1.44 \times A \ (\mu CI) \times T_{1/2} \ (hr).$$

The quality of nuclear radiation images is generally related to activity, whereas patient dose is more dependent on the amount of radioactive material or cumulated activity. Therefore, the "ratio" of image quality to patient dose is inversely proportional to radionuclide lifetime (half-life); a radionuclide with a short half-life yields more activity from less radioactive material and is generally desirable for clinical studies. The relationship of patient dose to half-life (and other factors) is explored in a later chapter.

ACTIVITY AND TIME

One of the most important characteristics of a radioactive material is that the quantity and activity constantly change with time. As each nucleus undergoes transition, it no longer belongs to the radioactive material. In each transition one atom is removed from the parent radioactive material and converted into the daughter product. Because the activity is proportional to the quantity of radioactive material at any instant in time, both quantity and activity decrease continuously with elapsed time. This decrease is generally referred to as radioactive decay.

The nature of radioactive decay is such that during a given time interval the same fraction (or percent) of radioactive nuclei will undergo transitions. The important point is that the fraction (but not the amount) per unit time remains constant. The fraction of nuclei that undergo transitions in a specified time period is different for each nuclide and depends on the nuclide lifetime (transformation constant or half-life). This characteristic of radioactive decay is illustrated in Figure 6-3.

Let us assume that we have a radioactive material with a transformation constant of 0.1 per hour. This means that approximately one-tenth of the nuclei will undergo transitions during a 1-hour time interval. If we begin with 100 units of radioactive material, 10 units will undergo transition during the first hour. At the beginning of the second hour there will be 90 units of material. During the second hour, one-tenth of 90 units will undergo transition which results in 81 units remaining at the end of the second hour. The relationship between amount of

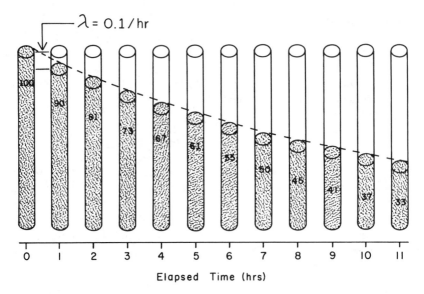

Figure 6-3 Relationship Between Amount of Radioactive Material and Elapsed Time

radioactivity and time is not linear, but is exponential. This relationship is encountered when the fraction of material undergoing change remains constant, but the amount decreases with time.

Remaining Fraction and Half-Life

It is often necessary to determine the fraction of radioactive material (or activity) that remains after a specific elapsed time. If the elapsed time is one half-life, the remaining fraction, f, is always 0.5. If the elapsed time is not one half-life, the remaining fraction is the fraction 0.5 multiplied by itself the number of times corresponding to the number of half-lives. For example,

    1 half-life, f = 0.5
    2 half-lives, f = (0.5) × (0.5) = 0.25
    3 half-lives, f = (0.5) × (0.5) × (0.5) = 0.125
    4 half-lives, f = (0.5) × (0.5) × (0.5) × (0.5) = 0.0625.

This can be expressed as

$$f = (0.5)^{t/T} = (0.5)^{n}$$

where t is the elapsed time, T is the half-life, and n is the number of half-lives. When the elapsed time is an integral number of half-lives, the remaining fraction can be easily calculated. If the elapsed time is not an integral number of half-lives, the computation requires a calculator that can perform exponential functions or a special mathematical table. Table 6-1 gives the remaining fractions for several elapsed time intervals expressed in terms of the number of half-lives.

Let us see how this table can be used to find the activity remaining after some elapsed time. Assume you have 100 μCi of a radioactive nuclide with a half-life of 6 hours. How much activity will remain after 33 hours? The first step is to express the elapsed time in terms of half-lives:

$$n = 33 \text{ hr}/6 \text{ hr} = 5.5.$$

The remaining fraction is

$$f = (0.5)^{5.5}.$$

Table 6-1 Tabulation of Remaining Fraction (f) After an Elapsed Time of n Half-Lives

n	f	n	f	n	f
0.0	1.0	1.25	0.42	2.5	0.175
0.05	0.97	1.3	0.41	2.55	0.17
0.1	0.93	1.35	0.39	2.6	0.165
0.15	0.90	1.4	0.38	2.65	0.16
0.2	0.87	1.45	0.37	2.7	0.15
0.25	0.84	1.5	0.35	2.75	0.145
0.3	0.81	1.55	0.34	2.8	0.14
0.35	0.78	1.6	0.33	2.85	0.135
0.4	0.76	1.65	0.32	2.9	0.13
0.45	0.73	1.7	0.31	2.95	0.129
0.5	0.71	1.75	0.3	3.0	0.125
0.55	0.68	1.8	0.29	3.5	0.088
0.6	0.66	1.85	0.28	4.0	0.063
0.65	0.64	1.9	0.27	4.5	0.044
0.7	0.62	1.95	0.26	5.0	0.031
0.75	0.59	2.0	0.25	5.5	0.022
0.8	0.57	2.05	0.24	6.0	0.016
0.85	0.55	2.1	0.23	6.5	0.011
0.9	0.54	2.15	0.225	7.0	0.008
0.95	0.52	2.2	0.22	7.5	0.006
1.0	0.50	2.25	0.21	8.0	0.004
1.05	0.48	2.3	0.2	8.5	0.003
1.1	0.47	2.35	0.195	9.0	0.002
1.15	0.45	2.4	0.19	9.5	0.0014
1.2	0.44	2.45	0.18	10.0	0.001

The value of this is obtained from Table 6-1 and is

$$f = 0.022 \ (2.2\%).$$

Therefore, if we started with 100 μCi, 2.2 μCi would remain after an elapsed time of 33 hours.

Another expression relating remaining fraction to elapsed time is

$$f = e^{-\lambda t}$$

where λ is the transformation constant and t is the elapsed time expressed in the same time units (hours, days, etc.) as the transformation constant. To determine the remaining fraction from this expression also requires a calculator that can perform exponential functions or special exponential tables.

RADIOACTIVE EQUILIBRIUM

We have considered fixed quantities of radioactive material that decay with elapsed time. If the radioactive material is being formed or replenished during the decay process, however, the relationship between activity and elapsed time is quite different from a simple exponential decay. The form of this relationship depends on the relationship of the rate of formation to the rate of decay. If we began by forming radioactive material, we would expect the activity to increase with elapsed time as illustrated in Figure 6-4. As the amount of radioactive

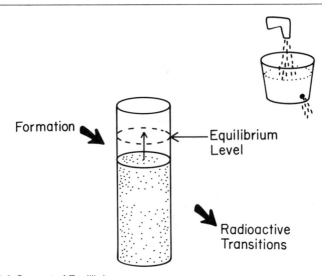

Figure 6-4 Concept of Equilibrium

material (and activity) increases, however, the rate of loss of material by radioactive transitions also increases.

Consider filling a bucket with a hole in it. As the water level rises in the bucket, the rate at which water flows out of the hole also increases. The water will usually reach a level at which the rate of loss is equal to the rate of filling, and the water level will remain constant. This could be described as a state of equilibrium between the rate of filling and rate of loss. The same process occurs with radioactive material. As the amount of material or activity builds up, the rate of loss by radioactive transitions can, under certain conditions, become the same as the rate of formation, and a state of equilibrium will be established. When the radioactive material being formed is the daughter of a radioactive parent, as illustrated in Figure 6-5, the type of activity-time relationship depends on the relationship of the two half-lives. If the half-life of the parent is shorter, no state of equilibrium will be reached. If the half-life of the parent is longer, and long enough that there is no noticeable decay during the time interval of interest, a condition of secular equilibrium will be reached. If the parent half-life is longer, but short enough so that there is a noticeable decay of the parent during the time interval of interest, a condition of transient equilibrium will be reached.

When a state of equilibrium is reached, the activity of the radioactive daughter is determined by the activity of the parent.

Secular Equilibrium

Assume that the radioactive material is forming at an almost constant rate. If, at the beginning, no radioactive daughter material is present, no nuclei will be undergoing transition. As soon as the radioactive material begins to accumulate, transitions will begin and some radioactive nuclei will be lost. As the number of

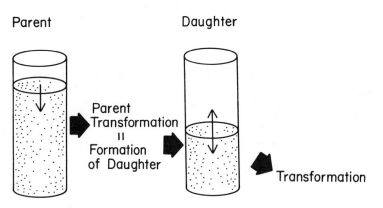

Figure 6-5 Factors Affecting Build-up of Daughter Activity

radioactive nuclei increases, the activity and rate of loss increase. Initially, the rate of loss is much less than the rate of formation. As the quantity of radioactive material builds, the activity or transition rate increases until it is equal to the rate of formation as shown in Figure 6-6. In other words, radioactive nuclei undergo transitions at exactly the same rate they are forming, and a condition of equilibrium is established. The amount of radioactive material will then remain constant regardless of elapsed time. Under this condition, the activity is equal to the rate of formation and is referred to as the saturation activity. The important point is that the maximum activity of a radioactive material is determined by the rate (nuclei per second) at which the material is being formed. Although it is true that the activity gradually builds with time, a point is reached at which build-up stops and the activity remains at the saturation level.

The time required to reach a specific activity depends on the half-life of the material being formed (daughter). After n half-lives the activity will be some fraction, f, of the rate of formation or saturation activity. The relationship is

$$f = 1 - \left(\frac{1}{2}\right)^n.$$

Activity values after a specific elapsed time can be obtained for this relationship by using Table 6-1 to find the value of $(1/2)^n$. It should be observed that the build-up of radioactivity is a mirror image of radioactive decay. Just as a radioactive material never decays to zero activity (at least theoretically), radioactive build-up never reaches saturation. However, for practical purposes, saturation is reached in approximately 5 half-lives when the activity is more than 96% of the saturation value.

After the activity reaches the saturation value it remains constant and is in a state of secular equilibrium. This occurs when the rate of formation does not change during the time period of interest because either the parent material has a very long half-life or the radioactive material is forming at a constant rate by another means such as a cyclotron or nuclear reactor.

Transient Equilibrium

When the half-life of the parent is only a few times greater than the half-life of the daughter, the condition of transient equilibrium will occur. During the period of interest the parent will undergo radioactive decay. Daughter activity will build and establish a state of equilibrium with the parent activity. Transient equilibrium differs from secular equilibrium in two respects.

First, the equilibrium or saturation activity of the daughter, A_d, is not equal to the activity of the parent, A_p. The relationship is

$$A_d = A_p \frac{T_p}{T_p - T_d}.$$

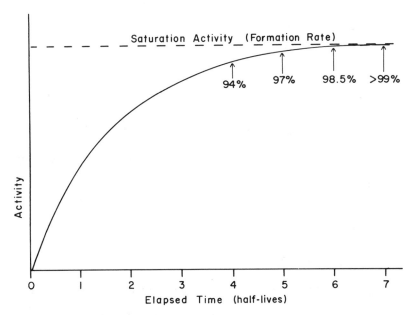

Figure 6-6 Build-up of Activity to Saturation Level During Transient Equilibrium

When the half-life of the parent, T_p, is much greater than that of the daughter, T_d, the term $(T_p/T_p - T_d)$ approaches a value of one, and daughter activity approaches parent activity, as in secular equilibrium. However, as daughter and parent half-lives become closer, this term becomes greater than one, which means that daughter activity is actually greater than parent activity under equilibrium conditions. The ratio of daughter to parent activity becomes greater as the half-lives become closer.

Second, with transient equilibrium the equilibrium activity of the daughter changes with time because the parent activity is changing. The relationship of parent and daughter activity for a transient condition is shown in Figure 6-7. After the condition of equilibrium is reached, the daughter appears to decay with the half-life of the parent.

Technetium-99m and molybdenum-99 are good examples of transient equilibrium. Technetium-99m is obtained from a generator that contains molybdenum-99. The molybdenum-99 undergoes an isobaric transition into technetium-99m (86%) and technetium-99 (14%). The technetium-99m is radioactive with a half-life of 6 hours. Molybdenum-99 has a half-life of approximately 67 hours. The relationship between technetium and molybdenum activity in a typical generator is shown in Figure 6-8. In this example it is assumed that all technetium is removed from the generator every 24 hours.

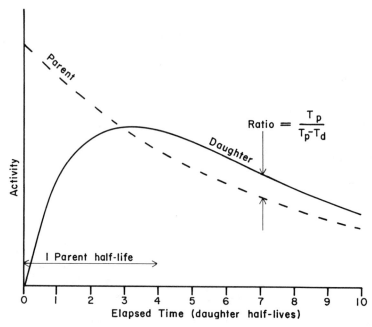

Figure 6-7 Transient Equilibrium

If all molybdenum nuclei changed into technetium-99m nuclei, the saturation activity would be

$$A_{Tc} = A_{mo} \frac{T_{mo}}{T_{mo} - T_{Tc}}$$

$$= \frac{67}{61\ A_{mo}}$$

$$= 1.1\ A_{mo}.$$

However, since only about 86% of the molybdenum-99 goes to technetium-99m, the saturation activity of technetium-99m will be only about 95% of the molybdenum-99 activity. In a 24-hour period (4 half-lives), the activity of technetium-99m will be approximately 94% of the saturation activity value. This would be only 84% of the molybdenum activity at that particular time.

EFFECTIVE LIFETIME

When a radioactive material is in a living organism, the material can be removed from a particular organ or location by two mechanisms, as illustrated in Figure 6-9. One is the normal radioactive decay, and the other is biological transport or elimination from the specific site.

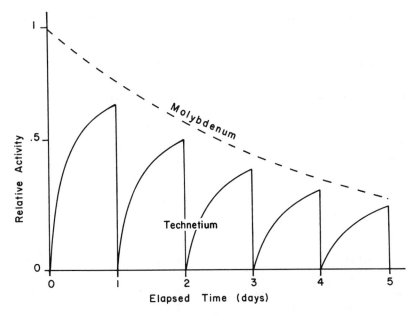

Figure 6-8 Molybdenum and Technetium Activity in a Generator

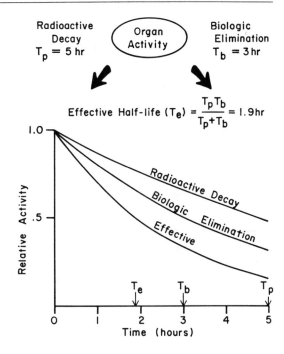

Figure 6-9 Relationship of Effective Lifetime to Rates of Radioactive Decay and Biologic Elimination

Half-life values can be used to express the rate of removal by both mechanisms. The half-life associated with normal radioactive decay is generally designated the physical half-life and has a characteristic value for each radionuclide. The rate of biological removal can generally be expressed in terms of the biological half-life. The value of the biological half-life is determined by such things as the chemical form of the radionuclide and the physiological function of the organ or organism considered.

When biological transport or elimination occurs, the lifetime of the radioactive material in the organ is reduced. This is generally expressed in terms of an effective half-life. The relationship between effective half-life (T_e), physical half-life (T_p), and biological half-life (T_b) is given by

$$T_e = \frac{T_p \times T_b}{T_p + T_b}.$$

When both radioactive decay and biological elimination are present, the effective half-life will always be less than either the physical or biological half-life. If the difference in the two half-life values is rather large, the effective half-life will be slightly less than the shorter half-life of the two; if the two are equal, the effective half-life will be one-half of the physical or biological half-life value.

Chapter 7

X-Ray Production

INTRODUCTION AND OVERVIEW

X-radiation is created by taking energy from electrons and converting it into photons with appropriate energies. This energy conversion takes place within the x-ray tube. The quantity and quality of the x-radiation produced can be controlled by adjusting the electrical quantities (KV, MA) and exposure time, S, applied to the tube. In this chapter we first become familiar with the design and construction of x-ray tubes, then look at the x-ray production process, and conclude by reviewing the quantitative aspects of x-ray production.

THE X-RAY TUBE

Function

An x-ray tube is an energy converter. It receives electrical energy and converts it into two other forms: x-radiation and heat. The heat is an undesirable byproduct. X-ray tubes are designed and constructed to maximize x-ray production and to dissipate heat as rapidly as possible.

The x-ray tube is a relatively simple electrical device typically containing only two elements: a cathode and an anode. As the electrical current flows through the tube from cathode to anode, the electrons undergo an energy loss, which results in the generation of x-radiation. A cross-sectional view of a typical x-ray tube is shown in Figure 7-1.

Anode

The anode is the component in which the x-radiation is produced. It is a relatively large piece of metal that connects to the positive side of the electrical

97

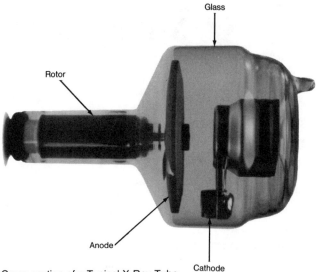

Figure 7-1 Cross-section of a Typical X-Ray Tube

circuit. The anode has two primary functions: (1) to convert electronic energy into x-radiation, and (2) to dissipate the heat created in the process. The material for the anode is selected to enhance these functions.

The ideal situation would be if most of the electrons created x-ray photons rather than heat. The fraction of the total electronic energy that is converted into x-radiation (efficiency) depends on two factors: the atomic number (Z) of the anode material and the energy of the electrons. Most x-ray tubes use tungsten, which has an atomic number of 74, as the anode material. In addition to a high atomic number, tungsten has several other characteristics that make it suited for this purpose. Tungsten is almost unique in its ability to maintain its strength at high temperatures, and it has a high melting point and a relatively low rate of evaporation. For many years, pure tungsten was used as the anode material. In recent years an alloy of tungsten and rhenium has been used as the target material but only for the surface of some anodes. The anode body under the tungsten-rhenium surface on many tubes is manufactured from a material that is relatively light and has good heat storage capability. Two such materials are molybdenum and graphite. The use of molybdenum as an anode base material should not be confused with its use as an anode surface material. Some x-ray tubes used for mammography have molybdenum-surface anodes. This material has an intermediate atomic number (Z = 42), which produces characteristic x-ray photons with energies well suited to this particular application.

The use of a rhenium-tungsten alloy improves the long-term radiation output of tubes. With x-ray tubes with pure tungsten anodes, radiation output is reduced with usage because of thermal damage to the surface.

Design

Most anodes are shaped as beveled disks and attached to the shaft of an electric motor that rotates them at relatively high speeds during the x-ray production process. The purpose of anode rotation is to dissipate heat and is considered in detail in Chapter 9.

Focal Spot

All of the anode is not involved in x-ray production. The radiation is produced in a very small area on the surface of the anode known as the focal spot. The dimensions of the focal spot are determined by the dimensions of the electron beam arriving from the cathode. In most x-ray tubes, the focal spot is rectangular. The dimensions of focal spots usually range from 0.2 mm to 2 mm. X-ray tubes are designed to have specific focal spot sizes; small focal spots produce sharper images, and large focal spots have a greater heat-dissipating capacity.

Focal spot size is one factor that must be considered when selecting an x-ray tube for a specific application. Tubes with small focal spots are used when high image quality is essential and the amount of radiation needed is relatively low. Most x-ray tubes have two focal spot sizes (small and large), which can be selected by the operator according to the imaging procedure.

Cathode

The basic function of the cathode is to expel the electrons from the electrical circuit and focus them into a well-defined beam aimed at the anode. The typical cathode consists of a small coil of wire (a filament) recessed within a cup-shaped region, as shown in Figure 7-2.

Electrons that flow through electrical circuits cannot generally escape from the conductor material and move into free space. They can, however, if they are given sufficient energy. In a process known as thermionic emission, thermal energy (or heat) is used to expel the electrons from the cathode. The filament of the cathode is heated in the same way as a light bulb filament by passing a current through it. This heating current is not the same as the current flowing through the x-ray tube that produces the x-radiation. During tube operation, the cathode is heated to a glowing temperature, and the heat energy expels some of the electrons from the cathode.

Envelope

The anode and cathode are contained in an airtight enclosure, or envelope. The envelope and its contents are often referred to as the tube insert, which is the part of the tube that has a limited lifetime and can be replaced within the housing. The

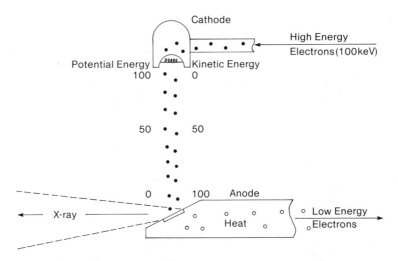

Figure 7-2 Energy Exchanges within an X-Ray Tube

majority of x-ray tubes have glass envelopes, although tubes for some applications have metal and ceramic envelopes.

The primary functions of the envelope are to provide support and electrical insulation for the anode and cathode assemblies and to maintain a vacuum in the tube. The presence of gases in the x-ray tube would allow electricity to flow through the tube freely, rather than only in the electron beam. This would interfere with x-ray production and possibly damage the circuit.

Housing

The x-ray tube housing provides several functions in addition to enclosing and supporting the other components. It absorbs radiation, except for the radiation that passes through the window as the useful x-ray beam. Its relatively large exterior surface dissipates most of the heat created within the tube. The space between the housing and insert is filled with oil, which provides electrical insulation and transfers heat from the insert to the housing surface.

ELECTRON ENERGY

The energy that will be converted into x-radiation (and heat) is carried to the x-ray tube by a current of flowing electrons. As the electrons pass through the x-ray tube, they undergo two energy conversions, as illustrated in Figure 7-2: The electrical potential energy is converted into kinetic energy that is, in turn, converted into x-radiation and heat.

Potential

When the electrons arrive at the x-ray tube, they carry electrical potential energy. The amount of energy carried by each electron is determined by the voltage or KV, between the anode and cathode. For each kV of voltage, each electron has 1 keV of energy. By adjusting the KV, the x-ray machine operator actually assigns a specific amount of energy to each electron.

Kinetic

After the electrons are emitted from the cathode, they come under the influence of an electrical force pulling them toward the anode. This force accelerates them, causing an increase in velocity and kinetic energy. This increase in kinetic energy continues as the electrons travel from the cathode to the anode. As the electron moves from cathode to anode, however, its electrical potential energy decreases as it is converted into kinetic energy all along the way. Just as the electron arrives at the surface of the anode its potential energy is lost, and all its energy is kinetic. At this point the electron is traveling with a relatively high velocity determined by its actual energy content. A 100-keV electron reaches the anode surface traveling at more than one half the velocity of light. When the electrons strike the surface of the anode, they are slowed very quickly and lose their kinetic energy; the kinetic energy is converted into either x-radiation or heat.

The electrons interact with individual atoms of the anode material, as shown in Figure 7-3. Two types of interactions produce radiation. An interaction with electron shells produces *characteristic* x-ray photons; interactions with the atomic nucleus produce *Bremsstrahlung* x-ray photons.

BREMSSTRAHLUNG

Production Process

The interaction that produces the most photons is the Bremsstrahlung process. Bremsstrahlung is a German word for "braking radiation" and is a good description of the process. Electrons that penetrate the anode material and pass close to a nucleus are deflected and slowed down by the attractive force from the nucleus. The energy lost by the electron during this encounter appears in the form of an x-ray photon. All electrons do not produce photons of the same energy.

Spectrum

Only a few photons that have energies close to that of the electrons are produced; most have lower energies. Although the reason for this is complex, a simplified model of the Bremsstrahlung interaction is shown in Figure 7-4. First,

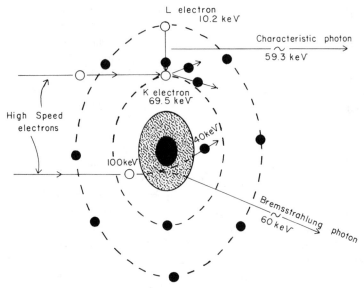

Figure 7-3 Electron-Atom Interactions that Produce X-Ray Photons

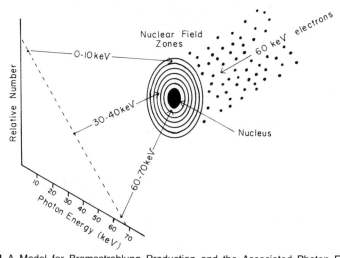

Figure 7-4 A Model for Bremsstrahlung Production and the Associated Photon Energy Spectrum

assume that there is a space, or field, surrounding the nucleus in which electrons experience the "braking" force. This field can be divided into zones, as illustrated. This gives the nuclear field the appearance of a target with the actual nucleus located in the center. An electron striking anywhere within the target experiences some braking action and produces an x-ray photon. Those electrons striking nearest the center are subjected to the greatest force and, therefore, lose the most energy and produce the highest energy photons. The electrons hitting in the outer zones experience weaker interactions and produce lower energy photons. Although the zones have essentially the same width, they have different areas. The area of a given zone depends on its distance from the nucleus. Since the number of electrons hitting a given zone depends on the total area within the zone, it is obvious that the outer zones capture more electrons and create more photons. From this model, an x-ray energy spectrum, such as the one shown in Figure 7-4, could be predicted.

The basic Bremsstrahlung spectrum has a maximum photon energy that corresponds to the energy of the incident electrons. This is 70 keV for the example shown. Below this point, the number of photons produced increases as photon energy decreases. The spectrum of x-rays emerging from the tube generally looks quite different from the one shown here because of selective absorption within the filter.

A significant number of the lower-energy photons are absorbed or filtered out as they attempt to pass through the anode surface, x-ray tube window, or added filter material. X-ray beam filtration is discussed more extensively in Chapter 11. The amount of filtration is generally dependent on the composition and thickness of material through which the x-ray beam passes and is generally what determines the shape of the low-energy end of the spectrum curve.

KV_p

The high-energy end of the spectrum is determined by the kilovoltage applied to the x-ray tube. This is because the kilovoltage establishes the energy of the electrons as they reach the anode, and no x-ray photon can be created with an energy greater than that of the electrons. The maximum photon energy, therefore, in kiloelectron volts is numerically equal to the maximum applied potential in kilovolts. In some x-ray equipment, the voltage applied to the tube might vary during the exposure. The maximum photon energy is determined by the maximum, or peak, voltage during the exposure time. This value is generally referred to as the kilovolt peak (KV_p) and is one of the adjustable factors of x-ray equipment.

In addition to establishing the maximum x-ray photon energy, the KV_p has a major role in determining the quantity of radiation produced for a given number of electrons, such as 1 mAs, striking the anode. Since the general efficiency of x-ray production by the Bremsstrahlung process is increased by increasing the energy of the bombarding electrons, and the electronic energy is determined by the KV_p, it follows that the KV_p affects x-ray production efficiency.

Changing the KV_p will generally alter the Bremsstrahlung spectrum, as shown in Figure 7-5. The total area under the spectrum curve represents the number of photons produced. If no filtration is present where the spectrum is essentially a triangle, the amount of radiation produced is approximately proportional to the KV squared. With the presence of filtration, however, increasing the KV also increases the relative penetration of the photons, and a smaller percentage is filtered out. This results in an even greater increase in radiation output with KV_p.

CHARACTERISTIC RADIATION

Production Process

The type of interaction that produces characteristic radiation, also illustrated in Figure 7-3, involves a collision between the high-speed electrons and the orbital electrons in the atom. The interaction can occur only if the incoming electron has a kinetic energy greater than the binding energy of the electron within the atom. When this condition exists, and the collision occurs, the electron is dislodged from the atom. When the orbital electron is removed, it leaves a vacancy that is filled by an electron from a higher energy level. As the filling electron moves down to fill the vacancy, it gives up energy emitted in the form of an x-ray photon. This is known as characteristic radiation because the energy of the photon is characteristic

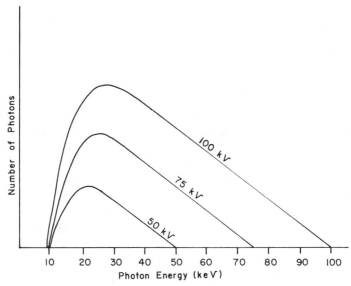

Figure 7-5 Comparison of Photon Energy Spectra Produced at Different KV_p Values

of the chemical element that serves as the anode material. In the example shown, the electron dislodges a tungsten K-shell electron, which has a binding energy of 69.5 keV. The vacancy is filled by an electron from the L shell, which has a binding energy of 10.2 keV. The characteristic x-ray photon, therefore, has an energy equal to the energy difference between these two levels, or 59.3 keV.

Actually, a given anode material gives rise to several characteristic x-ray energies. This is because electrons at different energy levels (K, L, etc.) can be dislodged by the bombarding electrons, and the vacancies can be filled from different energy levels. The electronic energy levels in tungsten are shown in Figure 7-6, along with some of the energy changes that give rise to characteristic photons. Although filling L-shell vacancies generates photons, their energies are too low for use in diagnostic imaging. Each characteristic energy is given a designation, which indicates the shell in which the vacancy occurred, with a subscript, which shows the origin of the filling electron. A subscript alpha (α) denotes filling with an L-shell electron, and beta (β) indicates filling from either the M or N shell.

Tungsten Spectrum

The spectrum of the significant characteristic radiation from tungsten is shown in Figure 7-6. Characteristic radiation produces a line spectrum with several discrete energies, whereas Bremsstrahlung produces a continuous spectrum of

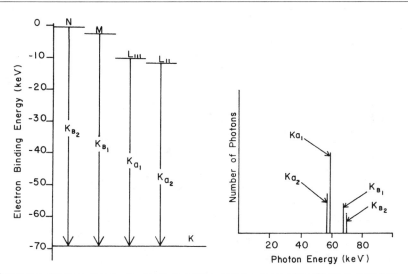

Figure 7-6 Electron Energy Levels in Tungsten and the Associated Characteristic X-Ray Spectrum

photon energies over a specific range. The number of photons created at each characteristic energy is different because the probability for filling a K-shell vacancy is different from shell to shell.

Molybdenum Spectrum

Molybdenum anode tubes produce two rather intense characteristic x-ray energies: K-alpha radiation, at 17.9 keV, and K-beta, at 19.5 keV.

KV_p

The KV_p value also strongly influences the production of characteristic radiation. No characteristic radiation will be produced if the KV_p is less (numerically) than the binding energy of the K-shell electrons. When the kilovoltage is increased above this threshold level, the quantity of characteristic radiation is generally proportional to the difference between the operating kilovoltage and the threshold kilovoltage.

The x-ray beam that emerges from a tube has a spectrum of photon energies determined by several factors. A typical spectrum is shown in Figure 7-7 and is made up of photons from both Bremsstrahlung and characteristic interactions.

The relative composition of an x-ray spectrum with respect to Bremsstrahlung and characteristic radiation depends on the anode material, kilovoltage, and filtration. In a tungsten anode tube, no characteristic radiation is produced when

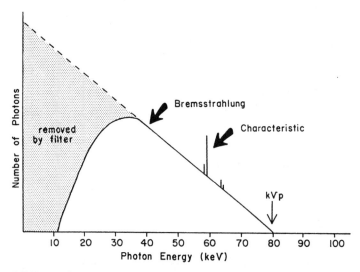

Figure 7-7 Typical Photon Energy Spectrum from a Machine Operating at kVp = 80

the KV_p is less than 69.5. At some higher kilovoltage values generally used in diagnostic examinations, the characteristic radiation might contribute as much as 25% of the total radiation. In molybdenum target tubes operated under certain conditions of KV_p and filtration, the characteristic radiation can be a major part of the total output.

EFFICIENCY

Concept

Only a small fraction of the energy delivered to the anode by the electrons is converted into x-radiation; most is absorbed and converted into heat. The efficiency of x-ray production is defined as the total x-ray energy expressed as a fraction of the total electrical energy imparted to the anode. The two factors that determine production efficiency are the voltage applied to the tube, KV, and the atomic number of the anode, Z. An approximate relationship is

$$\text{Efficiency} = \text{KV} \times \text{Z} \times 10^{-6}.$$

KV_p

The relationship between x-ray production efficiency and KV_p has a specific effect on the practical use of x-ray equipment. As we will see in Chapter 9, x-ray tubes have a definite limit on the amount of electrical energy they can dissipate because of the heat produced. This, in principle, places a limit on the amount of x-radiation that can be produced by an x-ray tube. By increasing KV_p, however, the quantity of radiation produced per unit of heat is significantly increased.

Anode Material

The relationship of x-ray production efficiency to anode material is only of academic interest because most tubes use tungsten. The exception is molybdenum used in mammography. The x-ray production efficiency of these tubes is significantly less than that of tungsten anode tubes.

EFFICACY (OUTPUT)

Concept

The x-ray efficacy of the x-ray tube is defined as the amount of exposure, in milliroentgens, delivered to a point in the center of the useful x-ray beam at a distance of 1 m from the focal spot for 1 mAs of electrons passing through the tube.

The efficacy value expresses the ability of a tube to convert electronic energy into x-ray exposure. Knowledge of the efficacy value for a given tube permits the determination of both patient and film exposures by methods discussed in later chapters. Like x-ray energy output, the efficacy of a tube depends on a number of factors including KV_p, voltage waveform, anode material, filtration, tube age, and anode surface damage. Figure 7-8 gives typical efficacy values for tungsten anode tubes with normal filtration.

KV_p

KV_p is very useful in controlling the radiation output of an x-ray tube. Figure 7-8 shows a nonlinear relationship. It is normally assumed that the radiation output is proportional to the square of the KV_p. Doubling KV_p quadruples the exposure from the tube.

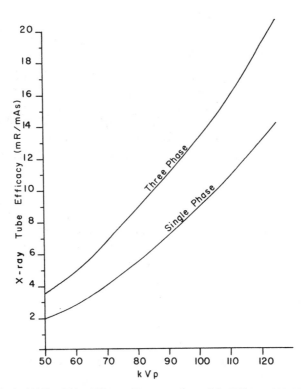

Figure 7-8 Typical X-Ray Tube Efficacy (Exposure Output) for Different kVp Values

Waveform

Waveform describes the manner in which the KV changes with time during the x-ray production process; several different KV waveforms are used. A general principle is that the waveform with the least KV variation during the exposure is the most effective x-ray producer. Single-phase and three-phase are two of the most common waveform types. Of these two, three-phase has the least fluctuation and produces more radiation per unit of MAS. Waveforms are described in more detail in the next chapter.

Chapter 8

Energizing and Controlling the X-Ray Tube

INTRODUCTION AND OVERVIEW

To produce x-radiation, the x-ray tube must be supplied with electrical energy. The electrical energy provided by a power company is not in the correct form for direct application to the x-ray tube. An x-ray machine has a number of components that rearrange, control, and perhaps store electrical energy before it is applied to the x-ray tube. These components are collectively referred to as either the power supply or the generator. The function of the generator is not to supply or generate energy, but to transform it into an appropriate form for x-ray production. The other major function of the generator is to permit the operator to control three quantities: (1) KV, (2) MA, and (3) exposure time.

The more specific functions of the generator are identified in Figure 8-1. These include:

- increase voltage (produce KV)
- convert AC to DC
- change waveform (filter)
- store energy (for portable machines)
- control kilovoltage (KV)
- control tube current (MA)
- control exposure time.

A simplified circuit diagram of an x-ray machine is shown in Figure 8-2. We now consider the functions of the components.

KV PRODUCTION

One requirement for x-ray production is that the electrons delivering energy to the x-ray tube must have individual energies at least equal to the energy of the

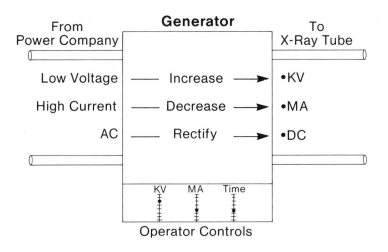

Figure 8-1 Functions Performed by an X-Ray Machine Generator

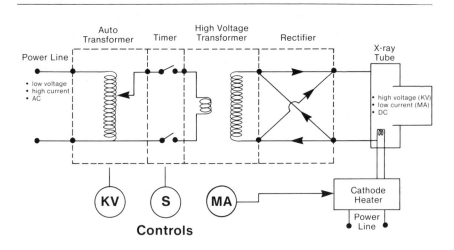

Figure 8-2 A Basic Circuit of an X-Ray Machine

x-ray photons; the x-ray photon energy (kiloelectron volts) is always limited by the electron energy, or voltage (kilovolts).

The electrical energy from a power company is generally delivered at 120, 240, or 440 V. This voltage must be increased to the range of 25,000 V to 150,000 V to produce diagnostic-quality x-rays.

Transformer Principles

The device that can increase voltage is the transformer, which is one of the major components of the generator. It is a relatively large device connected by cables to the x-ray tube. The basic function of a transformer is illustrated in Figure 8-3.

A transformer has two separate circuits. The input circuit, which receives the electrical energy, is designated the primary, and the output circuit is designated the secondary. Electrons do not flow between the two circuits; rather, energy is passed from the primary circuit to the secondary circuit by a magnetic field.

As electrons flow into the transformer and through the primary circuit, they transfer energy to the electrons in the secondary circuit. The voltage (individual electron energy) increases because the transformer collects the energy from a large number of primary-circuit electrons and concentrates it into a few secondary-circuit electrons. In principle, the transformer repackages the electron energy; the total energy entering and leaving the transformer is essentially the same. It enters in the form of high current, low voltage and leaves in the form of high voltage, low current.

Transformers are designed to produce specific changes in voltage. The transformer described above increases voltage and is therefore designated a ''step-up transformer.'' For some applications, transformers are designed to decrease voltage and are designated ''step-down transformers.''

Transformer Concept

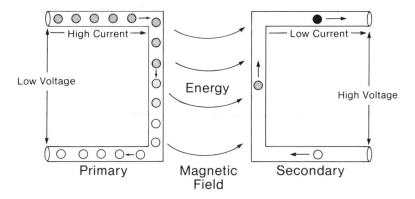

Figure 8-3 Electron-Energy Transfer in a Transformer

The High Voltage Transformer

The high voltage transformer in most x-ray machines has a voltage step-up ratio of approximately 1,000:1. The output of such a transformer would be 1,000 V (1 kV) for each volt applied to the primary.

In a step-up transformer, the current (electron flow) must be larger in the primary than in the secondary. The ratio of the currents is the same as the voltage ratio, except it is reversed. The larger current is in the primary, and the smaller current is in the secondary. For a transformer with a 1,000:1 ratio, the current flowing through the primary must be 1 A (1,000 mA) per 1 mA of current flowing through the secondary.

The high voltage transformer in an x-ray machine can be described in quantitative terms as a device that converts volts into kilovolts and converts amperes into milliamperes.

A transformer physically consists of two coils of wire, as shown in Figure 8-2. One coil forms the primary and the other the secondary circuit of the transformer. Each coil contains a specific number of loops or turns. The characteristic of the transformer that determines the voltage step-up ratio is the ratio of the number of turns (loops) in the secondary coil to the number in the primary. The voltage step-up ratio is determined by, and is the same as, the secondary-to-primary-turns ratio.

There is no direct flow of electrons between the primary and secondary coils; they are coupled by the magnetic field produced by current passing through the primary coil. The transformer is based on two physical principles involving the interaction between electrons and magnetic fields: (1) when electrons flow through a coil of wire, a magnetic field is created around the coil; (2) electrons within a coil of wire will receive energy if the coil is placed in a changing magnetic field.

The key to transformer operation is that the primary coil must produce a constantly changing, or pulsing, magnetic field to boost the energy of the electrons in the secondary coil. This occurs when the primary of the transformer is connected to an AC source. When AC is applied to the input of a transformer, the primary coil produces a pulsing magnetic field. It is this pulsing magnetic field that pumps the electrons through the secondary coil. An electron in the secondary coil gains a specific amount of energy each time it goes around one loop, or turn, on the coil. Therefore, the total energy gained by an electron as it passes through the secondary coil is proportional to the number of turns on the coil. Since the energy of an electron is directly related to voltage, it follows that the output voltage from a transformer is proportional to the number of turns on the secondary coil.

The Autotransformer

In most x-ray apparatus, it is desirable to change the voltage (KV) applied to the tube to accommodate clinical needs. This is generally done by using the type of transformer illustrated in Figure 8-2, the autotransformer, which has a movable contact on the secondary coil that permits the effective number of turns to be changed. Since the output voltage is proportional to the number of turns in the secondary, it can be adjusted by moving the contact. The typical system has an autotransformer that applies an adjustable voltage to the input of the high voltage (step-up) transformer. The autotransformer does not significantly increase voltage; in fact, most slightly reduce voltage. Autotransformers often use a combined primary-secondary coil, but the principle is the same as if the two coils were completely separated.

The question is often raised as to the possibility of putting an adjustable contact on the secondary of the high voltage transformer for the purpose of KV selection. Unfortunately, high voltage, such as that generated in the transformer, requires extensive insulation normally achieved by placing the high voltage transformer in an enclosed tank of oil. There is no practical way to connect the KV selector switch, located on the control console, to the high-voltage circuit without interfering with the insulation.

RECTIFICATION

The output voltage from the high voltage transformer is AC and changes polarity 60 times per second (60 Hz). If this voltage were applied to an x-ray tube, the anode would be positive with respect to the cathode only one half of the time. During the other half of the voltage cycle, the cathode would be positive and would tend to attract electrons from the anode. Although the anode does not emit electrons, unless it is very hot, this reversed voltage is undesirable. A circuit is needed that will take the voltage during one half of the cycle and reverse its polarity, as illustrated in Figure 8-4. This procedure is called rectification.

Rectifiers

The typical rectification circuit is made up of several rectifiers. A rectifier is a relatively simple two-terminal device that permits electrons to flow through it in one direction but not the other. It can be compared with the valves of the heart, which permit blood to flow in one direction but not the other. In fact, in some countries, rectifiers are referred to as valves. Earlier x-ray equipment used vacuum tube rectifiers, but most rectifiers are now solid state.

Rectifier Circuits

Notice that the circuit in Figure 8-4 has two input points, to which the incoming voltage from the transformer is applied, and two output points, across which the rectified output voltage will appear and be applied to the tube. The circuit contains

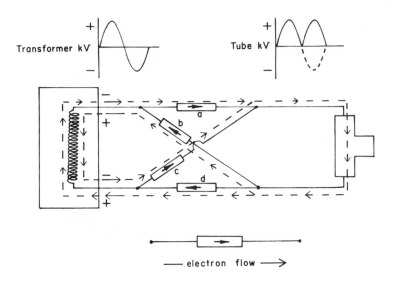

Figure 8-4 A Typical Full-Wave Rectifier Circuit

four rectifiers, labeled a, b, c, and d. Electrons (current) can flow through a rectifier only in the direction indicated by the arrow. The waveform shown indicates the polarity of the lower terminals with respect to the upper. The operation of this circuit can be easily understood by considering the following sequence of events.

During the first half of the voltage cycle, the upper transformer terminal is negative, and the electrons flow into the rectifier circuit at that point. From there, they flow only through rectifier a and on to the x-ray tube. They enter the tube at the cathode terminal, leave by means of the anode, and return by the lower conductor to the rectifier circuit. At that point, it would appear they have two possible pathways to follow. They flow, however, only through rectifier d because the lower transformer terminal is positive and is more attractive than the upper negative terminal. During this part of the voltage cycle, rectifiers b and c do not conduct. During the second half of the cycle, the polarity of the voltage from the transformer is reversed, and the lower terminal is negative. The electrons leave the transformer at this point and pass through rectifier c and on to the cathode. Electrons leaving the x-ray tube by means of the lower conductor pass through rectifier b because of the attraction of the upper transformer terminal, which is then positive.

Full-Wave

In effect, the rectifier circuit takes an alternating polarity voltage and reverses one half of it so that the outcoming voltage always has the same polarity. In this particular circuit, the cathode of the x-ray tube always receives a negative voltage with respect to the anode. This circuit, consisting of four rectifier elements connected as shown, is known as a bridge rectifier. Since it makes use of all of the voltage waveform, it is classified as a full-wave rectifier.

Half-Wave

A rectifier circuit can have only one rectifier element. The disadvantage is that it conducts during only one half of the cycle. This type is classified as a half-wave rectifier. This type of rectification is found in some smaller x-ray machines, such as those used in dentistry. In such apparatus, the x-ray tube itself often serves as the rectifier.

VOLTAGE WAVEFORM AND X-RAY PRODUCTION

Single-Phase and Constant Potential

Both the full-wave and half-wave circuits discussed up to this point use single high voltage transformers and are classified as single-phase apparatus. The basic disadvantage of single-phase operation is that the KV applied to the x-ray tube constantly changes, or pulses, throughout the exposure, as shown in Figure 8-5. This means that both the quantity and energy spectrum of the x-rays produced change constantly with time throughout the cycle. The output from the tube is a spectrum of photon energies that is an average of all instantaneous spectra.

Three principal KV values are associated with the typical single-phase wave-form. Each is related to an aspect of x-ray production. At any instant in time, the pulsing KV has an instantaneous value (KV_i), which determines the rate of x-ray production at each specific instant. During each cycle, the KV reaches a maximum or peak value (KV_p). It is the KV_p that is set by the operator as a control on x-ray

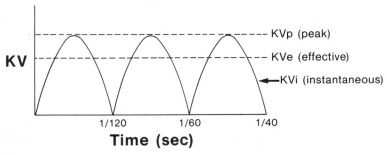

Figure 8-5 Relationship of KV Peak, Effective, and Instantaneous Values for a Single-Phase Generator

production. The ability of a voltage to transfer energy is related to its *effective value* (KV_e), which reflects the fact that the voltage varies with time and does not always produce energy at the peak value. For the typical sine-waveform voltage, as shown in Figure 8-5, the KV_e is 70.7% of the KV_p. Our primary interest in the KV_e is that it determines the rate at which heat is produced in the x-ray tube.

Some x-ray generators produce a constant KV; in these cases the KV_p, KV_e, and KV_i have the same value. These generators are called constant potential apparatus. The constant potential x-ray machine produces more photons with higher average or effective energy than are produced by the single-phase machine, as shown in Figure 8-6.

The rate at which exposure is delivered to the receptor varies significantly with time for single-phase equipment, as shown in Figure 8-6. Most of the exposure is produced during a small portion of the voltage cycle, when the voltage is near the KV_p value. Several factors contribute to this effect. One is that the efficiency of x-ray production increases with voltage and gives more exposure per milliampere-second at the higher voltage levels. Second, the photons produced at the higher tube voltages have higher average energies and are more penetrating. Third, the MA also changes with time during the voltage cycle.

When an x-ray machine is set at a certain MA value, the stated value is usually the average throughout the exposure time. In single-phase equipment, the MA value changes significantly during the voltage cycle. The effect is that the x-ray exposure is delivered to the receptor in a series of pulses. Between the pulses is a period of time during which no significant exposure is delivered. This means, generally, that the total exposure time must be longer for single-phase than for constant potential x-ray equipment, which can deliver a given film exposure in a much shorter total exposure time.

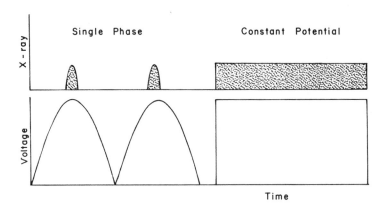

Figure 8-6 Comparison of Single-Phase and Constant Potential X-Ray Production

Three-Phase

One of the most practical means of obtaining essentially constant voltage and high average current is to use three-phase electrical power. The concept of three-phase electricity can best be understood by considering it as three separate incoming power circuits, as shown in Figure 8-7. Although this illustration shows six conductors coming in, this is not necessary in reality because the power lines can be shared by the circuits. Each circuit, or phase, delivers a voltage that can be transformed and rectified in the conventional manner. The important characteristic of a three-phase power system is that the waveforms or cycles in one circuit are out of step, or phase, with those in the other two. This means that the voltage in the three circuits peak at different times. In an actual circuit, the three voltage waveforms are combined, as shown in Figure 8-7. They are not added, but are combined so that the output voltage at any instant is equal to that of the highest phase at the time. Since the voltage drops only a few percent before it is picked up by another phase, the KV_i at all times is quite close to the KV_p.

The voltage variation over the period of a cycle is designated the ripple and is expressed as a percentage. The typical ripple levels for several power supply types are shown in Figure 8-8. One way to classify power supply circuits is according to the number of pulses they produce in the period of one cycle, ie, 1/60th of a second. By using a complex circuit of transformers and rectifiers, it is possible to produce a 12-pulse machine that has a ripple level of less than 4%.

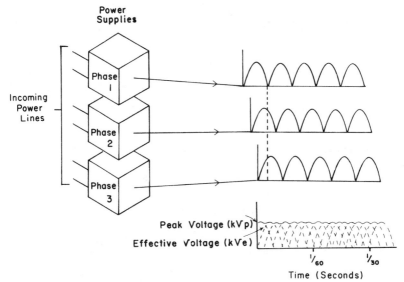

Figure 8-7 Concept of a Three-Phase Generator

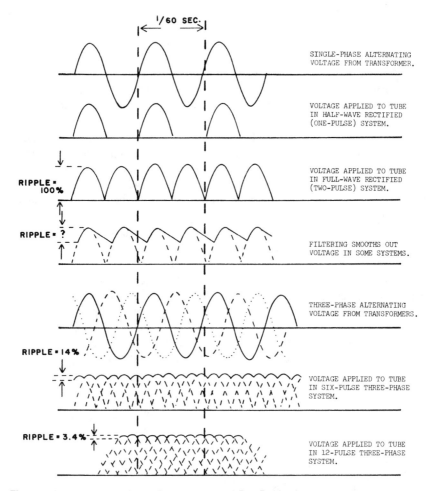

Figure 8-8 Voltage Waveforms Encountered in X-Ray Production

CAPACITORS

Capacitors (sometimes referred to as condensers) are electrical components used in many types of electronic equipment. They are used in some x-ray generators for two purposes. In capacitor discharge (or condenser discharge) portable x-ray machines, capacitors are used to accumulate and store electrical energy; in other types of equipment, they are used as a filtering device to produce constant potential KV.

A capacitor consists of two electrical conductors, such as metal foil, separated by a layer of insulation.

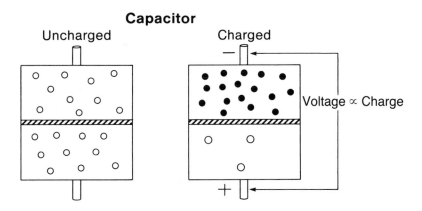

Figure 8-9 Concept of a Capacitor

Capacitor Principles

The basic function of a capacitor is illustrated in Figure 8-9. A capacitor can be described as a storage tank for electrons. When it is connected to a voltage source, electrons flow into the capacitor, and it becomes "charged." As the electrons flow in, the voltage of the capacitor increases until it reaches the voltage of the supply. Energy is actually stored in the capacitor when it is charged; the amount stored is proportional to the voltage and the quantity of stored electrons. If a charged capacitor is connected to another circuit, the capacitor becomes the source, and the electrons flow out and into the circuit.

Energy Storage

In the discussion of the high voltage transformer, it was pointed out that the current flowing into the power supply circuit must be greater than the tube current by a factor equal to the voltage step-up ratio. This is typically as high as 1,000:1, which would require 1 A of power line current for every 1 mA of tube current. The special circuits feeding permanently installed x-ray equipment can accommodate these high currents. In other areas of the hospital where portable x-ray equipment is used, the normal electrical circuits are limited to currents of about 15 A to 20 A. Many portable x-ray machines are now designed to overcome this limitation by using a capacitor as an electron-energy storage device.

A simplified capacitor storage-discharge power supply is shown in Figure 8-10. Step-up transformers and rectifiers are used to produce the high voltage and to charge the capacitor. The electrons are pumped into the capacitor. Charging times can be as long as 10 seconds to 20 seconds. The current flow into the capacitor is typically only a few milliamperes; when it is discharged to the tube over a short

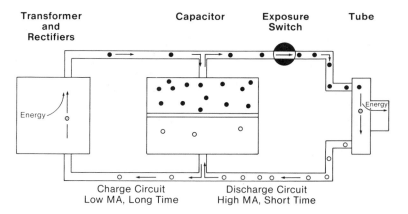

Figure 8-10 Basic Capacitor-Storage X-Ray Machine

period of time, ie, the exposure time, the current can be several hundred milli-amperes.

The voltage across a capacitor is proportional to the quantity of electrons stored (MAS); the actual relationship depends on the size, or capacity, of the capacitor. Many machines use 1-microfarad (μF) capacitors, which produce a voltage of 1 kV for each milliampere-second stored. As the electrons flow from the capacitor to the tube, the voltage drops at the rate of 1 kV/mAs. For example, if a machine is charged to 70 kV, and an exposure of 18 mAs is made, the voltage will have dropped to 52 kV at the end of the exposure.

Capacitor-storage x-ray equipment has a high-voltage waveform, unlike other power supplies. An attempt to obtain large milliampere-second exposures drops the kilovolts to very low values by the time the exposure terminates. Since low tube voltages produce very little film exposure, but increase patient exposure, this type of operation should be avoided. The total MAS should generally be limited to approximately one third of the initial KV value.

A means for turning the tube current on and off is included in the x-ray tube circuit. Most machines use a grid-control x-ray tube for this purpose.

Filtration

When a capacitor is used to produce a constant voltage, or potential, it is permanently connected between the rectifier circuit and the x-ray tube. As the voltage rises toward its peak, electrons from the rectifier circuit flow both to the x-ray tube and into the capacitor. When the voltage from the rectifier circuit begins to fall, electrons flow out of the capacitor and into the x-ray tube. Within certain operational limits, this can maintain a constant potential across the tube. Capacitors can be used on single-phase and three-phase equipment. On single-phase equipment, the maximum MA that can be used without introducing ripples is more limited.

HIGH-FREQUENCY POWER SUPPLIES

Another approach used for some machines producing relatively constant KV is to convert the 60-Hz (low frequency) electricity to a higher frequency before it is rectified. This function is performed by an electrical circuit known as an inverter. After the high-frequency voltage is rectified, the short-duration pulses are much easier to filter into an essentially constant potential.

MA CONTROL

The cathode is heated electrically by a current from a separate low-voltage power supply. The output of this supply is controlled by the MA selector. Increasing the MA selector setting passes more heating current through the cathode; this, in turn, increases the temperature, and the increased emission produces an increase in x-ray tube current. There are actually two currents flowing through portions of the x-ray tube: one, the MA, flows from the cathode to the anode and through the high voltage power supply; the other flows only through the filament of the cathode. It is this second current that controls the cathode-to-anode current.

The cathode temperature required to produce adequate thermionic emission, especially at high MA values, is relatively high. The temperature is sufficiently high, in many cases, to produce some evaporation of the tungsten cathode. Because of this, it is undesirable to keep the cathode at the high operating temperature except for the duration of the x-ray exposure. Most x-ray equipment operates with two levels of cathode heating. When the equipment is turned on, the cathode is heated to a standby level that should not produce significant evaporation. Just before the actual exposure is initiated, the cathode temperature is raised to a value that will give the appropriate tube current. In most radiographic equipment, this function is controlled by the same switch that activates the anode rotor. Unnecessarily maintaining the cathode temperature at full operating temperature can significantly shorten the x-ray tube lifetime.

Although it is true that the x-ray tube current is primarily controlled by cathode temperature, there are conditions under which it is influenced by the applied KV. At low KV values, some of the electrons emitted from the cathode are not attracted to the anode and form a space charge. In effect, this build-up of electrons in the vicinity of a cathode repels electrons at the cathode surface and reduces emission. Under this condition, the x-ray tube current is said to be space-charge limited. This can be especially significant at low KV, such as are used in mammography. This effect can be reduced by locating the cathode and anode closer together.

As the KV is increased, the space charge decreases, and the x-ray tube current rises to a value limited by the cathode emission. At that point the tube is said to be saturated. Many x-ray machines contain a compensation circuit to minimize the effect. The compensation is activated by the KV selector. As the KV is adjusted to higher values, the compensation circuit causes the cathode temperature to be decreased. The lower emission compensates for the decreased space charge.

The x-ray tube current can be read or monitored by a meter located in the high-voltage circuit; it must be placed in the part of the circuit that is near ground voltage, or potential. This permits the meter to be located on the control console without extensive high-voltage insulation.

EXPOSURE TIMING

Another function of the generator is to control the duration of the x-ray exposure. In radiography, the exposure is initiated by the equipment operator and then terminated either after a preset time has elapsed or when the receptor has received a specific level of exposure. In fluoroscopy, the exposure is initiated and terminated by the operator, but a timer displays accumulated exposure time and produces an audible signal at the end of each 5-minute exposure increment.

Operator-controlled switches and timers turn the radiation on and off by activating switching devices in the primary circuit of the x-ray generator.

Manual Timers

X-ray equipment with manual timers requires the operator to set the exposure time before initiating the exposure. The time is determined by personal knowledge, or from a technique chart, after the size of the patient and the KV and MA values being used are considered.

Exposure timers for single-phase equipment usually operate in increments of 1/120th of a second, which is the duration of one half of a 60-Hz voltage cycle. This is also the elapsed time between individual pulses of radiation. It is generally not practical to terminate an exposure during the actual radiation pulse.

A potential problem with this type of timer is its inability to make relatively small adjustments in exposure time. In a situation in which 1/120th of a second produces a slight underexposure, the next possible exposure value, 1/60th of a second, would double the amount of radiation and probably result in an overexposed film. This problem is especially significant for the shorter exposure times.

Three-phase and constant potential equipment produces radiation at a more constant rate, and the exposures can be timed and terminated with more precision.

Automatic Exposure Control

Automatic exposure control (AEC) is an x-ray machine function that terminates the exposure when a specific predetermined amount of radiation reaches the receptor. This function is also referred to as phototiming. AEC is used frequently in many general radiographic procedures and is always used in spot filming and cineradiography.

QUALITY ASSURANCE PROCEDURES

With all x-ray equipment, the operator can control the quantity and quality (penetrating ability) of the radiation with the KV, MA, and exposure-time controls. If the equipment is not properly calibrated, or is subject to periodic malfunction, it will not be possible to control the radiation output. This can result in reduced image quality and unnecessary patient exposure, especially when repeat images are required.

X-ray equipment is required to meet certain federal standards at the time of installation, and, in most states, periodic calibration and quality assurance inspections are required.

Chapter 9

X-Ray Tube Heating and Cooling

INTRODUCTION AND OVERVIEW

To produce x-radiation, relatively large amounts of electrical energy must be transferred to the x-ray tube. Only a small fraction (typically less than 1%) of the energy deposited in the x-ray tube is converted into x-rays; most appears in the form of heat. This places a limitation on the use of x-ray apparatus. If excessive heat is produced in the x-ray tube, the temperature will rise above critical values, and the tube can be damaged. This damage can be in the form of a melted anode or a ruptured tube housing. In order to prevent this damage, the x-ray equipment operator must be aware of the quantity of heat being produced and its relationship to the heat capacity of the x-ray tube.

Figure 9-1 identifies the factors that affect both heat production and heat capacity.

HEAT PRODUCTION

Heat is produced in the focal spot area by the bombarding electrons from the cathode. Since only a small fraction of the electronic energy is converted in x-radiation, it can be ignored in heat calculations. We will assume all of the electron energy is converted into heat. In a single exposure, the quantity of heat produced in the focal spot area is given by

$$\text{Heat (J)} = KV_e \times MAS$$

or

$$\text{Heat (J)} = w \times KV_p \times MAS.$$

In this relationship, w is the waveform factor; its value is determined by the waveform of the voltage applied to the x-ray tube. Values for most waveforms

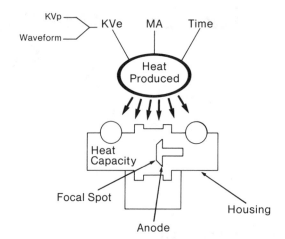

Figure 9-1 Factors That Determine the Amount of Heat Produced and the Three Areas of an X-Ray Tube That Have Specific Heat Capacities

---

encountered in diagnostic x-ray machines are constant potential, 1.0; three-phase, 12-pulse, 0.99; three-phase, 6-pulse, 0.96; single-phase, 0.71.

Although the joule is the basic unit for energy and heat, it is not always used to express x-ray tube heat. The heat unit was introduced for the purpose of expressing x-ray tube heat. The relationship between a quantity of heat expressed in heat units and in joules is given by

$$\text{Heat (HU)} = 1.4 \times \text{heat (J)}.$$

Since the product of the joules-to-heat unit conversion factor (1.4) and the waveform factor for single-phase (0.71) is equal to 1, the following relationship is obtained:

$$\text{Heat (HU)} = KV_p \times MAS.$$

Here it is seen that for single-phase operation, the heat produced in heat units is the product of the KV_p and MAS. In fact, this is why the heat unit is used. In the earlier days of radiology, when most equipment was single-phase, it was desirable to calculate heat quantities without having to use a waveform factor. This was achieved by introducing a new unit, the heat unit. For three-phase, six-pulse equipment, the heat in heat units is given by

$$\text{Heat (HU)} = 1.35 \times KV_p \times MAS.$$

The factor of 1.35 is the ratio of the waveform factors, 0.96/0.71.

The rate at which heat is produced in a tube is equivalent to the electrical power and is given by

$$\text{Power (watts)} = w \times KV_p \times MA.$$

The total heat delivered during an exposure, in joules or watt-seconds, is the product of the power and the exposure time.

HEAT CAPACITY

In order to evaluate the problem of x-ray tube heating, it is necessary to understand the relationship of three physical quantities: (1) heat, (2) temperature, and (3) heat capacity. Heat is a form of energy and can be expressed in any energy units. In x-ray equipment, heat is usually expressed in joules (watt-seconds) or heat units.

Temperature is the physical quantity associated with an object that indicates its relative heat content. Temperature is specified in units of degrees. Physical changes, such as melting, boiling, and evaporation, are directly related to an object's temperature rather than its heat content.

For a given object, the relationship between temperature and heat content involves a third quantity, heat capacity, which is a characteristic of the object. The general relationship can be expressed as follows:

$$\text{Temperature} = \text{heat/heat capacity}.$$

The heat capacity of an object is more or less proportional to its size, or mass, and a characteristic of the material known as the specific heat. As heat is added to an object, the temperature increases in proportion to the amount of heat added. When a given amount of heat is added, the temperature increase is inversely proportional to the object's heat capacity. In an object with a large heat capacity, the temperature rise is smaller than in one with a small heat capacity. In other words, the temperature of an object is determined by the relationship between its heat content and its heat capacity. This is illustrated in Figure 9-2.

In x-ray tube operation, the goal is never to exceed specific critical temperatures that produce damage. This is achieved by keeping the heat content below specified critical values related to the tube's heat capacity.

In most x-ray tubes there are three distinct areas with critical heat capacities, as shown in Figure 9-3. The area with the smallest capacity is the focal spot area, or track, and is the point at which heat is produced within the tube. From this area, the heat moves by conduction throughout the anode body and by radiation to the tube

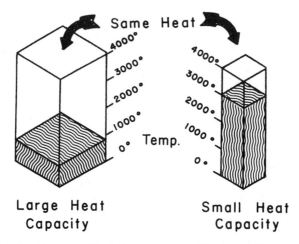

Figure 9-2 Relationship Among Heat, Temperature, and Heat Capacity

housing; heat is also transferred, by radiation, from the anode body to the tube housing. Heat is removed from the tube housing by transfer to the surrounding atmosphere. When the tube is in operation, heat generally flows into and out of the three areas shown. Damage can occur if the heat content of any area exceeds its maximum heat capacity.

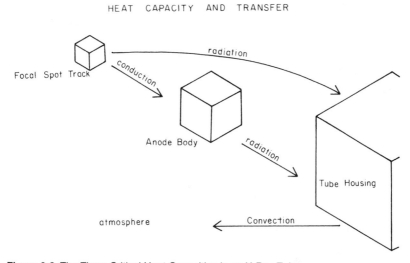

Figure 9-3 The Three Critical Heat Capacities in an X-Ray Tube

FOCAL SPOT AREA

The maximum heat capacity of the focal spot area, or track, is the major limiting factor with single exposures. If the quantity of heat delivered during an individual exposure exceeds the track capacity, the anode surface can melt, as shown in Figure 9-4. The capacity of a given focal spot track is generally specified by the manufacturer in the form of a curve, as shown in Figure 9-5. This type of curve shows the maximum power (KV and MA) that can be delivered to the tube for a given exposure time without producing overload. Graphs of this type are generally designated tube rating charts. From this graph, it is seen that the safe power limit of a tube is inversely related to the exposure time. This is not surprising, since the total heat developed during an exposure is the product of power and exposure time. It is not only the total amount of heat delivered to the tube that is crucial, but also the time in which it is delivered.

X-ray tubes are often given single power ratings. By general agreement, an exposure time of 0.1 second is used for specifying a tube's power rating. Although this does not describe a tube's limitations at other exposure times, it does provide a means of comparing tubes and operating conditions.

A number of different factors determine the heat capacity of the focal spot track. The focal spot track is the surface area of the anode that is bombarded by the electron beam. In stationary anode tubes, it is a small area with dimensions of a few millimeters. In the rotating anode tube, the focal spot track is much larger because of the movement of the anode with respect to the electron beam. Figure 9-6 shows a small section of a rotating anode.

Focal Spot Size

From the standpoint of producing x-ray images with minimum blur, a small focal spot is desired. However, a small focal spot tends to concentrate heat and give the focal spot track a lower heat capacity. The only advantage of a larger focal spot is increased heat capacity. Many x-ray tubes have two focal spot sizes that can be selected by the operator. The small focal spot is generally used at relatively low power (KV and MA) settings. The large focal spot is used when the machine must be operated at power levels that exceed the rated capacity of the small focal spot. The specified size of an x-ray tube focal spot is the dimensions of the effective or projected focal spot shown in Figure 9-6. Notice that the actual focal spot, the area bombarded by the electron beam, is always larger than the projected, or effective, focal spot. For a given anode angle, the width of the focal spot track is directly proportional to the size of the projected spot. The relationship between heat capacity and specified focal spot size is somewhat different. In many tubes, doubling the focal spot size increases the power rating by a factor of about 3.

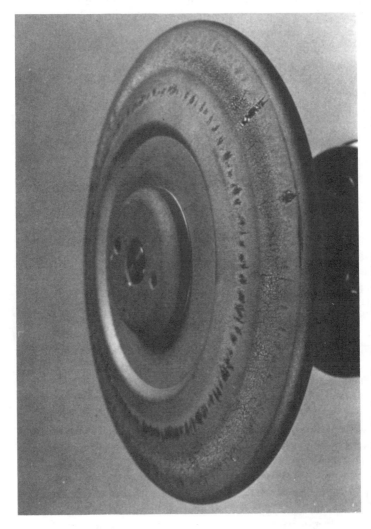

Figure 9-4 A Rotating Anode Damaged by Overheating

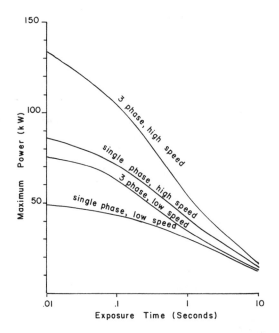

Figure 9-5 Rating Curves for an X-Ray Tube Operated under Different Conditions

Anode Angle

The actual relationship between focal spot width (and heat capacity) and the size of the projected focal spot is determined by the anode angle. Anode angles generally range from about 7° to 20°. For a given effective focal spot size, the track width and heat capacity are inversely related to anode angle. Although anodes with small angles give maximum heat capacity, they have specific limitations with respect to the area that can be covered by the x-ray beam. X-ray intensity usually drops off significantly toward the anode end because of the heel effect. In tubes with small angles, this is more pronounced and limits the size of the useful beam. Figure 9-7 shows the nominal field coverage for different anode angles. The x-ray tube anode angle should be selected by a compromise between heat capacity and field of coverage.

Anode Rotation Speed

In rotating tubes, the anode assembly is mounted on bearings and actually forms the rotor of an electric motor. The x-ray tube is surrounded by a set of coils that

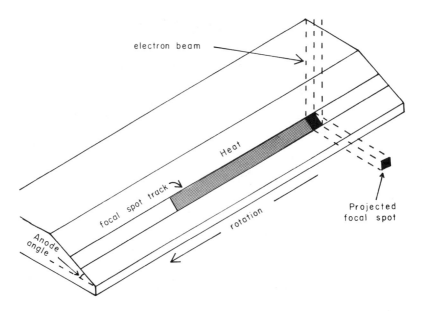

Figure 9-6 Section of a Rotating Anode Showing Relationship of Focal Spot Track to Electron Beam and Anode Angle

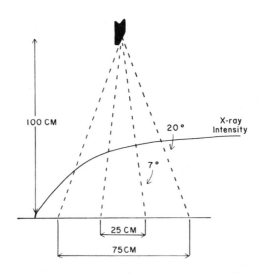

Figure 9-7 Variation of X-Ray Intensity Because of the Anode Heel Effect

form the stator of the motor. When the coils are energized from the power line, the rotor spins. The speed of rotation is determined by the frequency of the applied current. When the stator coils are operated from the 60-Hz power line, the speed of rotation is approximately 3,000 rpm. By using a power supply that produces 180-Hz current, rotation speeds of approximately 10,000 rpm can be obtained. This is commonly referred to as high-speed rotation.

The effective length of the focal spot track is proportional to the speed of rotation for a given exposure time. High-speed rotation simply spreads the heat over a longer track, especially in short exposure times. High-speed rotation generally increases the power capacity of a tube by approximately 60%.

Kilovoltage Waveform

Another factor that affects the heat capacity of the focal spot track is the waveform of the kilovoltage. Single-phase power delivers energy to the anode in pulses, as shown in Figure 9-8. Three-phase power delivers the heat at an essentially constant rate, as indicated. Figure 9-8 compares the temperatures produced by a single-phase and a three-phase machine delivering the same total heat. Because of the pulsating nature of single-phase power, some points on the anode surface are raised to higher temperatures than others. These hot spots exceed the temperature produced by an equal amount of three-phase energy. When an x-ray tube is operated from a single-phase power supply, the maximum power must be less than for three-phase operation to keep the hot spots from exceeding the critical temperature. In other words, three-phase operation increases the effective focal spot track heat capacity and rating of an x-ray tube.

The effect of kilovoltage waveform on tube rating should not be confused with the effect of waveform on heat production, which was discussed earlier. However, both factors should be considered to determine if there is any advantage, from the standpoint of tube heating, to using three-phase power. In comparing three-phase and single-phase operation, three factors should be considered:

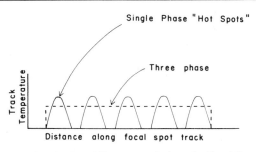

Figure 9-8 Approximate Distribution of Temperature along the Focal Spot Track for Single-Phase and Three-Phase Operation

1. Three-phase operation permits a tube to be operated at a higher power level because of the uniform distribution of heat.
2. Three-phase operation produces more x-radiation and increased penetration at a given KV_p and MAS setting.
3. Three-phase operation produces more heat for a given KV_p and MAS setting.

The real advantage of three-phase operation is related to the first two factors. Because of the increased efficiency of x-ray production, and the increased penetrating ability of the radiation, a lower KV_p or MAS value is required to produce a given film exposure. This more than compensates for the increased heat production associated with three-phase operation. The increased rating, or maximum permissible power, associated with the three-phase waveform also adds to the advantage. An x-ray tube can generally be operated at a higher power level when the power is supplied from a three-phase power supply, and it will also produce radiation more efficiently.

A rating chart for an x-ray tube operated at different waveforms and rotation speeds is shown in Figure 9-5. The highest power capacity is obtained by using three-phase power and high-speed rotation; notice that the real advantage occurs at relatively short exposure times. As exposure time is increased, overlapping of the focal spot track and the diffusion of heat make the difference in power capacity much less significant.

The rating charts supplied by x-ray tube manufacturers are usually different in format from the one shown in Figure 9-5. It is common practice for each of the four operating conditions (waveform and speed) to be on a separate chart. Each chart contains a number of different curves, each representing a different KV_p value. The vertical scale on such a rating chart is tube current. Although the format is different, a chart of this type is still a power rating chart. Each combination of KV_p and MA represents a constant power value. Such a chart is easier to use, since it is not necessary to calculate the power. The rating chart is used by the operator to determine if the technical factors, KV_p, MA, and exposure time, for a given exposure will exceed the tube's rated capacity.

Most rotating anode tubes contain two focal spots. As mentioned previously, the size of the focal spot significantly affects the heat capacity. Remember that a given x-ray tube has a number of different rating values, depending on focal spot size, rotation speed, and waveforms. Some typical values are shown in Table 9-1.

ANODE BODY

The heat capacity of the focal spot track is generally the limiting factor for single exposures. In a series of radiographic exposures, CT scanning, or fluoroscopy, the

Table 9-1 Heat Rating (in Joules) for Typical X-Ray Tube for Exposure Time of 0.1 sec and Focal Spot Sizes of 0.7 mm and 1.5 mm

	Single-phase	Three-phase
3,600 rpm	700 (0.7 mm)	1,050 (0.7 mm)
	2,300 (1.5 mm)	3,400 (1.5 mm)
10,800 rpm	1,100 (0.7 mm)	1,700 (0.7 mm)
	3.900 (1.5 mm)	5,800 (1.5 mm)

build-up of heat in the anode can become significant. Excessive anode temperature can crack or warp the anode disc. The heat capacity of an anode is generally described graphically, as shown in Figure 9-9. This set of curves, describing the thermal characteristics of an anode, conveys several important pieces of information. The maximum heat capacity is indicated on the heat scale. The heating curves indicate the build-up of heat within the anode for various energy input rates. These curves apply primarily to the continuous operation of a tube, such as in CT or fluoroscopy. For a given x-ray tube, there is a critical input rate that can cause the rated heat capacity to be exceeded after a period of time. This is generally indicated on the graph. If the heat input rate is less than this critical value, normal cooling prevents the total heat content from reaching the rated capacity.

The cooling curve can be used to estimate the cooling time necessary between sets of exposures. Suppose a rapid sequence of exposures has produced a heat

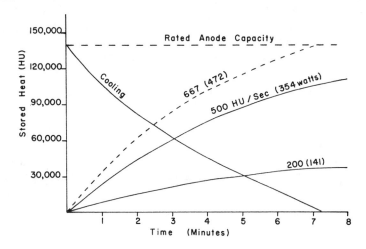

Figure 9-9 Anode Heating and Cooling Curves

input of 90,000 HU. This is well over 50% of the anode storage capacity. Before a similar sequence of exposures can be made, the anode must cool to a level at which the added heat will not exceed the maximum capacity. For example, after an initial heat input of 90,000 HU, a cooling time of approximately 3.5 minutes will decrease the heat content to 30,000 HU. At this point, another set of exposures producing 90,000 HU could be taken.

The cooling rate is not constant. An anode cools faster when it has a high heat content and a high temperature. In CT scanning, when anode heating is a limiting factor, a higher scan rate can be obtained by operating the anode with the highest safe heat content since the cooling rate is higher for a hot anode and more scans can be obtained in a specific time than with a cool anode. Most CT systems have a display that shows the anode heat content as a percentage of the rated capacity.

The anodes in most radiographic equipment are cooled by the natural radiation of heat to the surrounding tube enclosures. However, anodes in some high-powered equipment, such as that used in CT, are cooled by the circulation of oil through the anode to a heat exchanger (radiator).

Anode damage can occur if a high-powered exposure is produced on a cold anode. It is generally recommended that tubes be warmed up by a series of low-energy exposures to prevent this type of damage.

TUBE HOUSING

The third heat capacity that must be considered is that of the tube housing. Excessive heat in the housing can rupture the oil seals, or plugs. Like the anode, the housing capacity places a limitation on the extended use of the x-ray tube, rather than on individual exposures. Since the housing is generally cooled by the movement of air, or convection, its effective capacity can be increased by using forced-air circulation.

The housing heat capacity is much larger than that of the anode and is typically over 1 million HU. The time required for a housing to dissipate a given quantity of heat can be determined with cooling charts supplied by the manufacturer.

SUMMARY

The heat characteristics of x-ray tubes should be considered when tubes are selected for specific applications and should be used as a guide to proper tube operation.

Chapter 10

Interaction of Radiation with Matter

INTRODUCTION AND OVERVIEW

X-ray photons are created by the interaction of energetic electrons with matter at the atomic level. Photons (x-ray and gamma) end their lives by transferring their energy to electrons contained in matter. X-ray interactions are important in diagnostic examinations for many reasons. For example, the selective interaction of x-ray photons with the structure of the human body produces the image; the interaction of photons with the receptor converts an x-ray or gamma image into one that can be viewed or recorded. This chapter considers the basic interactions between x-ray and gamma photons and matter.

INTERACTION TYPES

Photon Interactions

Recall that photons are individual units of energy. As an x-ray beam or gamma radiation passes through an object, three possible fates await each photon, as shown in Figure 10-1:

1. It can penetrate the section of matter without interacting.
2. It can interact with the matter and be completely absorbed by depositing its energy.
3. It can interact and be scattered or deflected from its original direction and deposit part of its energy.

There are two kinds of interactions through which photons deposit their energy; both are with electrons. In one type of interaction the photon loses all its energy; in

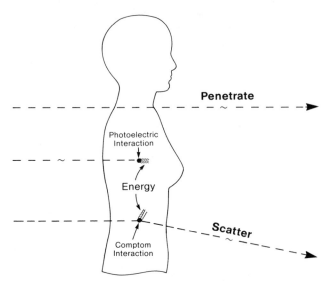

Figure 10-1 Photons Entering the Human Body Will Either Penetrate, Be Absorbed, or Produce Scattered Radiation

the other, it loses a portion of its energy, and the remaining energy is scattered. These two interactions are shown in Figure 10-2.

Photoelectric

In the photoelectric (photon-electron) interaction, as shown in Figure 10-2, a photon transfers all its energy to an electron located in one of the atomic shells. The electron is ejected from the atom by this energy and begins to pass through the surrounding matter. The electron rapidly loses its energy and moves only a relatively short distance from its original location. The photon's energy is, therefore, deposited in the matter close to the site of the photoelectric interaction. The energy transfer is a two-step process. The photoelectric interaction in which the photon transfers its energy to the electron is the first step. The depositing of the energy in the surrounding matter by the electron is the second step.

Photoelectric interactions usually occur with electrons that are firmly bound to the atom, that is, those with a relatively high binding energy. Photoelectric interactions are most probable when the electron binding energy is only slightly less than the energy of the photon. If the binding energy is more than the energy of the photon, a photoelectric interaction cannot occur. This interaction is possible only when the photon has sufficient energy to overcome the binding energy and remove the electron from the atom.

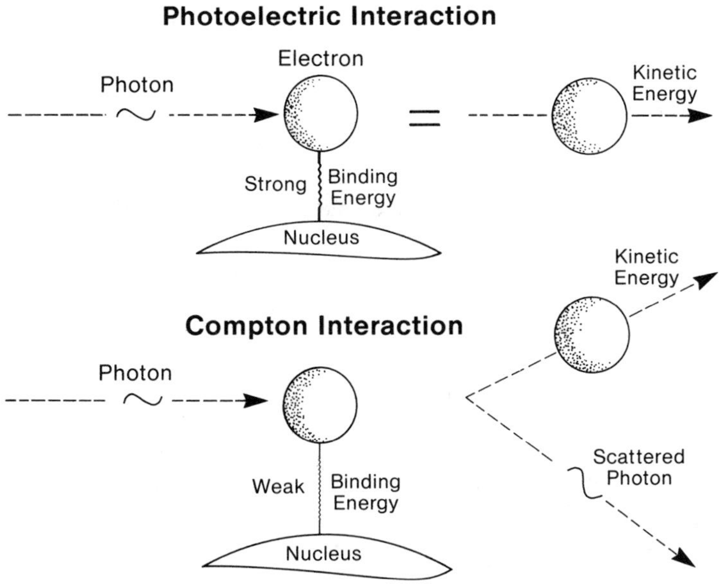

Photoelectric Interaction

Compton Interaction

Figure 10-2 The Two Basic Interactions Between Photons and Electrons

The photon's energy is divided into two parts by the interaction. A portion of the energy is used to overcome the electron's binding energy and to remove it from the atom. The remaining energy is transferred to the electron as kinetic energy and is deposited near the interaction site. Since the interaction creates a vacancy in one of the electron shells, typically the K or L, an electron moves down to fill in. The drop in energy of the filling electron often produces a characteristic x-ray photon. The energy of the characteristic radiation depends on the binding energy of the electrons involved. Characteristic radiation initiated by an incoming photon is referred to as fluorescent radiation. Fluorescence, in general, is a process in which some of the energy of a photon is used to create a second photon of less energy. This process sometimes converts x-rays into light photons. Whether the fluorescent radiation is in the form of light or x-rays depends on the binding energy levels in the absorbing material.

Compton

A Compton interaction is one in which only a portion of the energy is absorbed and a photon is produced with reduced energy. This photon leaves the site of the interaction in a direction different from that of the original photon, as shown in Figure 10-2. Because of the change in photon direction, this type of interaction is classified as a scattering process. In effect, a portion of the incident radiation "bounces off" or is scattered by the material. This is significant in some situations because the material within the primary x-ray beam becomes a secondary radiation source. The most significant object producing scattered radiation in an x-ray procedure is the patient's body. The portion of the patient's body that is within the primary x-ray beam becomes the actual source of scattered radiation. This has two undesirable consequences. The scattered radiation that continues in the forward direction and reaches the image receptor decreases the quality (contrast) of the image; the radiation that is scattered from the patient is the predominant source of radiation exposure to the personnel conducting the examination.

Coherent Scatter

There are actually two types of interactions that produce scattered radiation. One type, referred to by a variety of names, including coherent, Thompson, Rayleigh, classical, and elastic, is a pure scattering interaction and deposits no energy in the material. Although this type of interaction is possible at low photon energies, it is generally not significant in most diagnostic procedures.

Pair Production

Pair production is a photon-matter interaction that is not encountered in diagnostic procedures because it can occur only with photons with energies in excess of 1.02 MeV. In a pair-production interaction, the photon interacts with the nucleus in such a manner that its energy is converted into matter. The interaction produces a pair of particles, an electron and a positively charged positron. These two particles have the same mass, each equivalent to a rest mass energy of 0.51 MeV.

Electron Interactions

The interaction and transfer of energy from photons to tissue has two phases. The first is the "one-shot" interaction between the photon and an electron in which all or a significant part of the photon energy is transferred; the second is the transfer of energy from the energized electron as it moves through the tissue. This occurs as a series of interactions, each of which transfers a relatively small amount of energy.

Several types of radioactive transitions produce electron radiation including beta radiation, internal conversion (IC) electrons, and Auger electrons. These radiation electrons interact with matter (tissue) in a manner similar to that of electrons produced by photon interactions.

In photoelectric interactions, the energy of the electron is equal to the energy of the incident photon less the binding energy of the electron within the atom. In Compton interactions, the relationship of the electron energy to that of the photon

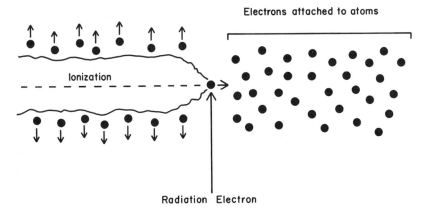

Figure 10-3 Ionization Produced by a Radiation Electron

depends on the angle of scatter and the original photon energy. The electrons set free by these interactions have kinetic energies ranging from relatively low values to values slightly below the energy of the incident photons.

As the electrons leave the interaction site, they immediately begin to transfer their energy to the surrounding material, as shown in Figure 10-3. Because the electron carries an electrical charge, it can interact with other electrons without touching them. As it passes through the material, the electron, in effect, pushes the other electrons away from its path. If the force on an electron is sufficient to remove it from its atom, ionization results. In some cases, the atomic or molecular structures are raised to a higher energy level, or excited state. Regardless of the type of interaction, the moving electron loses some of its energy. Most of the ionization produced by x- and gamma-radiation is not a result of direct photon interactions, but rather of interactions of the energetic electrons with the material. For example, in air, radiation must expend an average energy of 33.4 eV per ionization. Consider a 50-keV x-ray photon undergoing a photoelectric interaction. The initial interaction of the photon ionizes one atom, but the resulting energetic electron ionizes approximately 1,500 additional atoms.

Electron Range

The total distance an electron travels in a material before losing all its energy is generally referred to as its range. The two factors that determine the range are (1) the initial energy of the electrons and (2) the density of the material. One important characteristic of electron interactions is that all electrons of the same energy have the same range in a specific material, as illustrated in Figure 10-4. The general relationship between electron range and energy is shown in Fig-

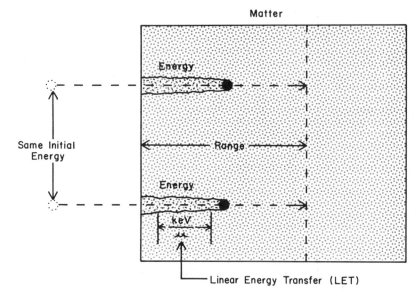

Figure 10-4 The Range of Electrons with the Same Initial Energies

ure 10-5. The curve shown is the range for a material with a density of 1 g/cm³. This is the density of water and the approximate density of muscle tissue.

The electron range in other materials can be determined by dividing the range given in Figure 10-5 by the density of the material. Let us now apply this procedure to determine the range of 300-keV beta particles in air. (Air has a density of 0.00129 g/cm³.) From Figure 10-5 we see that a 300-keV electron has a range of 0.76 mm in a material with a density of 1 g/cm³. When this value is divided by the density of air, we find the range to be 59 cm.

In general, the range of electron radiation in materials such as tissue is a fraction of a millimeter. This means that essentially all electron radiation energy is absorbed in the body very close to the site containing the radioactive material.

Linear Energy Transfer

The rate at which an electron transfers energy to a material is known as the linear energy transfer (LET), and is expressed in terms of the amount of energy transferred per unit of distance traveled. Typical units are kiloelectron volts per micrometer (keV/μm). In a given material, such as tissue, the LET value depends on the kinetic energy (velocity) of the electron. The LET is generally inversely related to the electron velocity. As a radiation electron loses energy, its velocity decreases, and the value of the LET increases until all its energy is dissipated. LET values in soft tissue for several electron energies are given below.

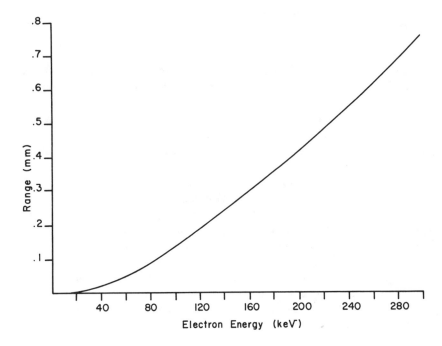

Figure 10-5 Relationship of Electron Range to Initial Energy in a Material with a Density of 1 g/cm³ (Soft Tissue)

Electron Energy (keV)	LET (keV/μm)
1000	0.2
100	0.3
10	2.2
1	12.0

The effectiveness of a particular radiation in producing biological damage is often related to the LET of the radiation. The actual relationship of the efficiency in producing damage to LET values depends on the biological effect considered. For some effects, the efficiency increases with an increase in LET, for some it decreases, and for others it increases up to a point and then decreases with additional increases in LET. For a given biological effect, there is an LET value that produces an optimum energy concentration within the tissue. Radiation with lower LET values does not produce an adequate concentration of energy. Radiations with higher LET values tend to deposit more energy than is needed to produce the effect; this tends to waste energy and decrease efficiency.

Positron Interactions

Recall that a positron is the same size as an electron, but has a positive charge. It is also different from the electron in that it is composed of what is referred to as antimatter. This leads to a type of interaction that is quite different from the interactions among electrons.

The interaction between a positron and matter is in two phases, as illustrated in Figure 10-6. These are ionization and annihilation. As the energetic positron passes through matter, it interacts with the atomic electrons by electrical attraction. As the positron moves along, it pulls electrons out of the atoms and produces ionization. A small amount of energy is lost by the positron in each interaction. In general, this phase of the interaction is not too unlike the interaction of an energetic electron, but the positron pulls electrons as it races by and electrons push electrons away from the path. Also, when the positron has lost most of its kinetic energy and is coming to a stop, it comes into close contact with an electron and enters into an annihilation interaction.

The annihilation process occurs when the antimatter positron combines with the conventional-matter electron. In this interaction, the masses of both particles are completely converted into energy. The relationship between the amount of energy and mass is given by

$$E = mc^2.$$

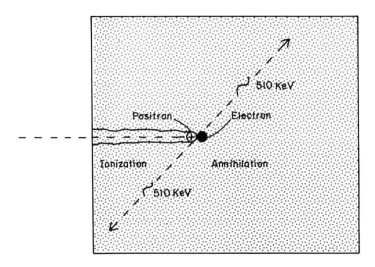

Figure 10-6 A Positron Interaction that Produces Annihilation Radiation

The energy equivalent of one electron or positron mass is 511 keV. The energy that results from the annihilation process is emitted from the interaction site in the form of two photons, each with an energy of 511 keV. The pair of photons leave the site in opposite directions. With special imaging equipment it is possible to capture both photons and to determine the precise three-dimensional location of the interaction site. Since the range of a positron, like that of an electron, is relatively short, the site of interaction is always very close to the location of the radioactive nuclei.

PHOTON INTERACTION RATES

Attenuation

As a photon makes its way through matter, there is no way to predict precisely either how far it will travel before engaging in an interaction or the type of interaction it will engage in. In clinical applications we are generally not concerned with the fate of an individual photon but rather with the collective interaction of the large number of photons. In most instances we are interested in the overall rate at which photons interact as they make their way through a specific material.

Let us observe what happens when a group of photons encounters a slice of material that is 1 unit thick, as illustrated in Figure 10-7. Some of the photons interact with the material, and some pass on through. The interactions, either photoelectric or Compton, remove some of the photons from the beam in a process known as *attenuation*. Under specific conditions, a certain percentage of the photons will interact, or be attenuated, in a 1-unit thickness of material.

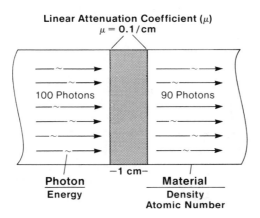

Figure 10-7 Linear Attenuation Coefficient

Linear Attenuation Coefficient

The linear attenuation coefficient (μ) is the actual fraction of photons interacting per 1-unit thickness of material. In our example the fraction that interacts in the 1-cm thickness is 0.1, or 10%, and the value of the linear attenuation coefficient is 0.1 per cm.

Linear attenuation coefficient values indicate the rate at which photons interact as they move through material and are inversely related to the average distance photons travel before interacting. The rate at which photons interact (attenuation coefficient value) is determined by the energy of the individual photons and the atomic number and density of the material.

Mass Attenuation Coefficient

In some situations it is more desirable to express the attenuation rate in terms of the mass of the material encountered by the photons rather than in terms of distance. The quantity that affects attenuation rate is not the total mass of an object but rather the area mass. Area mass is the amount of material behind a 1-unit surface area, as shown in Figure 10-8. The area mass is the product of material thickness and density:

$$\text{Area Mass (g/cm}^2) = \text{Thickness (cm)} \times \text{Density (g/cm}^3).$$

The mass attenuation coefficient is the rate of photon interactions per 1-unit (g/cm^2) area mass.

Figure 10-8 compares two pieces of material with different thicknesses and densities but the same area mass. Since both attenuate the same fraction of photons, the mass attenuation coefficient is the same for the two materials. They do not have the same linear attenuation coefficient values.

The relationship between the mass and linear attenuation coefficients is

$$\text{Mass Attenuation Coefficient } (\mu/\rho) = \text{Linear Attenuation Coefficient}(\mu) / \text{Density } (\rho).$$

Notice that the symbol for mass attenuation coefficient (μ/ρ) is derived from the symbols for the linear attenuation coefficient (μ) and the symbol for density (ρ).

We must be careful not to be misled by the relationship stated in this manner. Confusion often arises as to the effect of material density on attenuation coefficient values. Mass attenuation coefficient values are actually normalized with respect to material density, and therefore do not change with changes in density. Material density does have a direct effect on linear attenuation coefficient values.

The total attenuation rate depends on the individual rates associated with photoelectric and Compton interactions. The respective attenuation coefficients are related as follows:

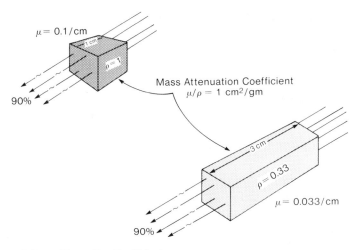

Figure 10-8 Mass Attenuation Coefficient

μ (total) = μ (photoelectric) + μ (Compton).

Let us now consider the factors that affect attenuation rates and the competition between photoelectric and Compton interactions. Both types of interactions occur with electrons within the material. The chance that a photon will interact as it travels a 1-unit distance depends on two factors.

One factor is the concentration, or density, of electrons in the material. Increasing the concentration of electrons increases the chance of a photon coming close enough to an electron to interact. In Chapter 4 we observed that electron concentration was determined by the physical density of the material. Therefore, density affects the probability of both photoelectric and Compton interactions.

All electrons are not equally attractive to a photon. What makes an electron more or less attractive is its binding energy. The two general rules are:

1. Photoelectric interactions occur most frequently when the electron binding energy is slightly less than the photon energy.
2. Compton interactions occur most frequently with electrons with relatively low binding energies.

In Chapter 4 we observed that the electrons with binding energies within the energy range of diagnostic x-ray photons were the K-shell electrons of the intermediate- and high-atomic-number materials. Since an atom can have, at the most, two electrons in the K shell, the majority of the electrons are located in the other shells and have relatively low binding energies.

Photoelectric Rates

The probability, and thus attenuation coefficient value, for photoelectric inter-actions depends on how well the photon energies and electron binding energies match, as shown in Figure 10-9. This can be considered from two perspectives. In a specific material with a fixed binding energy, a change in photon energy alters the match and the chance for photoelectric interactions. On the other hand, with photons of a specific energy, the probability of photoelectric interactions is affected by the atomic number of the material, which changes the binding energy.

Dependence on Photon Energy

In a given material, the probability of photoelectric interactions occurring is strongly dependent on the energy of the photon and its relationship to the binding energy of the electrons. Figure 10-10 shows the relationship between the attenuation coefficient for iodine ($Z = 53$) and photon energy. This graph shows two significant features of the relationship. One is that the coefficient value, or the probability of photoelectric interactions, decreases rapidly with increased photon energy. It is generally said that the probability of photoelectric interactions is inversely proportional to the cube of the photon energy ($1/E^3$). This general relationship can be used to compare the photoelectric attenuation coefficients at two different photon energies. The significant point is that the probability of photoelectric interactions occurring in a given material drops drastically as the photon energy is increased.

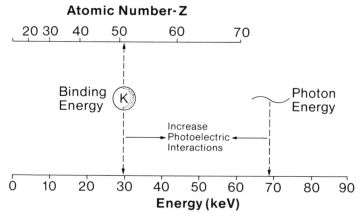

Figure 10-9 The Relationship Between Material Atomic Number and Photon Energy That Enhances the Probability of Photoelectric Interactions

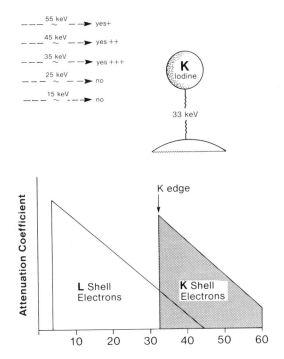

Figure 10-10 Relationship Between the Probability of Photoelectric Interactions and Photon Energy

---

The other important feature of the attenuation coefficient–photon energy relationship shown in Figure 10-10 is that it changes abruptly at one particular energy: the binding energy of the shell electrons. The K-electron binding energy is 33 keV for iodine. This feature of the attenuation coefficient curve is generally designated as the K, L, or M edge. The reason for the sudden change is apparent if it is recalled that photons must have energies equal to or slightly greater than the binding energy of the electrons with which they interact. When photons with energies less than 33 keV pass through iodine, they interact primarily with the L-shell electrons. They do not have sufficient energy to eject electrons from the K shell, and the probability of interacting with the M and N shells is quite low because of the relatively large difference between the electron-binding and photon energies. However, photons with energies slightly greater than 33 keV can also interact with the K-shell electrons. This means that there are now more electrons in the material that are available for interactions. This produces a sudden increase in the attenuation coefficient at the K-shell energy. In the case of iodine, the attenuation coefficient abruptly jumps from a value of 5.6 below the K edge to a value of 36, or increases by a factor of more than 6.

A similar change in the attenuation coefficient occurs at the L-shell electron binding energy. For most elements, however, this is below 10 keV and not within the useful portion of the x-ray spectrum.

Photoelectric interactions occur at the highest rate when the energy of the x-ray photon is just above the binding energy of the electrons.

Material Atomic Number

The probability of photoelectric interactions occurring is also dependent on the atomic number of the material. An explanation for the increase in photoelectric interactions with atomic number is that as atomic number is increased, the binding energies move closer to the photon energy. The general relationship is that the probability of photoelectric interactions (attenuation coefficient value) is proportional to Z^3. In general, the conditions that increase the probability of photoelectric interactions are low photon energies and high-atomic-number materials.

Compton Rates

Compton interactions can occur with the very loosely bound electrons. All electrons in low-atomic-number materials and the majority of electrons in high-atomic-number materials are in this category. The characteristic of the material that affects the probability of Compton interactions is the number of available electrons. It was shown earlier that all materials, with the exception of hydrogen, have approximately the same number of electrons per gram of material. Since the concentration of electrons in a given volume is proportional to the density of the materials, the probability of Compton interactions is proportional only to the physical density and not to the atomic number, as in the case of photoelectric interactions. The major exception is in materials with a significant proportion of hydrogen. In these materials with more electrons per gram, the probability of Compton interactions is enhanced.

Although the chances of Compton interactions decrease slightly with photon energy, the change is not so rapid as for photoelectric interactions, which are inversely related to the cube of the photon energy.

Direction of Scatter

It is possible for photons to scatter in any direction. The direction in which an individual photon will scatter is purely a matter of chance. There is no way in which the angle of scatter for a specific photon can be predicted. However, there are certain directions that are more probable and that will occur with a greater frequency than others. The factor that can alter the overall scatter direction pattern is the energy of the original photon. In diagnostic examinations, the most significant scatter will be in the forward direction. This would be an angle of scatter of only a few degrees. However, especially at the lower end of the energy spectrum, there is a significant amount of scatter in the reverse direction, ie, backscatter. For the diagnostic photon energy range, the number of photons that scatter at right angles to the primary beam is in the range of one-third to one-half of the number that scatter in the forward direction. Increasing primary photon energy causes a general shift of scatter to the forward direction. However, in diagnostic procedures, there is always a significant amount of back- and sidescatter radiation.

Energy of Scattered Radiation

When a photon undergoes a Compton interaction, its energy is divided between the scattered secondary photon and the electron with which it interacts. The electron's kinetic energy is quickly absorbed by the material along its path. In other words, in a Compton interaction, part of the original photon's energy is absorbed and part is converted into scattered radiation.

The manner in which the energy is divided between scattered and absorbed radiation depends on two factors—the angle of scatter and the energy of the original photon. The relationship between the energy of the scattered radiation and the angle of scatter is a little complex and should be considered in two steps. The photon characteristic that is specifically related to a given scatter angle is its change in wavelength. It should be recalled that a photon's wavelength (λ) and energy (E) are inversely related as given by:

$$E = \frac{12.4}{\lambda}.$$

Since photons lose energy in a Compton interaction, the wavelength always increases. The relationship between the change in a photon's wavelength, $\Delta\lambda$, and the angle of scatter is given by:

$$\Delta\lambda = 0.024(1 - \cos\theta).$$

For example, all photons scattered at an angle of 90 degrees, where the cosine has a value of 0, will undergo a wavelength change of 0.024 Å. Photons which scatter back at an angle of 180 degrees where the cosine has a value of -1 will undergo a wavelength change of 0.048 Å. This is the maximum wavelength change that can occur in a scattering interaction.

It is important to recognize the difference between a change in wavelength and a change in energy. Since higher energy photons have shorter wavelengths, a change of say 0.024 Å represents a larger energy change than it would for a lower energy photon. All photons scattered at an angle of 90 degrees will undergo a wavelength change of 0.0243 Å. The change in energy associated with 90-degree scatter is not the same for all photons and depends on their original energy. The change in energy can be found as follows. For a 110-keV photon, the wavelength is 0.1127 Å. A scatter angle of 90 degrees will always increase the wavelength by 0.0243. Therefore, the wavelength of the scattered photon will be 0.1127 plus 0.0243 or 0.1370. The energy of a photon with this wavelength is 91 keV. The 110-keV photons will lose 19 keV or 17% of their energy in the scattering process. Lower energy photons lose a smaller percentage of their energy.

COMPETITIVE INTERACTIONS

As photons pass through matter, they can engage in either photoelectric or Compton interactions with the material electrons. The photoelectric interaction captures all photon energy and deposits it within the material, whereas the Compton interaction removes only a portion of the energy, and the remainder continues as scattered radiation. The combination of the two types of interactions produces the overall attenuation of the x-ray beam. We now consider the factors that determine which of the two interactions is most likely to occur in a given situation.

The energy at which interactions change from predominantly photoelectric to Compton is a function of the atomic number of the material. Figure 10-11 shows this crossover energy for several different materials. At the lower photon energies, photoelectric interactions are much more predominant than Compton. Over most of the energy range, the probability of both decreases with increased energy. However, the decrease in photoelectric interactions is much greater. This is because the photoelectric rate changes in proportion to $1/E^3$, whereas Compton interactions are much less energy dependent. In soft tissue, the two lines cross at an energy of about 30 keV. At this energy, both photoelectric and Compton interactions occur in equal numbers. Below this energy, photoelectric interactions predominate. Above 30 keV, Compton interactions become the significant process of x-ray attenuation. As photon energy increases, two changes occur: the probability of both types of interactions decreases, but the decrease for Compton is less, and it becomes the predominant type of interaction.

In higher-atomic-number materials, photoelectric interactions are more probable, in general, and they predominate up to higher photon energy levels. The conditions that cause photoelectric interactions to predominate over Compton are the same conditions that enhance photoelectric interactions, that is, low photon energies and materials with high atomic numbers.

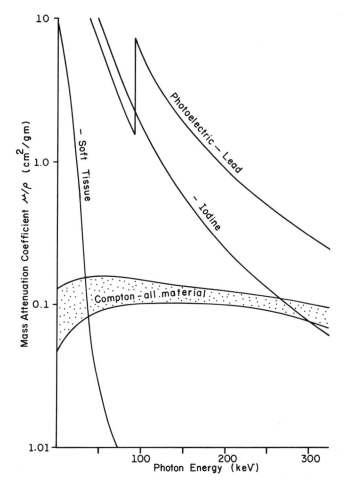

Figure 10-11 Comparison of Photoelectric and Compton Interaction Rates for Different Materials and Photon Energies

The total attenuation coefficient value for materials involved in x-ray and gamma interactions can vary tremendously if photoelectric interactions are involved. A minimum value of approximately 0.15 cm^2/g is established by Compton interactions. Photoelectric interactions can cause the total attenuation to increase to very high values. For example, at 30 keV, lead (Z = 82) has a mass attenuation coefficient of 30 cm^2/g.

Chapter 11

Radiation Penetration

INTRODUCTION AND OVERVIEW

One of the characteristics of x- and gamma radiation that makes them useful for medical imaging is their penetrating ability. When they are directed into an object, some of the photons are absorbed or scattered, whereas others completely penetrate the object. The penetration can be expressed as the fraction of radiation passing through the object. Penetration is the inverse of attenuation. The amount of penetration depends on the energy of the individual photons and the atomic number, density, and thickness of the object, as illustrated in Figure 11-1.

The probability of photons interacting, especially with the photoelectric effect, is related to their energy. Increasing photon energy generally *decreases* the probability of interactions (attenuation) and, therefore, *increases* penetration. As a rule, high-energy photons are better penetrators than low-energy photons, although there are limits and exceptions to this, which we discuss later.

PHOTON RANGE

It might be helpful in understanding the characteristics of radiation penetration to first consider the range, or distance, traveled by the individual photons before they are absorbed or scattered. When photons enter an object, they travel some distance before interacting. This distance can be considered the range of the individual photons.

A characteristic of radiation is that photons do not have the same range, even when they have the same energy. In fact, there is no way to predict the range of a specific photon. Let us consider a group of monoenergetic photons entering an object, as shown in Figure 11-2. Some of the photons travel a relatively short distance before interacting, whereas others pass through or penetrate the object. If we count the number of photons penetrating through each thickness of material,

157

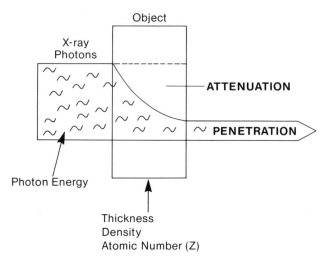

Figure 11-1 Factors that Affect the Penetration of Radiation through a Specific Object

we begin to see a fundamental characteristic of photon penetration. The relationship between the number of photons reaching a specific point and the thickness of the material to that point is exponential.

The nature of the exponential relationship is that each thickness of material attenuates the same fraction of photons entering it. This means that the first layer encountered by the radiation beam attenuates many more photons than the succeeding layers.

In a given situation a group of photons have different individual ranges which, when considered together, produce an average range for the group. The average range is the average distance traveled by the photons before they interact. Very few photons travel a distance exactly equal to the average range. The average range of a group of photons is inversely related to the attenuation rate. Increasing the rate of attenuation by changing photon energy or the type of material decreases the average range of photons. Actually, the average photon range is equal to the reciprocal of the attenuation coefficient (μ):

Average Range (cm) = 1/Attenuation Coefficient (cm^{-1}).

Therefore, the average distance (range) that photons penetrate a material is determined by the same factors that affect the rate of attenuation: photon energy, type of material (atomic number), and material density.

Average photon range is a useful concept for visualizing the penetrating characteristics of radiation photons. It is, however, not the most useful parameter for measuring and calculating the penetrating ability of radiation.

HALF VALUE LAYER

Half value layer (HVL) is the most frequently used factor for describing both the penetrating ability of specific radiations and the penetration through specific objects. HVL is the thickness of material penetrated by one half of the radiation and is expressed in units of distance (mm or cm).

Increasing the penetrating ability of a radiation increases its HVL. HVL is related to, but not the same as, average photon range. There is a difference between the two because of the exponential characteristic of x-ray attenuation and penetration. The specific relationship is

$$HVL = 0.693 \times \text{Average Range} = 0.693/\mu.$$

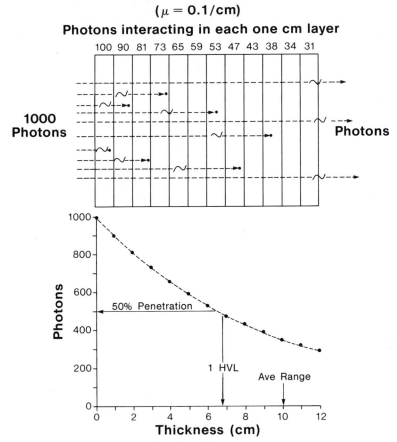

Figure 11-2 Penetration Range of Individual Photons

This shows that the HVL is inversely proportional to the attenuation coefficient. The number, 0.693, is the exponent value that gives a penetration of 0.5 ($e^{-0.693} = 0.5$).

Any factor that changes the value of the attenuation coefficient also changes the HVL. These two quantities are compared for aluminum in Figure 11-3. Aluminum has two significant applications in an x-ray system. It is used as a material to filter x-ray beams and as a reference material for measuring the penetrating ability (HVL) of x-rays. The value of the attenuation coefficient decreases rather rapidly with increased photon energy and causes the penetrating ability to increase.

Figure 11-4 illustrates an important aspect of the HVL concept. If the penetration through a thickness of 1 HVL is 0.5 (50%), the penetration through a thickness of 2 HVLs will be 0.5 × 0.5 or 25%. Each succeeding layer of material with a thickness of 1 HVL reduces the number of photons by a factor of 0.5. The relationship between penetration (P) and thickness of material that is n half value layers thick is

$$P = (0.5)^n.$$

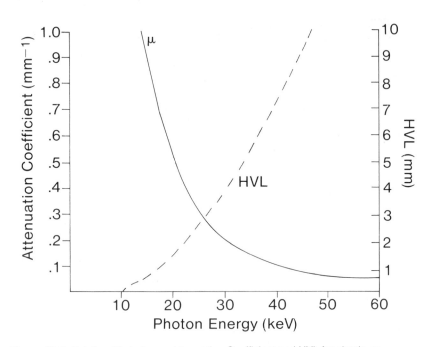

Figure 11-3 Relationship between Attenuation Coefficient and HVL for aluminum

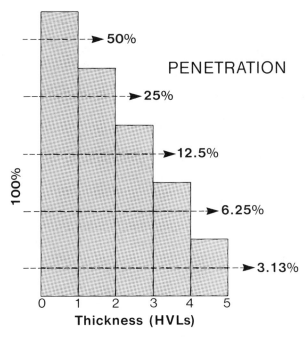

Figure 11-4 Relationship between Penetration and Object Thickness Expressed in HVLs

An example using this relationship is determining the penetration through lead shielding. Photons of 60 keV have an HVL in lead of 0.125 mm. The problem is to determine the penetration through a lead shield that is 0.5 mm thick. At this particular photon energy, 0.5 mm is 4 HVLs, and the penetration is

$$n = \text{thickness/HVL} = 0.5/0.125 = 4$$
$$P = (0.5)^4 = 0.0625.$$

Figure 11-5 summarizes two important characteristics of HVL. In a specific material, the HVL is affected by photon energy. On the other hand, for a specific photon energy, the thickness of 1 HVL is related to characteristics of the material, density, and/or atomic number.

The general procedure for determining the HVL value of an x-ray beam is illustrated in Figure 11-6. Two items are required. One is an instrument for measuring radiation exposure, and the second is a set of aluminum absorbers. Typically, the set includes absorbers with thicknesses of both 0.5 mm and 1 mm.

The exposure meter is positioned as shown, and a reading is made. Aluminum absorbers are then placed in the beam, typically in 0.5- or 1-mm increments, and an exposure reading is made. Dividing each exposure reading by the exposure with no absorber gives the penetration for each thickness of absorber. The penetration values are then plotted as a function of aluminum-absorber thickness. The absorber thickness corresponding to a penetration value of 0.5 is the HVL. This value is referred to as the first HVL. The second HVL value is the additional thickness required to reduce the penetration to 0.25. Generally, it is larger than the first value because the first aluminum absorbers added to the beam act as a filter and produce an increase in the equivalent energy and corresponding HVL value. In actual practice, it is usually more desirable to plot the penetration values on a logarithmic scale (by using semilogarithmic graph paper) so that the resulting graph is essentially a straight line.

X-RAY BEAM QUALITY

The general term "quality" refers to an x-ray beam's penetrating ability. It has been shown that, for a given material, the penetrating ability of an x-ray beam depends on the energy of the photons. Up to this point, the discussion has related

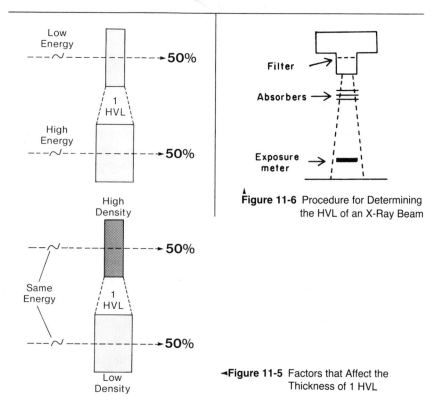

Figure 11-6 Procedure for Determining the HVL of an X-Ray Beam

◄**Figure 11-5** Factors that Affect the Thickness of 1 HVL

penetration to specific photon energies. For x-ray beams that contain a spectrum of photon energies, the penetration is different for each energy. The overall penetration generally corresponds to the penetration of a photon energy between the minimum and maximum energies of the spectrum. This energy is designated the effective energy of the x-ray spectrum. For example, the x-ray spectrum shown in Figure 11-7, which is produced by a machine operating at 70 kVp, has a penetrating ability that can be measured relatively easily. The HVL has a value of approximately 2.4 mm of aluminum. By referring to the HVL curve in Figure 11-3, it is seen that this value corresponds to a photon energy of 24 keV. This spectrum therefore has, with respect to penetrating ability, an effective energy of 24 keV. The effective energy of an x-ray spectrum is the energy of a mono-energetic beam of photons that has the same penetrating ability (HVL) as the spectrum of photons.

The effective energy is generally close to 30% or 40% of peak energy, but its exact value depends on the shape of the spectrum. For a given KV_p, two factors that can alter the spectrum are the amount of filtration in the beam and the high-voltage waveform used to produce the x-rays.

FILTRATION

As an x-ray beam made up of different photon energies passes through many materials, photons of certain energies penetrate better than others. This selective

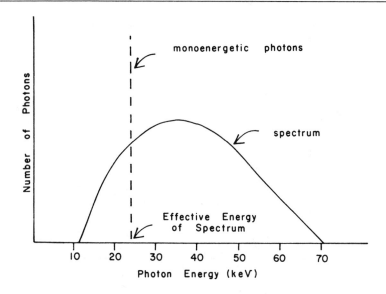

Figure 11-7 Effective Energy of an X-Ray Spectrum

attenuation of photons, according to their energy, is referred to as filtration. Figure 11-8 shows the penetration through two materials of special interest, a 1-cm thickness of muscle and a 1-mm thickness of aluminum. The penetration through the muscle, or soft tissue, is considered first. For photons with energies less than 10 keV, there is virtually no penetration; all the photons are attenuated by the tissue. The low penetration in tissue by photons of this energy is because of the high value for the attenuation coefficient. Recall that the high attenuation coefficient value is the result of photoelectric interactions, which are highly probable at this energy. In the range of 10 keV to 25 keV, penetration rapidly increases with energy. As photon energy increases to about 40 keV, penetration increases, but much more gradually. Of special interest is the very low penetrating ability of x-ray photons with energies below approximately 20 keV. At this energy, the penetration through 1 cm of tissue is 0.45, and the penetration through 15 cm of tissue is

$$P = (0.45)^{15} = 0.0000063.$$

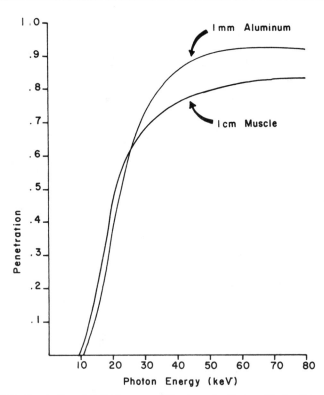

Figure 11-8 Penetration of Soft Tissue and Aluminum for Various Photon Energies

On the other hand, the penetration through 15 cm of tissue for photons with an energy of 50 keV is

$$P = (0.8)^{15} = 0.035.$$

A significant portion (3.5%) of photons with an energy near 50 keV penetrate a 15-cm-thick patient, whereas virtually no photons with energies of 20 keV or less make it through. This means that low-energy photons in an x-ray spectrum do not contribute to image formation; they contribute only to patient exposure. In other words, the tissue of the body selectively filters out the low-energy photons.

An obvious solution is to place some material in the x-ray beam, before it enters the patient, to filter out the low-energy photons. In diagnostic x-ray equipment, aluminum is normally used for this purpose. Figure 11-8 shows the penetration through a 1-mm thickness of aluminum. Typically, most x-ray machines contain the equivalent of several millimeters of aluminum filtration. This might not always be in the form of aluminum because several objects contribute to x-ray beam filtration: the x-ray tube window, the x-ray beam collimator mirror, and the table top in fluoroscopic equipment. The total amount of filtration in a given x-ray machine is generally specified in terms of an equivalent aluminum thickness.

The addition of filtration significantly alters the shape of the x-ray spectrum, as shown in Figure 11-9. Since filtration selectively absorbs the lower energy photons, it produces a shift in the effective energy of an x-ray beam. Figure 11-9 compares an unfiltered spectrum to spectra that passed through 1-mm and 3-mm filters. It is apparent that increasing the filtration from 1 mm to 3 mm of aluminum produces a noticeable decrease in the number of x-ray photons. It should be observed, however, that most of this decrease is in photons with energies less than approximately 40 keV. These are the photons with a low probability of penetrating a typical patient and contributing to image formation. They do, however, contribute to patient exposure.

Adding filtration increases the penetration (HVL) of an x-ray beam by removing the low-energy photons. HVL values are used to judge the adequacy of the filtration. Regulations that specify filtration requirements generally state a minimum acceptable HVL value. Typical values are shown in Table 11-1. It is assumed that if an x-ray beam has the minimum specified HVL value at a stated KV_p, the filtration is adequate.

PENETRATION WITH SCATTER

Up to this point, the x-ray photons that penetrate an object were assumed to be those that had escaped both photoelectric and Compton interactions. In situations in which Compton interactions are significant, it is necessary to modify this

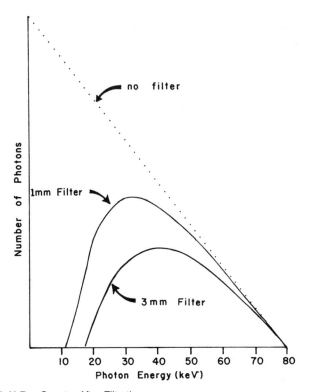

Figure 11-9 X-Ray Spectra After Filtration

concept because some of the radiation removed from the primary beam by Compton interactions is scattered in the forward direction and creates the appearance of increased penetration. A prime example is an x-ray beam passing through the larger portions of the human body, as illustrated in Figure 11-10. When significant forward-scattered radiation combines with the penetrated portion of the primary beam, the effective penetration, Pe, is given by:

$$Pe = P \times S$$

where S is the scatter factor. Its value ranges from 1 (no scatter) to approximately 6 for conditions encountered in some diagnostic examinations.

Several factors contribute to the amount of radiation scattered in the forward direction and hence to the value of S. One of the most significant factors is the x-ray beam area, or field size. Since the source of the scattered radiation is the volume of the patient within the primary x-ray beam, the source size is proportional to the beam area. Within limits, the value of S increases from a value of 1,

Table 11-1 Recommended Minimum Penetration (HVL) for Various KV_p Values

kVp	Minimum penetration (HVL) for aluminum (mm)
30	0.3
50	1.2
70	1.5
90	2.5
110	3.0

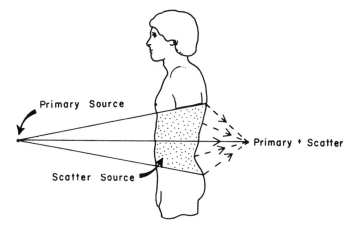

Figure 11-10 Scattered Radiation Adds to the Primary Radiation that Penetrates an Object

more or less, in proportion to field size. Another important factor is body section thickness, which affects the size of the scattered radiation source. A third significant factor is KV_p. As the KV_p is increased over the diagnostic range, several changes occur. A greater proportion of the photons that interact with the body are involved in Compton interactions, and a greater proportion of the photons created in Compton interactions scatters in the forward direction. Perhaps the most significant factor is that the scattered radiation produced at the higher KV_p values is more penetrating. A larger proportion of it leaves the body before being absorbed. When the scattered radiation is more penetrating, there is a larger effective source within the patient. At low KV_p values, most of the scattered radiation created near the entrance surface of the x-ray beam does not penetrate the body; at higher KV_p values, this scattered radiation contributes more to the radiation passing through the body.

PENETRATION VALUES

We have seen that the amount of radiation that penetrates through a specific thickness of material is determined by the energy of the individual photons and the characteristics (density and atomic number) of the material. HVL values provide useful information about the penetration of a specific radiation in a specific material. When an HVL value is known, the penetration through other thicknesses can be easily determined. Table 11-2 gives HVL values for several materials related to diagnostic imaging.

Table 11–2 HVL Values for Certain Materials

Material	HVL (mm)		
	30 keV	60 keV	120 keV
Tissue	20.	35.	45.
Aluminum	2.3	9.3	16.6
Lead	0.02	0.13	0.15

Chapter 12

X-Ray Image Formation and Contrast

INTRODUCTION AND OVERVIEW

There are two basic ways to create images with x-radiation. One method is to pass an x-ray beam through the body section and project a shadow image onto the receptor. The second method, used in CT, employs a digital computer to calculate (reconstruct) an image from x-ray penetration data. CT image formation is discussed in Chapter 23. At this time, we consider only projection imaging, which is the basic process employed in conventional radiography and fluoroscopy.

The contrast that ultimately appears in the image is determined by many factors, as indicated in Figure 12-1. In addition to the penetration characteristics to be considered, image contrast is significantly affected by scattered radiation (Chapter 13) and the contrast characteristics of the film (Chapter 16). The contrast of small objects within the body and anatomical detail are reduced by image blurring (Chapters 18 and 19). As the x-ray beam emerges from the patient's body, as shown in Figure 12-2, it contains an image in the form of variations in exposure across the image area. A significant characteristic of this invisible x-ray image is the amount of contrast it contains. Contrast is represented by the amount of variation in x-ray exposure between points within the image; the amount of contrast produced in a specific examination is determined by both the physical characteristics of the body section and the penetrating characteristics of the x-ray beam.

In this chapter we explore the characteristics of both the objects within a body and the x-ray beam and show how optimum image contrast can be achieved.

CONTRAST TYPES

Several types of contrast are encountered during x-ray image formation. The formation of a visible image involves the transformation of one type of contrast to another at two stages in the image-forming process, as shown in Figure 12-2.

169

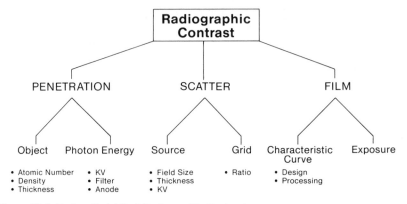

Figure 12-1 Factors that Affect Radiographic Contrast

Object Contrast

For an object to be visible in an x-ray image, it must have physical contrast in relationship to the tissue or other material in which it is embedded. This contrast can be a difference in physical density or chemical composition (atomic number).

When an object is physically different it absorbs either more or less x-radiation than an equal thickness of surrounding tissue and casts a shadow in the x-ray beam. If the object absorbs less radiation than the surrounding tissue (ie, gas surrounded by tissue), it will cast a negative shadow that appears as a dark area in a radiograph. The third factor that affects object contrast is its thickness in the direction of the x-ray beam. Object contrast is proportional to the product of object density and thickness. This quantity represents the mass of object material per unit area (cm^2) of the image. For example, a thick (large diameter) vessel filled with diluted iodine contrast medium and a thin (small diameter) vessel filled with undiluted medium will produce the same amount of contrast if the products of the diameters and iodine concentrations (densities) are the same.

The chemical composition of an object contributes to its contrast only if its effective atomic number (Z) is different from that of the surrounding tissue. Relatively little contrast is produced by the different chemical compositions found in soft tissues and body fluids because the effective atomic number values are close together. The contrast produced by a difference in chemical composition (atomic number) is quite sensitive to photon energy (KV_p).

Most materials that produce high contrast with respect to soft tissue differ from the soft tissue in both physical density and atomic number. The physical characteristics of most materials encountered in x-ray imaging are compared in Table 12-1.

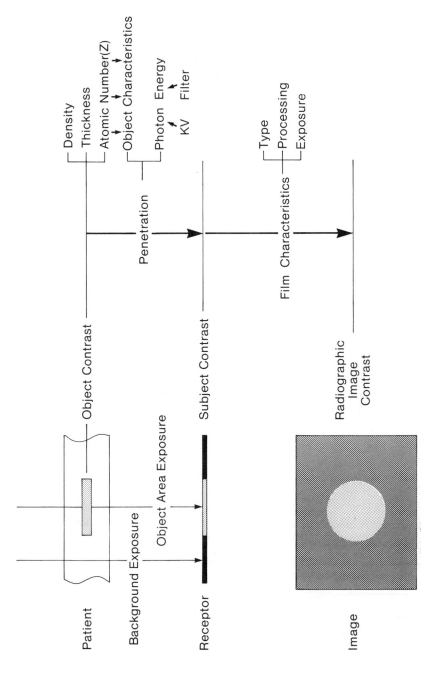

Figure 12-2 Stages of Contrast Development in Radiography

Table 12–1 Physical Characteristics of Contrast-Producing Materials

Material	Effective Atomic Number (Z)	Density (g/cm³)
Water	7.42	1.0
Muscle	7.46	1.0
Fat	5.92	0.91
Air	7.64	0.00129
Calcium	20.0	1.55
Iodine	53.0	4.94
Barium	56.0	3.5

Subject Contrast

The contrast in the invisible image emerging from the patient's body is traditionally referred to as subject contrast. Subject contrast is the difference in exposure between various points within the image area.

For an individual object, the significant contrast value is the difference in exposure between the object area and its surrounding background. This exposure difference is generally expressed as a percentage value relative to the background exposure level. Contrast will be present if the exposure in the object area is either more or less than in the surrounding background.

Subject contrast is produced because x-ray penetration through an object differs from the penetration through the adjacent background tissue. For objects that attenuate more of the radiation than the adjacent tissue, contrast is inversely related to object penetration. Maximum (100%) contrast is produced when no radiation penetrates the object. Metal objects (lead bullets, rods, etc.) are good examples. Contrast is reduced as x-ray penetration through the object increases. When object penetration approaches the penetration through an equal thickness of surrounding tissue, contrast disappears.

The amount of subject contrast produced is determined by the physical contrast characteristics (atomic number, density, and thickness) of the object and the penetrating characteristics (photon energy spectrum) of the x-ray beam.

Image Contrast

The third type of contrast is the contrast that appears in the visible image. The contrast in a radiograph (film) is in the form of differences in optical density between various points within the image, such as between an object area and the surrounding background. The amount of visible radiographic contrast produced in a specific procedure depends on the amount of x-ray beam exposure (subject) contrast delivered to the receptor and the contrast transfer characteristics of the film, which are discussed in Chapter 16.

The contrast in a visible fluoroscopic image is in the form of brightness ratios between various points within the image area. The amount of contrast in a fluoroscopic image depends on the amount of subject contrast entering the receptor system and the characteristics and adjustments of the components (image intensifier tube, video, etc.) of the imaging system. The contrast transfer characteristics of a fluoroscopic system are discussed in Chapter 20.

EFFECTS OF PHOTON ENERGY (KV_p)

Object penetration and the resulting contrast often depend on the photon energy spectrum. This, in turn, is determined by three factors: (1) x-ray tube anode material, (2) x-ray beam filtration, and (3) KV. Since most x-ray examinations are performed with tungsten anode tubes, the first factor cannot be used to adjust contrast. The exception is the use of molybdenum anode tubes in mammography. Most x-ray machines have essentially the same amount of filtration, which is a few millimeters of aluminum. Two exceptions are molybdenum filters used with molybdenum anode tubes in mammography and copper or brass filters, sometimes used in chest radiography.

In most procedures, KV_p is the only photon-energy controlling factor that can be changed by the operator to alter contrast. Radiographic examinations are performed with KV_p values ranging from a low of approximately 28 kVp, in mammography, to a high of approximately 140 kVp, in chest imaging. The selection of a KV for a specific imaging procedure is generally governed by the contrast requirement, but other factors, such as patient exposure (Chapters 17 and 33) and x-ray tube heating (Chapter 9), must be considered.

Both photoelectric and Compton interactions contribute to the formation of image contrast. It was shown in Chapter 10 that the rate of Compton interactions is primarily determined by tissue density and depends very little on either tissue atomic number or photon energy. On the other hand, the rate of photoelectric interactions is very dependent on the atomic number of the material and the energy of the x-ray photons. This means that when contrast is produced by a difference in the atomic numbers of an object and the surrounding tissue, the amount of contrast is very dependent on photon energy (KV_p). If the contrast is produced by a difference in density (Compton interactions), it will be relatively independent of photon energy. Changing KV_p produces a significant change in contrast when the conditions are favorable for photoelectric interactions. In materials with relatively low atomic numbers (ie, soft tissue and body fluids), this change is limited to relatively low KV_p values. However, the contrast produced by higher atomic number materials, such as calcium, iodine, and barium, has a KV_p dependence over a much wider range of KV_p values.

Soft Tissue Radiography

Two basic factors tend to limit the amount of contrast that can be produced between types of soft tissue and between soft tissue and fluid. One factor is the small difference in the physical characteristics (density and atomic number) among these materials, as shown in Table 12-1, and the second factor is the relatively low number of photoelectric interactions because of the low atomic numbers.

Mammography is a procedure that uses soft tissue contrast. The production of significant contrast requires the use of relatively low energy photons. Mammography is typically performed with equipment that uses the characteristic radiation produced in a molybdenum anode x-ray tube and filtered by a molybdenum filter. The spectrum of this radiation is shown in Figure 12-3. The range of photon energies contained within this spectrum represents a reasonable compromise between contrast production and overall breast penetration (patient exposure and machine loading).

Calcium

Calcium produces significant contrast relative to soft tissue because it differs in both density and atomic number. Because of its higher atomic number, photoelectric interactions predominate over Compton interactions up to a photon energy of approximately 85 keV. Above this energy, the photoelectric interactions contribute less to image contrast.

Figure 12-4 shows the relationship between calcium penetration (contrast) and photon energy. In principle, the optimum photon energy range (KV_p) for imaging

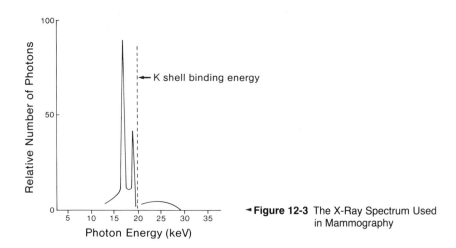

Figure 12-3 The X-Ray Spectrum Used in Mammography

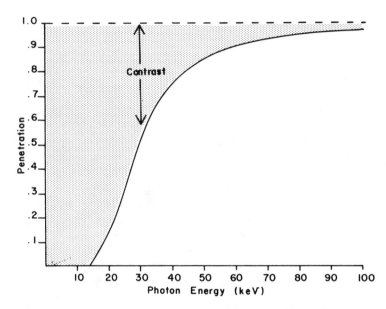

Figure 12-4 Relationship of Calcium Penetration and Contrast to Photon Energy

calcium depends, to some extent, on the thickness of the object. When imaging very small (thin) calcifications, as in mammography, a low photon energy must be used or the contrast will be too low for visibility. When the objective is to see through a large calcified structure (bone), relatively high photon energies (KV_p) must be used to achieve adequate object penetration.

Iodine and Barium Contrast Media

The two chemical elements iodine and barium produce high contrast with respect to soft tissue because of their densities and atomic numbers. The significance of their atomic numbers (Z = 53 for iodine, Z = 56 for barium) is that they cause the K-absorption edge to be located at a very favorable energy relative to the typical x-ray energy spectrum. The K edge for iodine is at 33 keV and is at 37 keV for barium. Maximum contrast is produced when the x-ray photon energy is slightly above the K-edge energy of the material. This is illustrated for iodine in Figure 12-5. A similar relationship exists for barium but is shifted up to slightly higher photon energies.

Since the typical x-ray beam contains a rather broad spectrum of photon energies, all of the energies do not produce the same level of contrast. In practice, maximum contrast is achieved by adjusting the KV_p so that a major part of the spectrum falls just above the K-edge energy. For iodine, this generally occurs when the KV_p is set in the range of 60–70.

AREA CONTRAST

We have considered a single object embedded in tissue. In this simple case an increase in contrast generally increases the visibility of the object. However, in most clinical applications one image contains many objects or anatomical structures. A problem arises when the different objects are located in different areas of the body and the thickness or density of the different areas is significantly different. A chest image that contains lung and mediastinal areas is a good example; a simple representation is shown in Figure 12-6. Because of the large difference in tissue density between the lungs and the mediastinum the contrast is significant between these two areas in the image. In this typical radiograph, the area of the mediastinum is very light (low film density), and the lung areas are much darker. Any objects within the mediastinum are imaged on a light background, and objects within the lung areas are imaged on dark backgrounds.

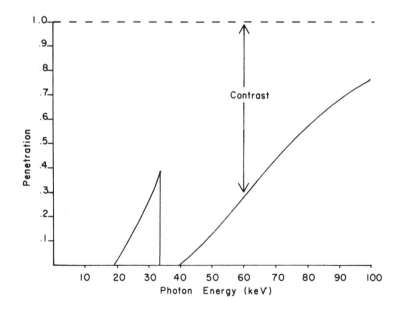

Figure 12-5 Relationship of Iodine Penetration and Contrast to Photon Energy; The Values Shown Are for a 1-mm Thickness of Iodine Contrast Medium

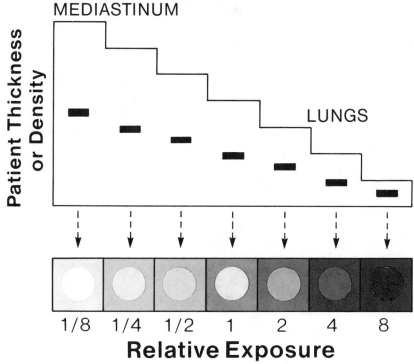

Figure 12-6 Physical Conditions that Produce Area Contrast

A characteristic of radiographic film is that its ability to display object contrast is reduced in areas that are either very light (mediastinum) or relatively dark (lungs). If there is a relatively high level of contrast between areas within an image, then the contrast of objects within these areas can be reduced because of film limitations. Three actions can be taken to minimize the problem. One is to use a wide latitude film that reduces area contrast and improves visibility within the individual areas in many situations; this is described in Chapter 16. A second approach is to place compensating filters between the x-ray tube and the patient's body. The filter has areas with different thicknesses and is positioned so that its thickest part is over the thinnest, or least dense, part of the body. The overall effect is a reduction in area contrast within the image. The third action is to use a very penetrating x-ray beam produced by high KV.

Figure 12-7 compares chest radiographs made at two KV_p values. The image on the left was made at 60 kVp. Although it has high contrast between the mediastinum and lung areas, visibility of structures within these areas is diminished. The high-KV radiograph, which has less area contrast, has increased object contrast, especially within the lung areas.

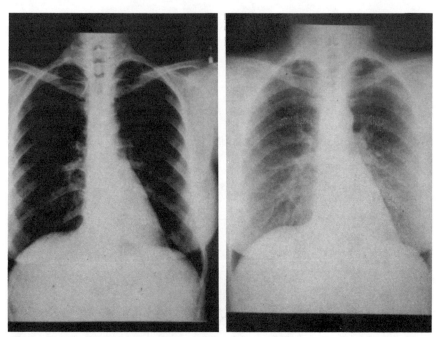

Figure 12-7 Radiographs Illustrating a Difference in Area Contrast Produced by Changing from 60 kVp (left image) to 140 kVp

Chapter 13

Scattered Radiation and Contrast

INTRODUCTION AND OVERVIEW

When an x-ray beam enters a patient's body, a large portion of the photons engage in Compton interactions and produce scattered radiation. Some of this scattered radiation leaves the body in the same general direction as the primary beam and exposes the image receptor. The scattered radiation reduces image contrast. The degree of loss depends on the scatter content of the radiation emerging from the patient's body. In most radiographic and fluoroscopic procedures, the major portion of the x-ray beam leaving the patient's body is scattered radiation. This, in turn, significantly reduces contrast.

Subject contrast was previously defined as the difference in exposure to the object area on a film expressed as a percentage of the exposure to the surrounding background. Maximum contrast, ie, 100%, is obtained when the object area receives no exposure with respect to the background. A previous chapter discussed the reduction of subject contrast because of x-ray penetration through the object being imaged. This chapter describes the further reduction of contrast by scattered radiation.

CONTRAST REDUCTION

The basic concept of contrast reduction by scattered radiation is illustrated in Figure 13-1. For simplicity, it is assumed that the object is not penetrated and, if it were not for scattered radiation, would produce 100% subject contrast. The object is assumed to be embedded in a larger mass of material, such as the human body, that produces the scattered radiation. The exposure to the background area of the receptor, or film, is produced by radiation that penetrates the body adjacent to the object plus the scattered radiation. For a given x-ray machine setting, the background area exposure is proportional to PS, the product of the penetration through

179

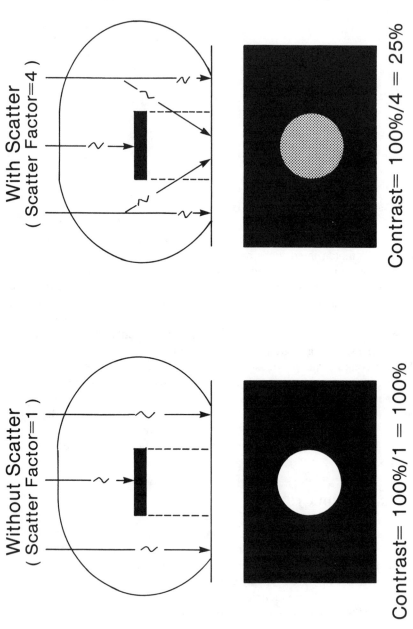

Figure 13-1 Reduction of Image Contrast by Scattered Radiation

the patient and the scatter factor. For the same exposure conditions, the exposure to the object area is proportional to P (S − 1). By combining these expressions for relative background and object area exposure, it can be shown that the contrast is inversely related to the value of the scatter factors, as follows:

$$Cs\ (\%)\ =\ 100/S.$$

This relationship shows that as the proportion of scattered radiation in the x-ray beam increases, contrast proportionally decreases. For example, if the scatter factor has a value of 4, the contrast between the object and background areas will be reduced to 25%. In other words, the object area exposure is 75% of the exposure reaching the surrounding background. The contrast can also be determined as follows. The ratio of scattered to primary radiation is always S − 1. For a scatter factor value of 4, the scatter-primary ratio is 3. The background area exposure is, therefore, composed of one unit of primary and three units of scattered radiation. The object area receives only the three units of scattered radiation. This yields an object area exposure of 75% of background and a contrast of 25%.

With respect to image contrast, the scatter factor, S, is also the contrast reduction factor. For example, if the scatter (contrast reduction) factor has a value of 2, the resulting contrast will be 50%. This is a reduction of 100% contrast by a factor of 2. A scatter factor value of 5 reduces contrast by a factor of 5, or down to 20%. Figure 13-2 shows the general relationship between contrast and scatter factor. The value of the scatter factor is primarily a function of patient thickness, field size, and KV_p. In examinations of relatively thick body sections, contrast reduction factors of 5 or 6 are common.

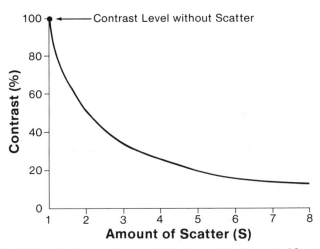

Figure 13-2 Relationship between Contrast Reduction and the Amount of Scatter

We developed our discussion of contrast reduction using an unpenetrated object that would produce 100% contrast in the absence of scatter. Most objects within the body are penetrated to some extent. Therefore, contrast is reduced by both object penetration and scattered radiation. For example, if an object is 60% penetrated (40% contrast), and the scatter factor, S, has a value of 4, the final contrast will be 10%.

Since scattered radiation robs an x-ray image of most of its contrast, specific actions must be taken to regain some of the lost contrast. Several methods can be used to reduce the effect of scattered radiation but none is capable of restoring the full image contrast. The use of each scatter reduction method usually involves compromises, as we will see below.

COLLIMATION

The amount of scattered radiation is generally proportional to the total mass of tissue contained within the primary x-ray beam. This is, in turn, determined by the thickness of the patient and the area or field size being exposed. Increasing the field size increases the total amount of scattered radiation and the value of the scatter contrast-reduction factors. Therefore, one method of reducing scattered radiation and increasing contrast is to reduce the field size with x-ray beam collimators, cones, or other beam-limiting devices, as illustrated in Figure 13-3. This method is limited by the necessity to cover a specific anatomical region. However, in most situations, contrast can be improved by reducing the field size to the smallest practical value.

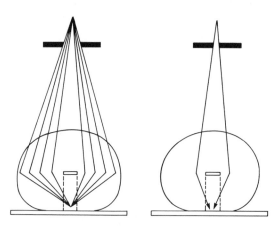

Figure 13-3 Contrast Improvement by Reducing X-Ray Beam Size

AIR GAP

The quantity of scattered radiation in an x-ray beam reaching a receptor can be reduced by separating the patient's body and receptor surface, as shown in Figure 13-4. This separation is known as an air gap. Scattered radiation leaving a patient's body is more divergent than the primary x-ray beam. Therefore, scattered radiation spreads out of the primary beam area. The reduction of scattered radiation in proportion to primary radiation increases with air-gap distance. Several factors must be considered when using this method of scatter reduction. Patient exposure is increased because of the inverse-square effect. The use of an air gap introduces magnification. Therefore, a larger receptor size is required to obtain the same patient area coverage. If the air gap is obtained by increasing the tube-to-receptor distance, the x-ray equipment must be operated at a higher output to obtain adequate receptor exposure.

Also, increasing the separation distance between the patient and the receptor increases focal spot blurring. It is usually necessary to use relatively small focal spots with an air-gap technique.

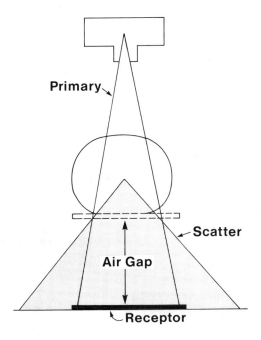

Figure 13-4 Contrast Improvement by Using an Air Gap

GRIDS

In most examinations, the most effective and practical method of removing a portion of the scattered radiation is to use a grid. The grid is placed between the patient's body and the receptor, as shown in Figure 13-5. It is constructed of alternate strips of an x-ray-absorbing material, such as lead, and a relatively nonabsorbing interspace material, such as fiber, carbon, or aluminum. Under normal operating conditions, the grid strips are aligned with the direction of the primary x-ray beam. In most grids, the interspaces are angled so as to align with a specific point in space. These are designated focused grids. The focal point of the grid should coincide with the focal spot of the x-ray tube, which is the source of the primary radiation. In an unfocused grid, the interspaces and strips are parallel and are not aligned with a single point in space. Because the x-ray beam direction is aligned with the grid, much of the primary radiation passes through the interspaces without encountering the lead strips. Scattered radiation, on the other hand, leaves the patient's body in a direction different from that of the primary beam, as shown in Figure 13-6. Since scattered radiation is not generally lined up with the grid strips, a large portion of it is absorbed by the grid. The ideal grid would absorb all scattered radiation and allow all primary x-rays to penetrate to the receptor. Unfortunately, there is no ideal grid, because all such devices absorb some primary radiation and allow some scattered radiation to pass through.

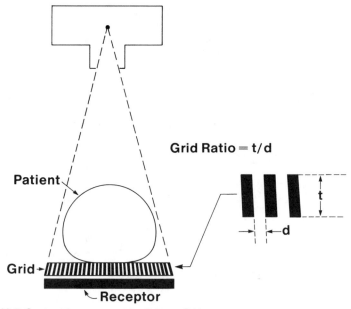

Figure 13-5 Contrast Improvement by Using a Grid

The penetration characteristics for scattered radiation are largely determined by the dimensions of the lead strips and the interspaces. The significant dimensions are illustrated in Figure 13-5. The height of the strips, *t,* is the thickness of the grid and is typically in the range of 2 mm to 5 mm. Another significant dimension is the width of the interspace, *d.* This dimension varies with grid design, but generally ranges from 0.25 mm to 0.4 mm. With respect to grid performance, the important variable is the ratio of these two dimensions, which is designated the grid ratio, *r.* Most grids have ratios ranging from 5:1 to 16:1. The selection of the appropriate grid ratio for a given examination involves the consideration of a number of factors. Although grids with higher ratios eliminate more scattered radiation, they tend to increase patient exposure and x-ray tube loading and require more precise positioning.

GRID PENETRATION

A knowledge of the total penetration of primary and scattered radiation through a grid is necessary to select appropriate exposure factors for the x-ray machine.

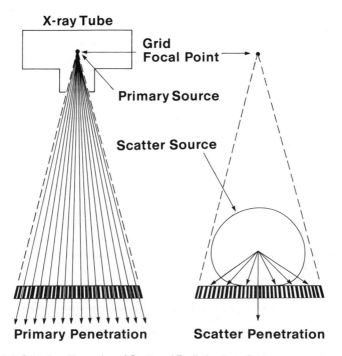

Figure 13-6 Selective Absorption of Scattered Radiation by a Grid

The total grid penetration is a function of scattered-radiation penetration and penetration of primary radiation. The relationship also involves the proportion of scattered radiation in the beam, S. Figure 13-7 shows the general relationship between the two components (primary radiation and scatter) of grid penetration and grid ratio. In general, the penetration of both types of radiation decreases as the grid ratio is increased.

Primary penetration does not change with the amount of scattered radiation, but does change with grid ratio. On the other hand, scattered-radiation penetration is strongly dependent on grid ratio and the amount of scattered radiation in the beam. Because the typical grid removes more scattered than primary radiation, total penetration decreases as the scattered-radiation content of the beam increases. The two major factors, therefore, that determine total grid penetration are the grid ratio and the scatter factor, S.

It is common to express grid penetration in terms of the Bucky factor, named after Dr. Gustave Bucky, who constructed the first grid in 1913. The Bucky factor is the reciprocal of the total grid penetration, or

$$1/\text{Bucky factor} = \text{Grid penetration.}$$

Grid penetration and Bucky factor values are shown in Figure 13-8 for various grid ratios and scatter factors.

It should be recalled that, in most cases, there is a correlation between S and KV_p. Since high KV_p values are generally used for thick body sections, and both

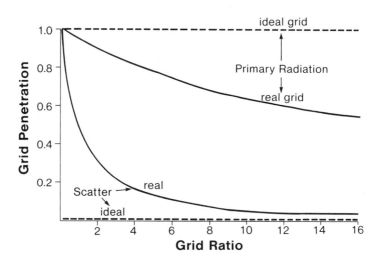

Figure 13-7 General Relationship between Radiation Penetration and Grid Ratio

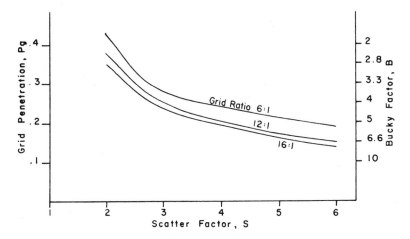

Figure 13-8 Grid Penetration and Bucky Factor Values

factors increase S, grid penetration appears to decrease as KV_p increases. This is because scatter radiation content at the higher KV_p values is generally greater than for primary radiation.

The amount of radiation delivered to a patient's body must be increased to compensate for the radiation absorbed by the grid. Patient exposure is directly proportional to the Bucky factor. For example, if a grid with a Bucky factor of 3 is replaced by one with a Bucky factor of 6, the exposure to the patient must be doubled to compensate for the additional grid absorption.

Scatter Penetration

The relationship between the quantity of scattered radiation that passes through the grid and the grid ratio can be visualized by referring to Figure 13-9. Consider the exposure that reaches a point on the receptor located at the bottom of an interspace. Since no radiation penetrates the lead strips, radiation can reach the point on the receptor only from the directions indicated. The amount of radiation reaching this point is generally proportional to the volume of the patient's body in direct ''view'' from this point. As grid ratio is increased, this volume becomes smaller, and the amount of radiation reaching this point is reduced. In effect, with a high-ratio grid, each point on the receptor surface is exposed to a smaller portion of the patient's body, which is the source of scattered radiation. Using basic geometrical relationships, the theoretical penetration of scattered radiation through grids of various ratios can be determined. This is shown graphically in Figure 13-7. In actual usage, the relationship can differ from the one shown, especially for certain grid ratio-KV_p combinations.

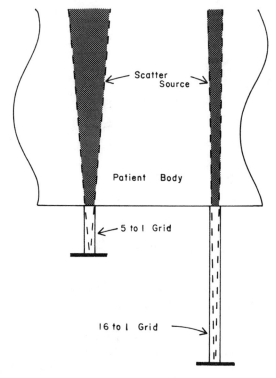

Figure 13-9 Relationship of Receptor Exposure to Grid Ratio

Primary Penetration

Because of the presence of the lead strips, grids attenuate part of the primary radiation. The penetration of primary radiation through the grid is generally in the range of 0.6 to 0.7. This value depends on grid design and is generally inversely related to grid ratio.

Contrast Improvement

It has been shown that as the grid ratio is increased, a greater proportion of the scattered radiation is removed from the beam. By using the scattered-radiation penetration shown in Figure 13-7 and an average primary penetration of 0.65, it is possible to calculate the expected contrast for various combinations of grid ratio and scatter factors, S. Some values are shown in Figure 13-10.

For a grid ratio of 0, that is, no grid, the contrast percentage is equal to 100 divided by S. As grid ratio is increased and scatter penetration decreases, contrast

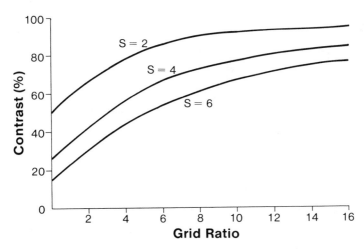

Figure 13-10 Relationship of Image Contrast to Scatter Factor and Grid Ratio

improves. For relatively small amounts of scattered radiation, that is, S = 2, a grid ratio of 8:1 restores the contrast to 90%. The additional improvement in contrast with higher grid ratios is relatively small. It should be noticed, however, that even with high grid ratios, all contrast is not restored. When the proportion of scattered radiation in the beam is higher, for example, when S has a value of 6, the situation is significantly different. At each grid ratio value, the contrast is much less than for lower scatter factor values. Even with a high-ratio grid, such as 16:1, the contrast is restored to only about 76%. This graph illustrates that contrast is not only a function of grid ratio, but is also determined by the quantity of scattered radiation in the beam, the value of S.

It might appear that the data in Figure 13-10 indicate that grids do not remove as much scattered radiation when the amount of scattered radiation in the beam is relatively large, such as for a value of S of 5 or 6. The relatively lower contrast obtained with large amounts of scattered radiation is because of the very low contrast values present without the grid. Actually, grids improve contrast by larger factors when the proportion of scattered radiation in the beam is higher. This can be illustrated by observing values of the contrast improvement factor, K, as shown in Figure 13-11. The contrast improvement factor is the ratio of the contrast when a specific grid is used compared with the contrast without the grid. It is a function of the grid penetration characteristics and the amount of scattered radiation, S.

The value of the contrast improvement factor, K, generally increases both with grid ratio and with the quantity of scattered radiation in the beam, S. Although it is true that grids improve contrast by larger factors under conditions of high levels of scattered radiation, one significant fact should not be overlooked: the total restora-

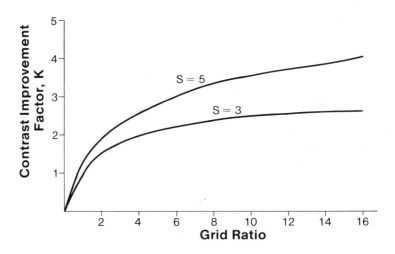

Figure 13-11 Relationship of Contrast Improvement Factor to Scatter Factor and Grid Ratio

tion of contrast for a given grid is always less for the higher values of scattered radiation. This becomes apparent by comparing the value of the contrast improvement factor to the value of the contrast reduction factor, which is equal to the value of S. This expresses the ability of a grid under various scatter conditions to recover lost contrast. For example, in Figure 13-11 it is shown that when S is equal to 5 (contrast reduced to one fifth) a 16:1-ratio grid produces a contrast improvement factor of 4. The contrast recovery, K/S, is four fifths, or 80%. However, at a lower level of scattered radiation, such as S = 3, the same grid produces a contrast improvement factor of 2.7, which represents a contrast recovery of 2.7/3, or 90%.

The relationship between the improvement in contrast and grid ratio strongly depends on the proportion of scattered radiation in the beam emerging from the patient's body. This, in turn, is a function of patient thickness, field size, and KV_p. Under conditions that produce high scatter radiation values, a given grid improves contrast by a greater factor, but cannot recover as much contrast as is possible at lower scattered radiation levels.

Artifacts

Since the grid is physically located between the patient and the receptor, there is always a possibility that it will interfere with the formation of the image. This interference can be in the form of an image of the grid strips (lines) on the film, or the abnormal attenuation of radiation in certain portions of the field.

Grid Lines

To some extent, the appearance of grid lines in the image depends on the thickness of the strips and the interspaces. This is usually specified in terms of the number of strips, or lines, per unit distance. The spacing of lines in grids normally encountered ranges from approximately 24 lines to 44 lines per centimeter (60 to 110 lines per inch). The grid lines are generally less distracting for the higher spacing densities.

A method frequently used to eliminate grid lines in the image is to blur them by moving the grid during the exposure. The mechanism for accomplishing this was first introduced by Dr. Hollis Potter, and a moving grid system is often referred to as a Potter-Bucky diaphragm. In a Potter-Bucky system the grid moves at right angles to the grid lines. The speed at which the grid moves determines the shortest exposure time that will not produce grid lines.

Grid motion during exposure also helps eliminate image patterns created by the irregular spacing of grid strips. This type of interference is generally less when grids with aluminum interspaces are used.

Grid Cutoff

The basic function of a grid is to absorb radiation that is moving along a path that is not aligned with the grid interspaces. It is desirable that the primary radiation from the x-ray tube focal spot pass through the grid with a minimum of absorption. Maximum grid penetration by primary radiation can occur only if the x-ray tube focal spot is located at the grid focal point. If these two points are not properly aligned, as shown in Figure 13-12, the direction of the primary radiation might be such that the radiation does not adequately penetrate certain sections of the grid.

Misalignment of the x-ray tube focal spot with respect to the focal point of the grid can be either lateral or vertical, or a combination of both. Lateral misalignment causes the x-ray beam to be misaligned with all interspaces, and grid penetration is decreased over the entire beam area. The amount of penetration reduction is related to the amount of misalignment and the grid ratio. Alignment becomes more critical for higher ratio grids. That is, the loss of grid penetration because of a specific misalignment is much greater for a high-ratio grid.

Vertical misalignment does not alter penetration in the center of the grid, but decreases penetration near the edges. The loss of penetration is related to the degree of misalignment and the grid ratio. The reduction in penetration for a given degree of misalignment increases with grid ratio. Focused grids are labeled with either a focal distance or a focal range, which should be carefully observed to prevent this type of grid cutoff. Cutoff toward the edges of the image area will also occur if a focused grid is turned upside down because the primary radiation will be unable to penetrate except near the center. This produces an artifact similar to vertical misalignment but usually much more pronounced.

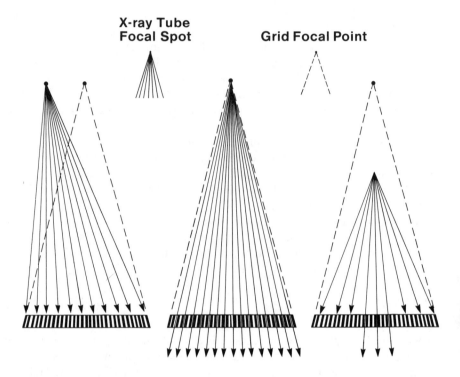

Figure 13-12 Two Forms of Grid Misalignment that Can Produce Artifacts

GRID SELECTION

A number of factors must be considered when selecting a grid for a specific application. In most cases, a grid is selected that provides a reasonable compromise between contrast improvement and patient exposure, machine loading, and positioning.

The advantages of a 5:1-ratio grid are that it is easy to use and does not require critical positioning. Its use must be restricted, however, to situations in which the amount of scattered radiation is relatively small (thin body section, low KV_p) or in which maximum image contrast is not necessary. On the other hand, a 16:1-ratio grid produces high-contrast recovery but significantly increases patient exposure. With a high-ratio grid of this type, there is very little latitude in positioning. Many applications are best served by grid ratio values between these two extremes. Such grids generally represent compromises between image quality and the other factors discussed.

Some grids have strips running at right angles to each other, generally designated crossed grids. This design generally increases contrast improvement but cannot be used in examinations in which the x-ray tube is tilted.

In stationary grid applications in which lines in the image are undesirable, grids with a high spacing density (lines per centimeter) can be used. An increase in the spacing density generally requires a higher ratio grid to produce the same contrast improvement.

Chapter 14

Radiographic Receptors

INTRODUCTION AND OVERVIEW

In conventional radiography, the receptor consists of the film mounted in contact with either one or two intensifying screens, as shown in Figure 14-1. Intensifying screens are thin sheets, or layers, of fluorescent materials. The screen-film combination is housed in either a cassette or a film changer. The x-ray energy is absorbed by the intensifying screen material, and a portion of it is converted into light. The light, in turn, exposes the film. Intensifying screens are used because film is much more sensitive to light than to x-radiation; approximately 100 times as much x-radiation would be required to expose a film without using intensifying screens. Unfortunately, intensifying screens introduce blurring into the imaging process.

A variety of intensifying screens is available for clinical use. The selection of a screen for a specific procedure is usually based on a compromise between the requirements for image detail and patient exposure.

The receptor used for most radiographic procedures contains two intensifying screens mounted on each side of double-emulsion film. Using two screens in this manner increases x-ray absorption and receptor sensitivity. In some procedures that require high image detail, such as mammography, one intensifying screen is used in conjunction with a single-emulsion film.

SCREEN FUNCTIONS

X-Ray Absorption

The first function performed by the intensifying screen is to absorb the x-ray beam (energy) emerging from the patient's body. The ideal intensifying screen would absorb all x-ray energy that enters it; real intensifying screens are generally

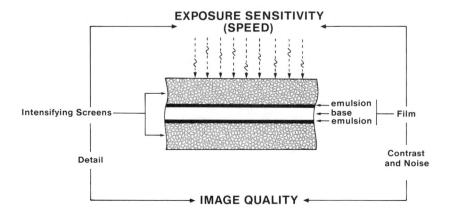

Figure 14-1 A Conventional Radiographic Receptor

not thick enough to absorb all of the photons. As we discuss later, increasing the thickness of an intensifying screen to increase its absorption capabilities degrades image quality.

In most cases, a significant portion of x-ray energy is not absorbed by the screen material and penetrates the receptor. This is wasted radiation since it does not contribute to image formation and film exposure. The absorption efficiency is the percentage of incident radiation absorbed by the screen material. An ideal screen would have a 100% absorption efficiency; actual screens generally have absorption efficiencies in the range of 20 to 70%. Absorption efficiency is primarily determined by three factors: (1) screen material, (2) screen thickness, and (3) the photon energy spectrum.

Light Production

The second function performed by the intensifying screen is to convert a portion of the absorbed x-ray energy into light. This is the fluorescent process. Fluorescence is the property of a material that enables it to absorb radiation energy in one portion of the photon-energy spectrum and emit some of the energy in the form of lower energy photons. Materials that glow, or emit visible light, when exposed to high-photon energy ultraviolet light have this property. Figure 14-2 illustrates what happens to the x-ray energy that is absorbed by an intensifying screen. In the intensifying screen, the fluorescent process creates visible light when such material is exposed to high-energy x-ray photons. The intensifying screen is an energy converter; it converts approximately 5 to 20% of the absorbed x-ray energy into light. This percentage is the conversion efficiency of the screen, and depends on the type of material used in the screen.

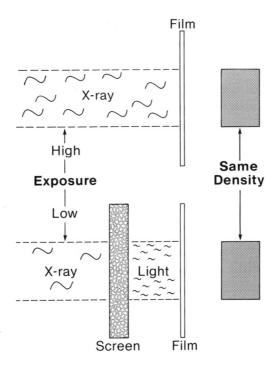

Figure 14-2 Conversion of X-Ray Energy in an Intensifying Screen

Although the total energy of the light emitted by a screen is much less than the total x-ray energy the screen receives, the light energy is much more efficient in exposing film because it is "repackaged" into a much larger number of photons. If we assume a 5% energy conversion efficiency, then one 50-keV x-ray photon can produce 1,000 blue-green light photons with an energy of 2.5 eV each.

Exposure Reduction

Since film is more sensitive to light than to x-ray exposure, film can be exposed with much less radiation if an intensifying screen is used. Conventional x-ray film has an x-ray exposure sensitivity in the range of 50 mR to 150 mR. When the film is combined with intensifying screens, the sensitivity ranges from approximately 0.1 mR to 10 mR, depending on the type of screen and film used.

RECEPTOR SENSITIVITY

The sensitivity of a receptor, such as an intensifying screen-film combination, is expressed in terms of the exposure required to produce a film density of 1 unit above the base plus fog level. Some manufacturers do not provide sensitivity values for their receptor systems, but most provide speed values such as 100, 200, 400, etc. The speed scale compares the relative exposure requirements of different receptor systems. Most speed numbers are referenced to a so-called par speed system that is assigned a speed value of 100. Whereas sensitivity is a precise receptor characteristic that expresses the amount of exposure the receptor requires, speed is a less precise value used to compare film-screen combinations. There is, however, a general relationship between exposure requirements (sensitivity) and receptor speed values:

$$\text{Sensitivity (mR)} = 128/\text{speed}.$$

For example, a receptor with a true speed value of 100 requires an exposure of 1.28 mR to produce a 1-unit film density. Sensitivity and speed values are inversely related. A more sensitive receptor has a higher speed value than a less sensitive receptor. The range of receptor sensitivity and speed values used in radiography is shown below.

Speed	Sensitivity (mR)
1200	0.1
800	0.16
400	0.32
200	0.64
100	1.28
50	2.56
25	5.
12	10.

Most receptors are given a nominal speed rating by the manufacturer. The actual speed varies, especially with KV_p and film processing conditions.

The sensitivity (speed) of an intensifying screen-film receptor depends on the type of screen and film used in addition to the conditions under which they are used and the film is processed.

We now consider characteristics of the screen that contribute to its sensitivity.

Materials

Several compounds are used to make intensifying screens. The two major characteristics the material must have are (1) high x-ray absorption and (2) fluorescence. Because of their fluorescence, intensifying screen materials are often referred to as phosphors.

Soon after the discovery of x-rays, calcium tungstate became the principal material in intensifying screens and continued to be until the 1970s. At that time, a variety of new phosphor materials were developed; many contain one of the rare earth chemical elements. Phosphor compounds now used as intensifying screen materials include:

- barium lead sulfate
- barium strontium sulfate
- barium fluorochloride
- yttrium oxysulfide
- lanthanum oxybromide
- lanthanum oxysulfide
- gadolinium oxysulfide.

Each compound contains one element that is the primary x-ray absorber.

You will recall that the probability of x-ray absorption is higher when the photon energy is just slightly higher than the K energy of the absorbing material. The K-edge energy is, in turn, determined by the atomic number of the material.

Calcium tungstate, the most common screen material for many years, uses tungsten as the absorbing element. The K edge of tungsten is at 69.4 keV. For most x-ray examinations, a major portion of the x-ray beam spectrum falls below this energy. For this reason, screens containing tungsten are limited with respect to x-ray absorption. Today, most intensifying screens contain either barium, lanthanum, gadolinium, or yttrium as the absorbing element. The K edge of these elements is below a major portion of the typical x-ray beam spectrum. This increases the chance of x-ray interaction and absorption.

Spectral Characteristics

The other elements in the compound contribute to the fluorescent properties of the material. Each compound produces light of a color (wavelength) that is specific to the particular material. The light from intensifying screens is produced in either the blue or green portion of the light spectrum, and intensifying screens are generally classified as either blue or green emitters. The significance of this is that a screen must be used with a film that has adequate sensitivity to the color of light the screen emits. Some radiographic films are sensitive only to blue light; others (orthochromatic) are also sensitive to green light. If screen and film spectral characteristics are not properly matched, receptor sensitivity is severely reduced.

Thickness

The selection of a screen is generally a compromise between exposure and image quality, as illustrated in Figure 14-3. Thin screens absorb a relatively small

Small Objects

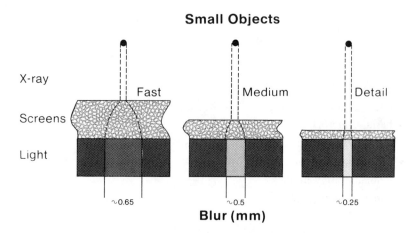

Blur (mm)

Figure 14-3 Effect of Screen Thickness on Image Blur

fraction of the x-ray photons; thicker screens absorb a greater fraction and thus require less x-radiation to produce the same film exposure. Unfortunately, increasing screen thickness also increases image blur.

Photon Energy (KV_p)

The sensitivity of intensifying screens varies with x-ray photon energy because sensitivity is directly related to absorption efficiency. Absorption efficiency and screen sensitivity are maximum when the x-ray photon energy is just above the K edge of the absorbing material. Each intensifying screen material generally has a different sensitivity-photon energy relationship because the K edge is at different energies.

The spectrum of photon energies within an x-ray beam is most directly affected and controlled by the KV_p; the sensitivity and speed of a specific intensifying screen is not constant but changes with KV_p.

Significant exposure errors can occur if technical factors (KV_p and MAS) are not adjusted to compensate for the variation in screen sensitivity. This often occurs when the same technique charts are used with screens composed of different materials. Also, the KV_p response characteristics of automatic exposure control (AEC) sensors should be matched to those of the intensifying screens.

IMAGE BLUR

The most significant effect of intensifying screens on image quality is that they produce blur. The reason for this is illustrated in Figure 14-3. Let us consider the imaging of a very small object, such as a calcification. The x-ray photons passing through the object are absorbed and produce light along the vertical path extending through the intensifying screen. Before exiting the screen, the light spreads out of the absorption path, as illustrated. The light image of the object that appears on the surface of the intensifying screen is therefore blurred; the degree of blurring by this process is related to the thickness and transparency of the intensifying screen.

The major issue in selecting intensifying screens for a particular clinical application is arriving at an appropriate compromise between patient exposure and image quality or, more specifically, between receptor sensitivity (speed) and image blurring (visibility of detail). Screens that produce maximum visibility of detail generally have a low absorption efficiency (sensitivity) and require a relatively high exposure. On the other hand, screens with a high sensitivity (speed) cannot produce images with high visibility of detail because of the increased blurring.

Intensifying screens are usually identified by brand names, which do not always indicate specific characteristics. Most screens, however, are of five generic types:

1. mammographic
2. detail
3. par speed
4. medium speed
5. high speed.

Figure 14-4 shows how these general screen types fit into the relationship between image blur and required exposure.

Screen-Film Contact

If the film and intensifying screen surfaces do not make good contact, the light will spread, as shown in Figure 14-5, and will produce image blurring. This is an abnormal condition that occurs when a cassette or film changer is defective and does not apply sufficient pressure over the entire film area. Inadequate film-screen contact usually produces blurring in only a portion of the image area.

The conventional test for film-screen contact is to radiograph a wire mesh. Areas within the image where contact is inadequate will appear to have a different density than the other areas. This variation in image density is most readily seen when the film is viewed from a distance of approximately 10 ft and at an angle.

Crossover

If the film emulsion does not completely absorb the light from the intensifying screen, the unabsorbed light can pass through the film base and expose the emulsion on the other side. This is commonly referred to as crossover. As the light

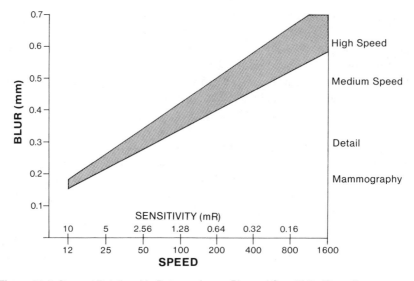

Figure 14-4 General Relationship Between Image Blur and Sensitivity (Speed)

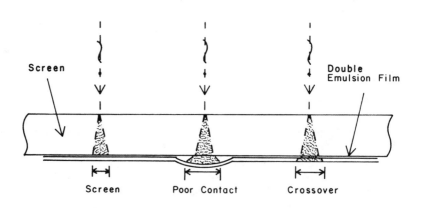

Figure 14-5 Sources of Blur in Screen-Film Receptors

passes through the film base, it can spread and introduce image blur, as illustrated in Figure 14-5. Some films are designed to minimize crossover blurring. Crossover can be decreased by placing a light-absorbing layer between the film emulsion and film base, using a base material that selectively absorbs the light wavelengths emitted by the intensifying screens, and designing the film emulsion to increase light absorption.

Halation

When light encounters a boundary between materials, reflection can occur at the boundary surface. Reflections at boundaries between film emulsion, film base, intensifying screens, and cassette surfaces are known as halation and contribute to image blur. Single-emulsion films generally have a light-absorbing layer coated on the other side of the base to prevent halation.

IMAGE NOISE

The amount of noise in radiographic images is affected, to some extent, by the characteristics of the intensifying screen; the crystal structure of the screen material produces a relatively small amount of image noise. Quantum noise is generally the most significant type of noise in radiographs. Intensifying screens with high conversion efficiencies generally produce more quantum noise than other screens for reasons discussed in Chapter 21. Also, the visibility of noise is decreased, to some extent, by the blurring created within screens.

ARTIFACTS

Intensifying screens can be significant sources of image artifacts. Artifacts can be produced by scratches, stains, and foreign objects, such as hair, dust, and cigarette ashes, on the screen surface.

Intensifying screens should be cleaned periodically according to the manufacturer's instructions.

Chapter 15

The Photographic Process and Film Sensitivity

INTRODUCTION AND OVERVIEW

Most medical images are recorded on photographic film. The active component of film is an emulsion of radiation-sensitive crystals coated onto a transparent base material. The production of an image requires two steps, as illustrated in Figure 15-1. First, the film is exposed to radiation, typically light, which activates the emulsion material but produces no visible change. The exposure creates a so-called latent image. Second, the exposed film is processed in a series of chemical solutions that convert the invisible latent image into an image that is visible as different optical densities or shades of gray. The darkness or density of the film increases as the exposure is increased. This general relationship is shown in Figure 15-2.

The specific relationship between the shades of gray and exposure depends on the characteristics of the film emulsion and the processing conditions. The basic principles of the photographic process and the factors that affect the sensitivity of film are covered in this chapter.

FILM FUNCTIONS

Film performs several functions in the medical imaging process. A knowledge of these functions and how they are affected by the characteristics of different types of film aids in selecting film for a specific clinical procedure and in perfecting radiographic techniques.

Image Recording

In principle, film is an image converter. It converts radiation, typically light, into various shades of gray. An important characteristic of film is that it records, or

EXPOSURE

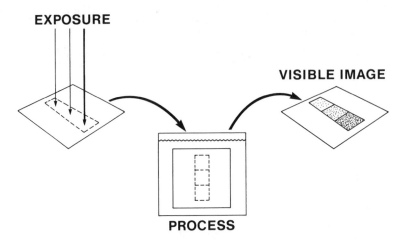

VISIBLE IMAGE

PROCESS

Figure 15-1 The Two Steps in the Formation of a Film Image

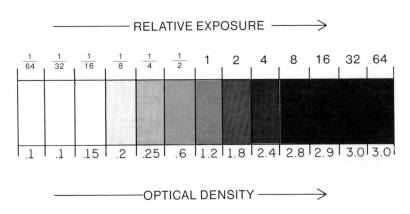

RELATIVE EXPOSURE ⟶

OPTICAL DENSITY ⟶

Figure 15-2 The General Relationship between Film Density (Shades of Gray) and Exposure

retains, an image. An exposure of a fraction of a second can create a permanent image. The amount of exposure required to produce an image depends on the sensitivity, or speed, of the film being used. Some films are more sensitive than others because of their design or the way they are processed. The sensitivity of radiographic film is generally selected to provide a compromise between two very important factors: patient exposure and image quality. A highly sensitive film reduces patient exposure but decreases image quality.

Image Display

Most medical images are recorded as transparencies. In this form they can be easily viewed by transillumination from a viewbox. The overall appearance and quality of a radiographic image depends on a combination of factors, including the characteristics of the particular film used, the way in which it was exposed, and the processing conditions. When a radiograph emerges from the film processor, the image is permanent and cannot be changed. It is, therefore, important that all factors associated with the production of the image are adjusted to produce optimum image quality.

Image Storage

Film has been the traditional medium for medical image storage. If a film is properly processed it will have a lifetime of many years and will, in most cases, outlast its clinical usefulness. The major disadvantages of storing images on film are bulk and inaccessibility. Most clinical facilities must devote considerable space to film storage. Retrieving films from storage generally requires manual search and transportation of the films to a viewing area.

Because film performs so many of the functions that make up the radiographic examination, it will continue to be an important element in the medical imaging process. Because of its limitations, however, it will gradually be replaced by digital imaging media in many clinical applications.

OPTICAL DENSITY

Optical density is the darkness, or opaqueness, of a transparency film and is produced by film exposure and chemical processing. An image contains areas with different densities that are viewed as various shades of gray.

Light Penetration

The optical density of film is assigned numerical values related to the amount of light that penetrates the film. Increasing film density decreases light penetration. The relationship between density values and light penetration is exponential, as illustrated in Figure 15-3.

A clear piece of film that allows 100% of the light to penetrate has a density value of 0. Radiographic film is never completely clear. The minimum film density is usually in the range of 0.1 to 0.2 density units. This is designated the base plus fog density and is the density of the film base and any inherent fog not associated with exposure.

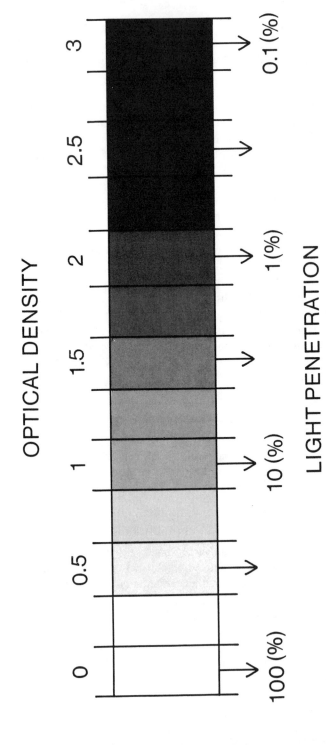

Figure 15-3 Relationship between Light Penetration and Film Density

Each unit of density decreases light penetration by a factor of 10. A film area with a density value of 1 allows 10% of the light to penetrate and generally appears as a medium gray when placed on a conventional viewbox. A film area with a density value of 2 allows 10% of 10% (1.0%) light penetration and appears as a relatively dark area when viewed in the usual manner. With normal viewbox illumination, it is possible to see through areas of film with density values of up to approximately 2 units.

A density value of 3 corresponds to a light penetration of 0.1% (10% of 10% of 10%). A film with a density value of 3 appears essentially opaque when trans-illuminated with a conventional viewbox. It is possible, however, to see through such a film using a bright "hot" light. Radiographic film generally has a maximum density value of approximately 3 density units. This is designated the D^{max} of the film. The maximum density that can be produced within a specific film depends on the characteristics of the film and processing conditions.

Measurement

The density of film is measured with a densitometer. A light source passes a small beam of light through the film area to be measured. On the other side of the film, a light sensor (photocell) converts the penetrated light into an electrical signal. A special circuit performs a logarithmic conversion on the signal and displays the results in density units.

The primary use of densitometers in a clinical facility is to monitor the performance of film processors.

FILM STRUCTURE

Conventional film is layered, as illustrated in Figure 15-4. The active component is an emulsion layer coated onto a base material. Most film used in radiography has an emulsion layer on each side of the base so that it can be used with two intensifying screens simultaneously. Films used in cameras and in selected radiographic procedures, such as mammography, have one emulsion layer and are called single-emulsion films.

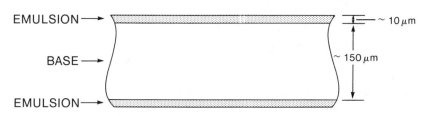

Figure 15-4 Cross-Section of Typical Radiographic Film

Base

The base of a typical radiographic film is made of a clear polyester material about 150 μm thick. It provides the physical support for the other film components and does not participate in the image-forming process. In some films, the base contains a light blue dye to give the image a more pleasing appearance when illuminated on a viewbox.

Emulsion

The emulsion is the active component in which the image is formed and consists of many small silver halide crystals suspended in gelatin. The gelatin supports, separates, and protects the crystals. The typical emulsion is approximately 10 μm thick.

Several different silver halides have photographic properties, but the one typically used in medical imaging films is silver bromide. The silver bromide is in the form of crystals, or grains, each containing on the order of 10^9 atoms.

Silver halide grains are irregularly shaped like pebbles, or grains of sand. Two grain shapes are used in film emulsions. The conventional form approximates a cubic configuration with its three dimensions being approximately equal. More recently, tabular-shaped grains were developed. The tabular grain is relatively thin in one direction, and its length and width are much larger than its thickness, giving it a relatively large surface area. The primary advantage of tabular grain film in comparison to cubic grain film is that sensitizing dyes can be used more effectively to increase sensitivity and reduce cross-over exposure.

THE PHOTOGRAPHIC PROCESS

The production of film density and the formation of a visible image is a two-step process. The first step in this photographic process is the exposure of the film to light, which forms an invisible latent image. The second step is the chemical process that converts the latent image into a visible image with a range of densities, or shades of gray.

Film density is produced by converting silver ions into metallic silver, which causes each processed grain to become black. The process is rather complicated and is illustrated by the sequence of events shown in Figure 15-5.

Each film grain contains a large number of both silver and bromide ions. The silver ions have a one-electron deficit, which gives them a positive charge. On the other hand, the bromide ions have a negative charge because they contain an extra electron. Each grain has a structural ''defect'' known as a sensitive speck. A film grain in this condition is relatively transparent.

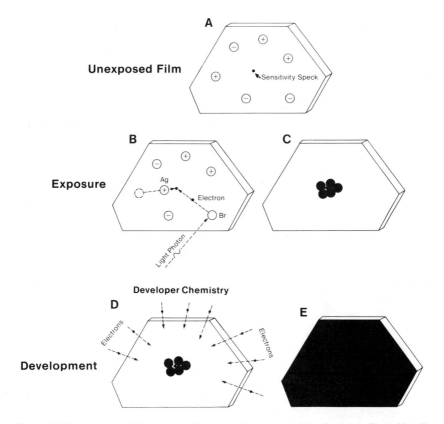

Figure 15-5 Sequence of Events that Convert a Transparent Film Grain into Black Metallic Silver

Latent Image Formation

The first step in the formation of the latent image is the absorption of light photons by the bromide ions, which frees the extra electron. The electron moves to the sensitivity speck, causing it to become negatively charged. The speck, in turn, attracts one of the positively charged silver ions. When the silver ion reaches the speck, its positive charge is neutralized by the electron. This action converts the silver ion into an atom of black metallic silver. If this process is repeated several times within an individual grain, the cluster of metallic silver at the sensitive speck will become a permanent arrangement. The number of grains in the emulsion that reach this status depends on the overall exposure to the film. The grains that received sufficient exposure to form a permanent change are not visually distinguishable from the unexposed grains, but are more sensitive to the action of the developer chemistry. The distribution of these activated, but "invisible," grains throughout the emulsion creates the latent image.

Development

The invisible latent image is converted into a visible image by the chemical process of development. The developer solution supplies electrons that migrate into the sensitized grains and convert the other silver ions into black metallic silver. This causes the grains to become visible black specks in the emulsion.

Radiographic film is generally developed in an automatic processor. A schematic of a typical processor is shown in Figure 15-6. The four components correspond to the four steps in film processing. In a conventional processor, the film is in the developer for 20 to 25 seconds.

When a film is inserted into a processor, it is transported by means of a roller system through the chemical developer. Although there are some differences in the chemistry of developer solutions supplied by various manufacturers, most contain the same basic chemicals. Each chemical has a specific function in the development process.

Reducer

Chemical reduction of the exposed silver bromide grains is the process that converts them into visible metallic silver. This action is typically provided by two chemicals in the solution: phenidone and hydroquinone. Phenidone is the more active and primarily produces the mid to lower portion of the gray scale. Hydroquinone produces the very dense, or dark, areas in an image.

Activator

The primary function of the activator, typically sodium carbonate, is to soften and swell the emulsion so that the reducers can reach the exposed grains.

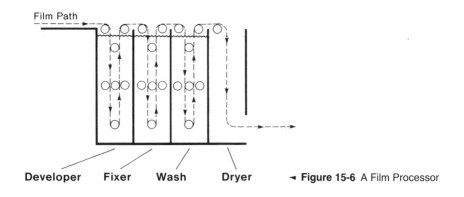

Film Path

Developer   Fixer   Wash   Dryer   ◄ **Figure 15-6** A Film Processor

Restrainer

Potassium bromide is generally used as a restrainer. Its function is to moderate the rate of development.

Preservative

Sodium sulfite, a typical preservative, helps protect the reducing agents from oxidation because of their contact with air. It also reacts with oxidation products to reduce their activity.

Hardener

Glutaraldehyde is used as a hardener to retard the swelling of the emulsion. This is necessary in automatic processors in which the film is transported by a system of rollers.

Fixing

After leaving the developer the film is transported into a second tank, which contains the fixer solution. The fixer is a mixture of several chemicals that perform the following functions.

Neutralizer

When a film is removed from the developer solution, the development continues because of the solution soaked up by the emulsion. It is necessary to stop this action to prevent over-development and fogging of the film. Acetic acid is in the fixer solution for this purpose.

Clearing

The fixer solution also clears the undeveloped silver halide grains from the film. Ammonium or sodium thiosulfate is used for this purpose. The unexposed grains leave the film and dissolve in the fixer solution. The silver that accumulates in the fixer during the clearing activity can be recovered; the usual method is to electro-plate it onto a metallic surface within the silver recovery unit.

Preservative

Sodium sulfite is used in the fixer as a preservative.

Hardener

Aluminum chloride is typically used as a hardener. Its primary function is to shrink and harden the emulsion.

Wash

Film is next passed through a waterbath to wash the fixer solution out of the emulsion. It is especially important to remove the thiosulfate. If thiosulfate (hypo) is retained in the emulsion, it will eventually react with the silver nitrate and air to form silver sulfate, a yellowish brown stain. The amount of thiosulfate retained in the emulsion determines the useful lifetime of a processed film. The American National Standard Institute recommends a maximum retention of 30 $\mu g/in^2$.

Dry

The final step in processing is to dry the film by passing it through a chamber in which hot air is circulating.

SENSITIVITY

One of the most important characteristics of film is its sensitivity, often referred to as film speed. The sensitivity of a particular film determines the amount of exposure required to produce an image. A film with a high sensitivity (speed) requires less exposure than a film with a lower sensitivity (speed).

The sensitivities of films are generally compared by the amount of exposure required to produce an optical density of 1 unit above the base plus fog density. The sensitivity of radiographic film is generally not described with numerical values but rather with a variety of generic terms such as "half speed," "medium speed," and "high speed." Radiographic films are usually considered in terms of their relative sensitivities rather than their absolute sensitivity values. Although it is possible to choose films with different sensitivities, the choice is limited to a range of not more than four to one by most manufacturers.

Figure 15-7 compares two films with different sensitivities. Notice that a specific exposure produces a higher density in the high sensitivity film; therefore, the production of a specific density value (ie, 1 density unit) requires less exposure.

High sensitivity (speed) films are chosen when the reduction of patient exposure and heat loading of the x-ray equipment are important considerations.

Low sensitivity (speed) films are used to reduce image noise. The relationship of film sensitivity to image noise is considered in Chapter 21.

The sensitivity of film is determined by a number of factors, as shown in Figure 15-8, which include its design, the exposure conditions, and how it is processed.

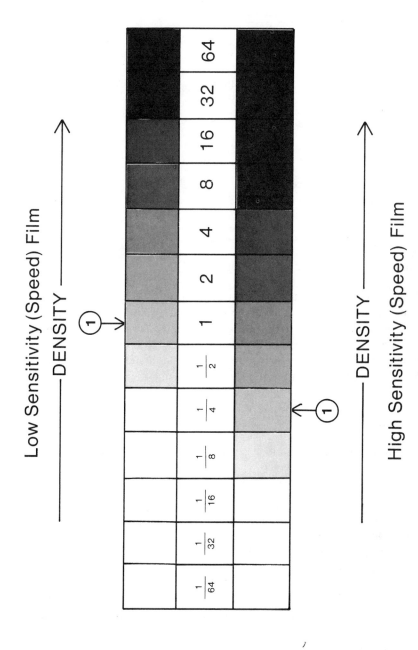

Figure 15-7 Comparison of Two Films with Different Sensitivities

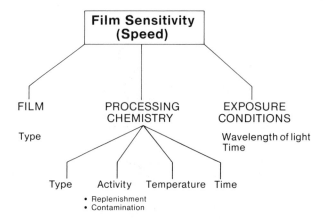

Figure 15-8 Factors that Affect Film Sensitivity

Composition

The basic sensitivity characteristic of a film is determined by the composition of the emulsion. The size and shape of the silver halide grains have some effect on film sensitivity. Increasing grain size generally increases sensitivity. Tabular-shaped grains generally produce a higher sensitivity than conventional grains. Although grain size may vary among the various types of radiographic film, most of the difference in sensitivity is produced by adding chemical sensitizers to the emulsion.

Processing

The effective sensitivity of film depends on several factors associated with the development:

- the type of developer
- developer concentration
- developer replenishment rates
- developer contamination
- development time
- development temperature.

In most medical imaging applications, the objective is not to use these factors to vary film sensitivity, but rather to control them to maintain a constant and predictable film sensitivity.

Developer Composition

The processing chemistry supplied by different manufacturers is not the same. It is usually possible to process a film in a variety of developer solutions, but they will not all produce the same film sensitivity. The variation in sensitivity is usually relatively small, but must be considered when changing from one brand of developer to another.

Developer Concentration

Developer chemistry is usually supplied to a clinical facility in the form of a concentrate that must be diluted with water before it is pumped into the processor. Mixing errors that result in an incorrect concentration can produce undesirable changes in film sensitivity.

Developer Replenishment

The film development process consumes some of the developer solution and causes the solution to become less active. Unless the solution is replaced, film sensitivity will gradually decrease.

In radiographic film processors, the replenishment of the developer solution is automatic. When a sheet of film enters the processor, it activates a switch that causes fresh solution to be pumped into the development tank. The replenishment rate can be monitored by means of flow meters mounted in the processor. The appropriate replenishment rate depends on the size of the films being processed. A processor used only for chest films generally requires a higher replenishment rate than one used for smaller films.

Developer Contamination

If the developer solution becomes contaminated with another chemical, such as the fixer solution, abrupt changes in film sensitivity can occur in the form of either an increase or decrease in sensitivity, depending on the type and amount of contamination. Developer contamination is most likely to occur when the film transport rollers are removed or replaced.

Development Time

When an exposed film enters the developer solution, development is not instantaneous. It is a gradual process during which more and more film grains are developed, resulting in increased film density. The development process is terminated by removing the film from the developer and placing it in the fixer. To some extent, increasing development time increases film sensitivity, since less exposure is required to produce a specific film density. In radiographic film processors, the development time is usually fixed and is approximately 20–25 seconds.

Development Temperature

The activity of the developer changes with temperature. An increase in temperature speeds up the development process and increases film sensitivity because less exposure is required to produce a specific film density.

The temperature of the developer is thermostatically controlled in an automatic processor. It is usually set within the range of 90–95 °F. Specific processing temperatures are usually specified by the film manufacturers.

Light Color (Wavelength)

Film is not equally sensitive to all wavelengths (colors) of light. The spectral sensitivity is a characteristic of film that must be taken into account in selecting film for use with specific intensifying screens and cameras. In general, the film should be most sensitive to the color of the light that is emitted by the intensifying screens, intensifier tubes, cathode ray tubes (CRTs), or lasers.

Blue Sensitivity

A basic silver bromide emulsion has its maximum sensitivity in the ultraviolet and blue regions of the light spectrum. For many years most intensifying screens contained calcium tungstate, which emits a blue light and is a good match for blue-sensitive film. Although calcium tungstate is no longer widely used as a screen material, several contemporary screen materials emit blue light.

Green Sensitivity

Several image light sources, including image intensifier tubes, CRTs, and some intensifying screens, emit most of their light in the green portion of the spectrum. Film used with these devices must, therefore, be sensitive to green light.

Silver bromide can be made sensitive to green light by adding sensitizing dyes to the emulsion. Users must be careful not to use the wrong type of film with intensifying screens. If a blue-sensitive film is used with a green-emitting intensifying screen, the combination will have a drastically reduced sensitivity.

Red Sensitivity

Many lasers produce red light. Devices that transfer images to film by means of a laser beam must, therefore, be supplied with a film that is sensitive to red light.

Safelighting

Darkrooms in which film is loaded into cassettes and transferred to processors are usually illuminated with a safelight. A safelight emits a color of light the eye can see but that will not expose film. Although film has a relatively low sensitivity to the light emitted by safelights, film fog can be produced with safelight illumination under certain conditions. The safelight should provide sufficient illumination for darkroom operations but not produce significant exposure to the film being handled. This can usually be accomplished if certain factors are controlled. These include safelight color, brightness, location, and duration of film exposure.

The color of the safelight is controlled by the filter. The filter must be selected in relationship to the spectral sensitivity of the film being used. An amber-brown safelight provides a relatively high level of working illumination and adequate protection for blue-sensitive film; type 6B filters are used for this application. However, this type of safelight produces some light that falls within the sensitive range of green-sensitive film.

A red safelight is required when working with green-sensitive films. Type GBX filters are used for this purpose.

Selecting the appropriate safelight filter does not absolutely protect film because film has some sensitivity to the light emitted by most safelights. Therefore, the brightness of the safelight (bulb size) and the distance between the light and film work surfaces must be selected so as to minimize film exposure.

Since exposure is an accumulative effect, handling the film as short a time as possible minimizes exposure. The potential for safelight exposure can be evaluated in a darkroom by placing a piece of film on the work surface, covering most of its area with an opaque object, and then moving the object in successive steps to expose more of the film surface. The time intervals should be selected to produce exposures ranging from a few seconds to several minutes. After the film is processed, the effect of the safelight exposure can be observed. Film is most sensitive to safelight fogging after the latent image is produced but before it is processed.

Exposure Time

In radiography it is usually possible to deliver a given exposure to film by using many combinations of radiation intensity (exposure rate) and exposure time. Since radiation intensity is proportional to x-ray tube MA, this is equivalent to saying that a given exposure (in milliampere-seconds) can be produced with many combinations of MA and time. This is known as the law of reciprocity. In effect, it means that it is possible to swap radiation intensity (in milliamperes) for exposure time and produce the same film exposure. When a film is directly exposed to x-radiation, the reciprocity law holds true. That is, 100 mAs will produce the same film density whether it is exposed at 1,000 mA and 0.1 seconds or 10 mA and 10 seconds. However, when a film is exposed by light, such as from intensifying screens or image intensifiers, the reciprocity law does not hold. With light exposure, as opposed to direct x-ray interactions, a single silver halide grain must absorb more than one photon before it can be developed and can contribute to image density. This causes the sensitivity of the film to be somewhat dependent on the intensity of the exposing light. This loss of sensitivity varies to some extent from one type of x-ray film to another. The clinical significance is that MAS values that give the correct density with short exposure times might not do so with long exposure times.

QUALITY CONTROL

One objective of a quality control program is to reduce exposure errors that cause either underexposed or overexposed film, because of variation in sensitivity. Variations in processing conditions can produce significant fluctuations in film sensitivity. Processors should be monitored several times each week to detect fluctuations in processing. This is done by exposing a test film to a fixed amount of light exposure in a sensitometer, running the film through the processor, and then measuring its density with a densitometer. The density values are recorded on a chart so that fluctuations can be easily detected. If abnormal variations in film density are observed, possible contributing factors, such as developer temperature, replenishment rates, and contamination, should be evaluated.

If more than one processor is used for films from the same imaging device, the level of development by the different processes should be matched.

Artifacts

A variety of artifacts can be produced during the storage, handling, and processing of film.

Bending unprocessed film can produce artifacts or "kink marks," which can appear as either dark or light areas in the processed image. Handling film, especially in a dry environment, can produce a build-up of static electricity; the discharge produces dark spots and streaks.

Artifacts can be produced during processing by factors such as uneven roller pressure or the accumulation of a substance on the rollers. This type of artifact is often repeated at intervals corresponding to the circumference of the roller.

Chapter 16

Film Contrast Characteristics

INTRODUCTION AND OVERVIEW

Contrast is perhaps the most significant characteristic of an image recorded on film. Contrast is the variation in film density (shades of gray) that actually forms the image. Without contrast there is no image. The amount of contrast in an image depends on a number of factors, including the ability of the particular film to record contrast.

Film can be considered as a contrast converter. One of its functions is to convert differences in exposure (subject contrast) into film contrast (differences in density), as shown in Figure 16-1. The amount of film contrast resulting from a specific exposure difference can vary considerably.

The exposure contrast between two areas can be expressed as a percentage difference, as illustrated in Figure 16-1. The film contrast between two areas is expressed as the difference between the density values. The ability of the film to convert exposure contrast into film contrast can be expressed in terms of the *contrast factor*. The value of the contrast factor is the amount of film contrast resulting from an exposure contrast of 50%. The amount of contrast produced by medical imaging films depends on four basic factors: (1) type of emulsion, (2) amount of exposure, (3) processing, and (4) fog.

In this chapter we consider the basic contrast characteristics of film, how these characteristics are affected by the factors listed above, and how contrast characteristics relate to clinical applications.

CONTRAST TRANSFER

The ability of a film to produce contrast can be determined by observing the difference in density between two areas receiving a specified difference in exposure, as shown in Figure 16-1. However, since the amount of contrast is

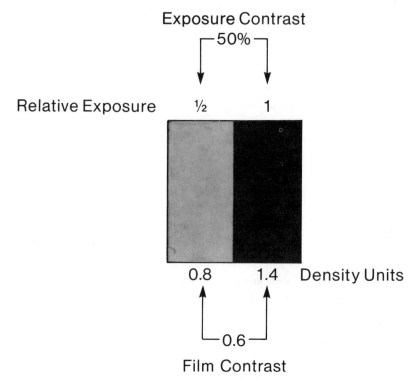

Figure 16-1 The General Relationship between Exposure Contrast and Film Contrast

affected by the level of exposure, a range of exposure values must be delivered to a film to demonstrate fully its contrast characteristics.

One method of doing this is illustrated in Figure 16-2; this type of exposure pattern is usually produced by a device known as a sensitometer. In this method, a strip of film is divided into a number of individual areas, and each area is exposed to a different level of radiation. In this particular illustration, the exposure is changed by a factor of 2 (50% contrast) between adjacent areas. When considering contrast characteristics, we are usually not interested in the actual exposure to a film but rather the relative exposure among different areas of film. In Figure 16-2 the exposures to the different areas are given relative to the center area, which has been assigned a relative exposure value of 1. We will use this relative exposure scale throughout our discussion of film contrast characteristics. Note that each interval on the scale represents a 2:1 ratio. This is a characteristic of a logarithmic scale. When the film is processed, each area will have density values, as shown directly below the area. The amount of contrast between any two adjacent areas is the difference in density, as shown. In this illustration we can observe one of the

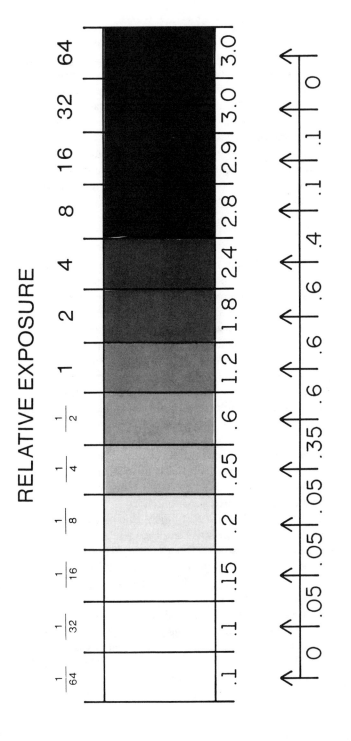

Figure 16-2 The Variation in Contrast with Exposure

very important characteristics of film contrast. Notice how the contrast is not the same between each pair of adjacent areas throughout the exposure range: there is no contrast between the first two areas, but the contrast gradually increases with exposure, reaches a maximum, and then decreases for the higher exposure levels. In other words, a specific type of film does not produce the same amount of contrast at all levels of exposure. This important characteristic must be considered when using film to record medical images.

All films have a limited exposure range in which they can produce contrast: if areas of a film receive exposures either below or above the useful exposure range, contrast will be diminished, or perhaps absent. Image contrast is reduced when a film is either underexposed or overexposed.

The Characteristic Curve

The relationship between film density and exposure is often presented in the form of a graph, as shown in Figure 16-3. This graph shows the relationship between the density and relative exposure for the values shown in Figure 16-2. This type of graph is known as either a film characteristic curve or an H and D (Hurter and Driffield) curve. The precise shape of the curve depends on the characteristics of the emulsion and the processing conditions. The primary use of a characteristic curve is to describe the contrast characteristics of the film throughout a wide exposure range. At any exposure value, the contrast characteristic of the film is represented by the slope of the curve. At any particular point, the slope represents the density difference (contrast) produced by a specific exposure difference. A specific interval on the relative exposure scale represents the amount of contrast delivered to the film during the exposure process. An interval along the density scale represents the amount of contrast that actually appears in the film. The slope of the characteristic curve at any point can be expressed in terms of the contrast factor because the contrast factor is the density difference (contrast) produced by a 2:1 exposure ratio (50% exposure contrast).

A film characteristic curve has three distinct regions with different contrast transfer characteristics. The part of the curve associated with relatively low exposures is designated the toe, and also corresponds to the light or low density portions of an image. When an image is exposed so that areas fall within the toe region, little or no contrast is transferred to the image. In the film shown in Figure 16-2, the areas on the left correspond to the toe of the characteristic curve.

A film also has a reduced ability to transfer contrast in areas that receive relatively high exposures. This condition corresponds to the upper portion of the characteristic curve in which the slope decreases with increasing exposure. This portion of the curve is traditionally referred to as the shoulder. In Figure 16-2 the dark areas on the right correspond to the shoulder of the characteristic curve. The two significant characteristics of image areas receiving exposure within this range

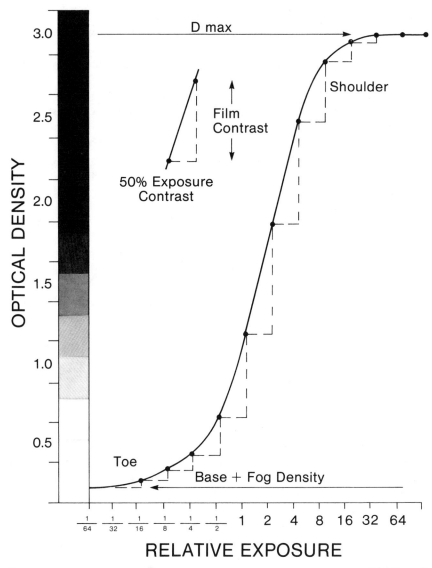

Figure 16-3 A Film Characteristic Curve Showing the Relationship between Density and Relative Exposure

are that the film is quite dark (dense) and contrast is reduced. In many instances, image contrast is present that cannot be observed on the conventional viewbox because of the high film density. This contrast can be made visible by viewing the film with a bright "hotlight."

The highest level of contrast is produced within a range of exposures falling between the toe and the shoulder. This portion of the curve is characterized by a relatively straight and very steep slope in comparison to the toe and shoulder regions. In most imaging applications, it is desirable to expose the film within this range so as to obtain maximum contrast.

The minimum density, in the toe, is the residual density, which is observed after processing unexposed film, and is typically in the range of 0.1 to 0.2 density units. This density is produced by the inherent density of the film base material and the low-level fog in the film emulsion; it is therefore commonly referred to as the base plus fog density. The maximum density, in the shoulder, is determined by the design of the film emulsion and the processing conditions and is typically referred to as the D^{max}.

Contrast Curve

It is easier to see the relationship between film contrast and exposure by using a contrast curve, as shown in Figure 16-4. The contrast curve corresponds to the slope of the characteristic curve. It clearly shows that the ability of a film to transfer exposure contrast into film contrast changes with exposure level, and that maximum contrast is produced only within a limited exposure range.

The exposure range over which a film produces useful contrast is designated the *latitude*. An underexposed film area contains little or no image contrast. Exposure values above the latitude range also produce areas with very little contrast and have the added disadvantage of being very dark or dense.

Since the contrast transfer characteristics of film change with exposure, a specific film characteristic can be described only by using either a characteristic curve or contrast curve, as illustrated in Figure 16-4. There are occasions, however, when it would be desirable to use a single-parameter value to describe the general contrast characteristics of a film. Two parameters are often used for this purpose: the *average gradient* expresses the average contrast transferring ability, and the *gamma* expresses the maximum contrast.

Gamma

The gamma value of a film is the maximum slope of the characteristic curve, as shown in Figure 16-5. By tradition, the gamma value is the slope expressed in terms of the density difference associated with an exposure ratio of 10:1. The relationship between the film gamma value and the maximum contrast factor is given by

$$\text{Gamma} = 3.32 \text{ Maximum contrast factor.}$$

The factor 3.32 converts a slope based on an exposure ratio of 2:1 to a slope expressed with respect to a 10:1 exposure ratio.

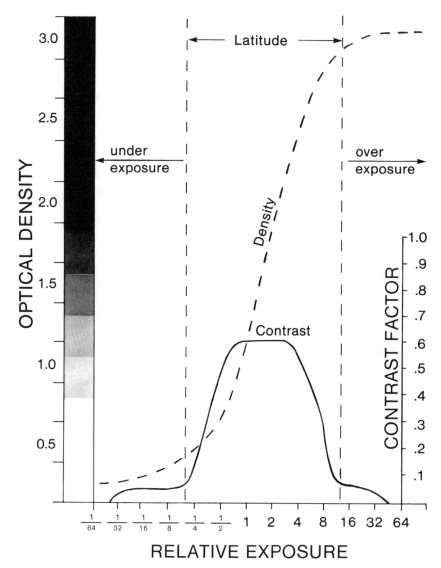

Figure 16-4 The Relationship of Film Contrast (Solid Line) to Relative Exposure and the Characteristic Curve (Dotted Line)

Average Gradient

The average gradient is the average slope between two designated density values, as illustrated in Figure 16-5. For medical imaging film the density values of 0.25 and 2.0 above the base plus fog density are used to determine average gradient. Average gradient values, like gamma values, are based on an exposure ratio of 10:1. The relationship between the average gradient and the average contrast factor is therefore:

$$\text{Average gradient} = 3.32 \text{ Average contrast factor.}$$

FILM LATITUDE

In Figure 16-4 we saw that film contrast is limited to a specific range of exposure values. The exposure range in which a film can produce useful contrast is known as its latitude. The latitude of a specific film is determined primarily by the composition of the emulsion and, to a lesser extent, by processing conditions. The significance of film latitude is that it represents the limitations of the exposure range that will yield useful image contrast.

The exposure to any given area of a film falls within one of three general ranges, as shown in Figure 16-4. Two general conditions can cause film exposure to fall outside the latitude range: an incorrect exposure setting of the equipment, which can produce either an underexposure or an overexposure, and an anatomical structure, which produces a wide range of exposure values within an image that exceed the latitude range.

Exposure Error

In every imaging procedure it is necessary to set the exposure to match the sensitivity (speed) of the film being used. This is not always an easy task.

Exposure error is generally a much more significant problem in radiography than in other imaging procedures. It is not always possible to predict the amount of x-ray exposure required in every procedure because of subtle variations in body size and composition. In any radiographic practice, a significant number of films must be repeated because of exposure error.

Subject Contrast Range

When an x-ray beam passes through certain body areas, the penetration of the areas varies considerably because of differences in tissue thickness and composition. Under these conditions it is possible for the range of exposures from the patient's body (subject contrast range) to exceed the latitude of the film. This typically produces a high level of area contrast, as discussed in a previous chapter.

When the exposure to some image areas falls outside the film latitude, details within the areas are recorded with reduced contrast, as illustrated in Figure 16-6. Notice that the objects located within the very thick and thin body sections are not

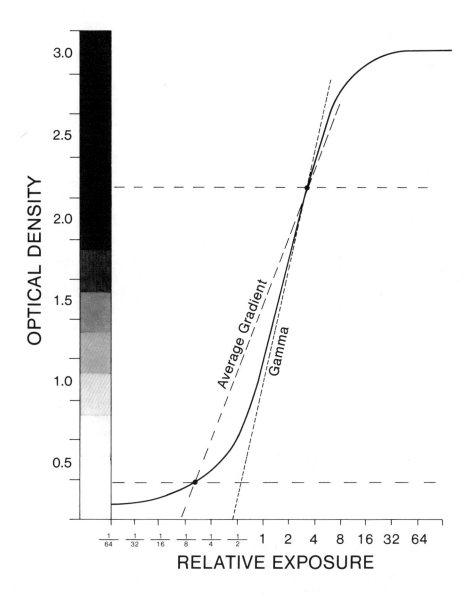

Figure 16-5 The Relationship of Average Gradient and Gamma to the Characteristic Curve

recorded because they are located in areas outside the film latitude. Radiography of the chest illustrates this problem: the area of the mediastinum receives a relatively low exposure whereas the lung areas receive a much higher level.

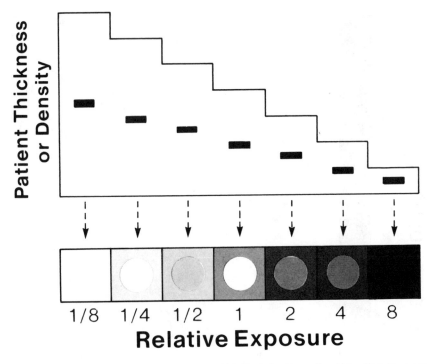

Figure 16-6 Loss of Contrast in Both Thick and Thin Body Sections when Using High Contrast Film

One possible solution to the problem is to decrease the subject contrast range by using increased KV_p, spacial filtration, bolus, or compression. Another possible solution is to use a film with a longer latitude.

FILM TYPES

The overall contrast characteristic of a film (shape of characteristic curve and latitude) is determined by the composition of the emulsion. Radiographic film is usually designated as either high contrast or medium contrast film. Medium contrast film is often referred to as latitude film.

When selecting a film for a particular medical imaging application, contrast characteristics should be considered. Figure 16-7 compares the contrast characteristics of two general types of radiographic film. The high contrast film can produce higher contrast. Notice the contrast of 0.6 between the areas with relative exposure values of 1 and 2. The contrast is limited, however, to a relatively small exposure range, or latitude. The medium contrast, or latitude, film

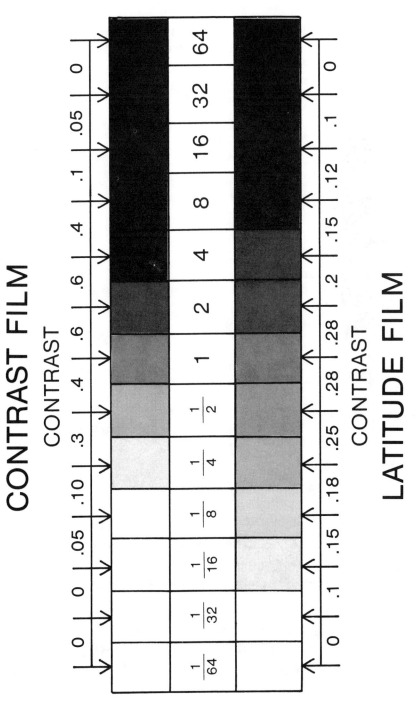

Figure 16-7 A Comparison of High Contrast and Medium Contrast or Latitude Film

produces less contrast but can produce contrast over a much larger range of exposure values. The corresponding characteristic and contrast curves are shown in Figures 16-8 and 16-9.

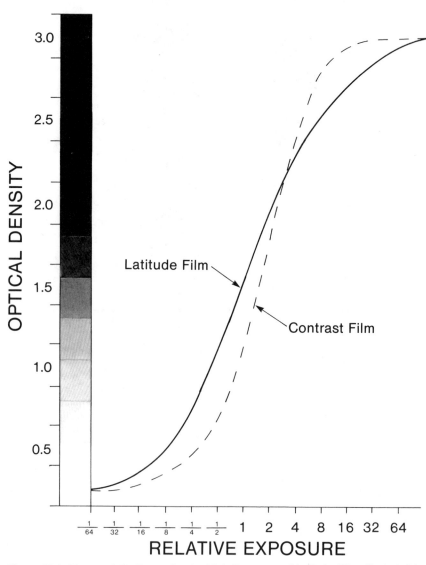

Figure 16-8 Characteristic Curves for the High Contrast and Latitude Films Illustrated in Figure 16-7

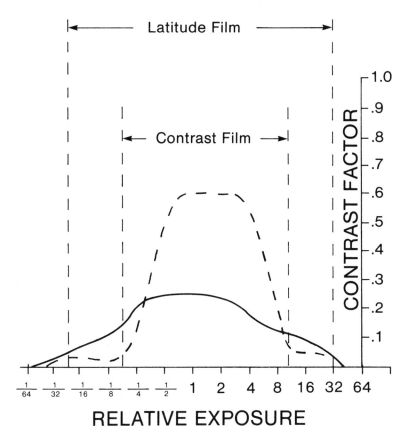

Figure 16-9 Contrast Curves for the High Contrast and Latitude Films Illustrated in Figure 16-7 (Compare with Characteristic Curves in Figure 16-8)

Figure 16-10 illustrates how using a medium contrast, or latitude, film actually increases object contrast within certain areas because of the overall reduction in area contrast.

EFFECTS OF PROCESSING

Both the sensitivity and the contrast characteristics of a given film type are affected by processing. The degree of processing received by film generally depends on three factors: (1) the chemical activity of the developer solution, (2) the temperature of the developer, and (3) the period of immersion in the developer. In most applications it is usually desirable to maintain a constant developer activity by replenishment and to control the degree of development by

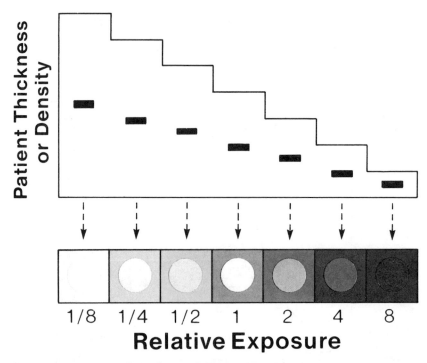

Figure 16-10 Increase in Object Contrast in Thick and Thin Body Sections with a Latitude Film (Compare with Figure 16-6.)

varying the temperature or, in some cases, the amount of development time. Varying the amount of development by changing either the chemical activity, the time period, or the temperature produces a shift in the characteristic curve.

The optimum performance of most film types is obtained by using the recommended degree of development. Deviation in either direction generally results in a loss of contrast. Although the sensitivity of film can usually be increased by over-developing, this is usually accompanied by an increase in undesirable fog.

Over-processing

Increasing development will cause the curve to shift to the left with a rise in the toe. The movement of the curve to the left indicates an increase in sensitivity because a given density value is produced with a lower exposure. As the toe of the curve rises, the general slope of the curve decreases, which results in less contrast. The increased density value of the toe also indicates an increased fog level. This fog density occurs because more of the unexposed silver grains are developed by the excess processing.

Under-processing

Under-processing causes the curve to shift to the right, indicating a decrease in sensitivity. The shoulder also begins to drop, and the slope of a curve decreases. This results in less contrast and less density.

FILM FOG

Any density in a film that is not produced as part of the image-forming exposure is generally referred to as fog. There are several potential sources of film fog.

Inherent

All film, even under the best conditions, shows some density even if it has received no radiation exposure. This density comes from the film base and from the unexposed emulsion, and is the density observed if a piece of unexposed film is processed. This is typically referred to as the base plus fog density and is generally in the range of 0.15 to 0.2 density units for radiographic film.

Chemical

If a film is over-processed, abnormally high densities will be developed by chemical action in image areas that received little or no exposure. This results from chemicals in the developer solution interacting with some of the film grains that were not sensitized by exposure.

Heat and Age

Fog will gradually develop in unprocessed film with age; therefore, film should not be stored for long periods of time. Each box of film is labeled with an expiration date by the manufacturer. When stored under proper conditions, film should not develop appreciable fog before the expiration date. When film is stored in a clinical facility, the stock should be rotated on a first-in, first-out basis.

The development of film fog with age is accelerated by heat; therefore, film should not be stored in hot areas. Refrigeration can extend the useful life of unprocessed film.

Radiation Exposure

It is not uncommon for film to be fogged by accidental exposure to either x-radiation or light. Light-exposure fogging can result from light leaks in a darkroom, the use of incorrect safelights, and cassettes with defective light seals around the edges.

Film darkrooms and storage areas should be properly shielded from nearby x-ray sources.

Chapter 17

Radiographic Density Control

INTRODUCTION AND OVERVIEW

Maximum visibility in a radiograph requires that the optical density be within a range that produces adequate contrast, as discussed in Chapter 16. This is achieved by setting the exposure to fit the conditions established by the receptor system and the patient. The exposure can be selected by either manually adjusting the KV, MA, and exposure time or using the AEC circuit of the x-ray machine. Neither method produces a perfect exposure each time. A number of sources of exposure error must be considered during the production of a radiograph.

A proper film density is obtained when the radiation exposure penetrating the patient's body (receptor exposure) matches the sensitivity (speed) requirements of the receptor system. Both receptor sensitivity and receptor exposure are affected by many factors, as shown in Figure 17-1. Film density is optimal when all of these factors are properly balanced.

After a radiographic system is installed, the films, screens, and grids are selected, and the processor is adjusted, the major task is selecting KV_p and MAS values to compensate for variations in patient thickness and composition. If the KV_p and MAS are to be selected manually, technique charts should be used for reference. The most common chart form gives KV_p and MAS values in relation to the thickness of different parts of the body. It should be emphasized that a given technique chart should be used only if it has been calibrated for the specific machine and film-screen-grid combination being used.

Exposure errors are produced by variations in any of the factors listed in Figure 17-1 that are not properly compensated for. When it is necessary to change certain factors, such as focal-film distance (FFD) or KV_p, to meet a specific examination objective, the change can usually be compensated for by changing another factor according to established relationships, such as the inverse-square law and the 15% rule.

237

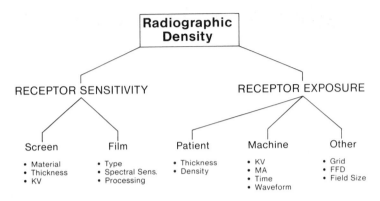

Figure 17-1 Factors that Affect Radiographic Density

In this chapter we consider the specific factors that relate to exposure (density) control, exposure error, and technique compensation.

THE X-RAY GENERATOR

The exposure delivered by an x-ray generator can be controlled by selecting appropriate values for KV_p, MA, and exposure time. In principle, several combinations of these three parameters produce the same film density; therefore, other factors, such as patient exposure, x-ray tube heat production, generator capabilities, image contrast, and image blur, must be considered in setting technical factors.

MA

The intensity (exposure rate) of an x-ray beam is directly proportional to the MA value. The typical radiographic generator provides several MA values (25, 50, 100, 200, 500, etc.) to choose from. The selection of an MA value is usually coupled with the selection of focal spot size. The use of the small focal spot (for better image detail) is typically limited to the lower MA values. The highest available MA value on a particular machine is determined by the capacity of the generator, as discussed in Chapter 8.

No one specific MA value must be used for a given procedure; the MA value must be selected in conjunction with the exposure time and KV_p. Some general rules governing the selection of MA are:

- Select low MA values to permit use of the small focal spot when image detail is important.
- Select large MA values to reduce exposure time when motion blurring is a problem.

- Select high MA values when it is desirable to reduce the KV_p to increase image contrast.

Two types of exposure errors are associated with the MA selection: one is primarily a human error and the other is an error associated with the calibration of the x-ray generator.

An exposure error can occur when the operator selects an MA value that is inappropriate in relation to the exposure time and KV_p value. This can occur if patient size and condition are not properly evaluated or if the technique charts are not correctly calibrated for the specific x-ray generator.

Exposure errors will occur if the output exposure rate of the x-ray machine is not proportional to the indicated MA value at a particular setting. It is not uncommon for the actual MA value to be different from the value indicated by the MA selector. This error source can be minimized by the periodic calibration of the x-ray generator. Calibration consists of measuring the x-ray exposure rate at each MA value that can be selected.

Exposure Time

Since the exposure produced by an x-ray tube is directly proportional to exposure time, it can be controlled by selecting an appropriate exposure time value. In radiography, exposure times are selected either by the operator, who sets the timer before initiating the exposure, or by the AEC circuit, which terminates the exposure after the selected exposure has reached the receptor.

As with MA, no one exposure time value is correct for a specific procedure. Remember that it is the combination of exposure time, MA, and KV_p that determines exposure. Some general rules for selecting an appropriate exposure time are:

- Select short exposure times to minimize motion blurring and improve image detail.
- Select longer exposure time when motion is not a problem and it is necessary to reduce either MA or KV_p.

Exposure errors can result from the selection of an inappropriate exposure time by the operator or from the failure of the generator to produce the exposure time indicated on the time selector.

X-ray machine timers should be calibrated periodically to determine if the machine produces an exposure that is proportional to the indicated exposure time. Timers can be calibrated by several methods including the use of a spinning top, an electronic timer, or the measurement and comparison of actual exposure output produced by each timer setting.

Exposure errors encountered in the use of AEC are discussed later.

KV$_p$

Film exposure is more sensitive to changes in KV$_p$ than to changes in either MA or exposure time. This is because the KV$_p$ affects several independent factors that contribute to film exposure. In Chapter 7 we saw that x-ray beam intensity increased exponentially with an increase in KV$_p$. A good approximation is that doubling the KV$_p$ increases exposure from an x-ray tube by a factor of 4. In Chapter 11 we observed that the penetration of radiation through an object, such as a patient's body, increases with KV$_p$. The increase in both x-ray production and penetration with KV$_p$ means that a relatively small change in KV$_p$ produces a relatively large change in the exposure penetrating the patient's body and reaching the receptor. It should be recalled (Chapter 14) that the sensitivity of intensifying screens changes with KV$_p$. Both the direction and amount of change depend on the specific screen material.

A general rule of thumb in radiography is that a 15% increase in KV$_p$ will double the exposure to the film. In other words, it takes only a 15% increase in KV$_p$ to produce the same increase in film exposure as a 100% increase in either MA or exposure time. The 15% rule is useful for comparing change in KV$_p$ and MAS, but it by no means expresses a precise relationship.

Figure 17-2 shows the approximate relationship between MAS and KV$_p$ values that would produce the same film exposure. The KV$_p$-MAS values represented by

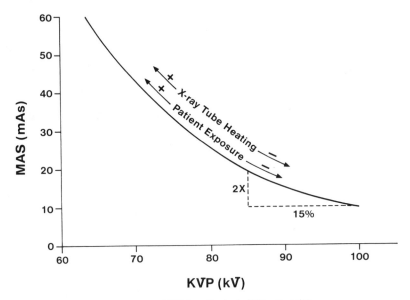

Figure 17-2 Relationship of KV$_p$ and MAS to Control of Film Density

points along this curve apply to a specific x-ray generator, patient, and receptor system. If either of these factors is changed, the position of the curve would be shifted.

Although it is true that KV_p-MAS values represented by any point along the curve produce the same film exposure, they will not produce the same image quality, patient exposure, and demands on the x-ray equipment. Moving down the curve (higher KV_p values) generally decreases patient exposure, x-ray tube heating, and motion blurring when the MAS is decreased by a shorter exposure time. The major reason for moving up the curve (higher MAS values) is to increase image contrast with the lower KV_p values, as discussed in Chapter 12.

The range of KV_p values for a specific procedure is selected on the basis of contrast requirements, patient exposure, and the limitations of the x-ray generator. However, small changes in KV_p within each range can be used to adjust film exposure.

Exposure errors can occur if the actual KV_p produced by an x-ray generator is different from the value indicated by the KV_p selector. Periodic calibration of an x-ray generator helps reduce this potential source of error.

Waveform

An x-ray generator that produces a relatively constant KV (ie, three-phase) requires less KV_p and/or MAS than a single-phase generator to produce the same film exposure. The constant potential, or three-phase, generator produces more radiation exposure per unit of MAS, as discussed in Chapter 7. For a specific KV_p value, the radiation is more penetrating because of the higher average KV during the exposure.

Technique charts designed for use with a single-phase generator would lead to considerable overexposure if used with a constant potential, or three-phase, generator.

X-Ray Tubes

All x-ray tubes do not produce the same exposure (for a specific KV_p-MAS value), and the exposure output sometimes decreases with aging. A difference in tube output among tubes is often caused by variations in the amount of filtration. The significance of the tube-to-tube variation is that technique factors for one x-ray machine might not produce proper film exposure if used with another machine.

RECEPTOR SENSITIVITY

The overall sensitivity (speed) of the radiographic receptor is determined by the characteristics of both the film and the intensifying screens. The sensitivity of a specific film-screen combination is usually specified in terms of a speed value, as described in Chapter 14. If either the film or screen type is changed so that the combined sensitivity (speed) changes, it will be necessary to change either the MAS or KV_p to compensate. If the speed is increased, less radiation will be required, so MAS or KV_p must be reduced. The relationship is

$$MAS \text{ (new)} = (\text{Speed (old)}/\text{Speed (new)}) \times MAS \text{ (old)}.$$

For example, if we change from a 200- to a 400-speed system,

$$MAS \text{ (new)} = 200 \text{ (old)}/400 \text{ (new)} \times MAS \text{ (old)} = 1/2 \times MAS \text{ (old)}.$$

A change in KV_p can also be selected to compensate for changes in receptors by using the 15% rule.

Many exposure errors are caused by undetected variations in receptor sensitivity from examination to examination, or over a period of time. When a receptor is described as having a specific speed value, such as 200, 400, etc., the value is nominal and applies to specific exposure and processing conditions. When these conditions change, so does the receptor sensitivity, as discussed in Chapters 14 and 15.

One of the major factors that produce variations in receptor sensitivity and, therefore, exposure error is variation in developer temperature and activity. The inherent sensitivity of film varies somewhat from one batch to another, but this is usually not sufficient to produce significant exposure error. Variations in screen sensitivity with KV_p can be a problem, especially when techniques appropriate for one type of screen (phosphor material) are used for another type.

Grids

When a grid is changed, the exposure factors must be changed. The approximate relationship between the old and new MAS values depends on the Bucky factors, B, or penetration values of the grids and is

$$MAS \text{ (new)} = (B \text{ (new)}/B \text{ (old)}) \times MAS \text{ (old)}.$$

The grid penetration is the reciprocal of the Bucky factor. If the condition being considered does not involve a grid, then the value of the Bucky factor or grid penetration will be 1. The value of these factors generally depends on grid ratio and the quantity of scattered radiation in the beam, as discussed in Chapter 13. Values of grid penetration range from 1 (no grid) to approximately 0.2 for a high-ratio grid. Changing from an examination condition without a grid to one with a grid penetration of 0.2 (Bucky factor of 5) requires the MAS to be increased by a factor of 5. Approximate grid penetration and Bucky factor values for different grids are given in Chapter 13.

PATIENT

For a given type of examination, the factor subject to the greatest variation from patient to patient is the penetration of the body section. For a given x-ray beam quality, or KV_p, the penetration depends on the thickness of the body part being examined and the composition of the body section. Changes in body thickness from one patient to another can be compensated for by changing either KV_p or MAS. An approximate relationship between KV_p and body thickness, t, is given by

$$KV_p = 50 + 2t \text{ (cm)}.$$

For example, a 15-cm thickness would require a KV_p of approximately 80, whereas a 20-cm thickness would require a KV_p of 90.

When a change in patient thickness is compensated for by changing MAS, a change of a factor of 2 is generally required for a thickness difference of approximately 5 cm. This varies, however, with KV_p. A given thickness difference requires a smaller MAS change when higher KV_p values are used.

The presence of various pathological conditions can also alter body penetration and require appropriate exposure adjustments. Muscular patients generally require an additional increase in exposure factors, whereas elderly patients require a reduction.

DISTANCE AND AREA

As the area covered by the x-ray beam, or field size, is increased, more scattered radiation is produced and contributes to film exposure. Although much of the scattered radiation is removed by the grid, it is often necessary to change exposure factors to get the same density with different field sizes.

Because of the inverse-square effect, the exposure that reaches the receptor is related to the focal spot-receptor distance, d. If this distance is changed, the new MAS value required to obtain the same film exposure will be given by

$$MAS \text{ (new)} = (d^2 \text{ (new)}/d^2 \text{ (old)}) \times MAS \text{ (old)}.$$

A characteristic of the relationship is that if the distance is doubled, the required MAS will increase by a factor of 4. Long focal spot-receptor distances generally decrease image blur, patient exposure, and distortion; however, a significantly higher MAS is required.

AUTOMATIC EXPOSURE CONTROL

Many radiographic systems are equipped with an AEC circuit. The AEC is often referred to as the phototimer. The basic function of an AEC is illustrated in Figure 17-3.

The principal component of the AEC is a radiation-measuring device, or sensor, located near the receptor. A common type of sensor contains an intensifying screen that converts the x-ray exposure into light. The sensor also contains a component, typically a photomultiplier tube, that converts the light into an electrical signal. Another type of sensor is an ionization chamber (described in Chapter 34) that also converts x-ray exposure into an electrical signal.

Within the AEC circuit, the exposure signal is compared to a reference value. When the accumulated exposure to the sensor (receptor) reaches the predetermined reference value, the exposure is terminated when the x-ray tube automatically turns off.

The reference exposure level is determined by two variables: one is the calibration of the AEC. A service engineer must adjust the basic reference level to match the sensitivity (speed) of the receptor. If either the intensifying screen or film is changed so that the overall receptor sensitivity changes, it will usually be necessary to recalibrate the AEC.

The other variable found on most systems is the density control, which can be adjusted by the operator. In general, the density control can be used to vary

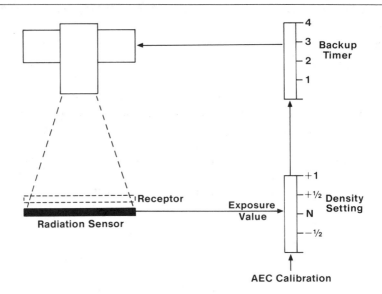

Figure 17-3 Basic Automatic Exposure Control System

receptor exposure (film density) within a limited range. The density control is usually marked with the factors by which the nominal (zero setting) exposure will be changed.

The AEC contains a back-up timer, which will terminate an exposure if there is a malfunction in the normal operation and is a safety feature to prevent excessive patient exposure. In most systems, the manual timer also serves as the back-up timer for the AEC. The back-up timer should be set to a value somewhat larger than the expected exposure time. If it is set at a value that is too low, it will terminate the exposure before adequate receptor exposure has accumulated. The result will be an underexposed film.

When using AEC, the location of the sensor with respect to patient anatomy must be considered. The sensitive area of the sensor has a definite size and shape. Typically, different sensor areas can be selected by the operator. The function of the AEC is to control the average density within the sensitive area of the sensor. If the sensitive area is incorrectly positioned relative to the patient's anatomy, exposure errors can be significant. For example, if, in chest radiography, the sensor field is placed over the mediastinum, the AEC will attempt to produce a density of approximately 1 unit (medium gray) in that area. Under this condition, the lung areas will be overexposed.

The use of AEC does not eliminate exposure error. Some possible sources of error that must be considered are the following:

- AEC not calibrated for a specific receptor
- Density control not set to proper value
- Back-up timer not set to proper value
- Sensor field incorrectly positioned with respect to anatomy.

Chapter 18

Blur, Resolution, and Visibility of Detail

INTRODUCTION AND OVERVIEW

An important characteristic of any medical imaging method is its ability to show the anatomical detail of the human body. Detail, as used here, refers to the small structures, features, and objects associated with normal anatomy and various pathological conditions. The smallest detail that can be visualized is determined, to a large extent, by the amount of blur produced by the imaging procedure. There is some blur in all medical images. Some methods, however, produce images with significantly less blur than others, and the result is images that show much greater detail. Each imaging method also has certain associated factors that control the amount of blurring and the ultimate visibility of detail.

In this chapter we consider the general characteristics of image blur and its relationship to other image characteristics.

BLUR

Blurring is present, to some extent, in all imaging processes, including vision, photography, and medical imaging methods. The basic concept of blur is illustrated in Figure 18-1. An image is a visual representation of a specific physical object, such as a patient's body. In an ideal situation, each small point within the object would be represented by a small, well-defined point within the image. In reality, the "image" of each object point is spread, or blurred, within the image. The amount of blurring can be expressed as the dimension of the blurred image of a very small object point. Blur values range from approximately 0.15 mm, for mammography, to approximately 15 mm, for imaging with a gamma camera.

The blur of a small object point can have a variety of shapes, as shown in Figure 18-2. The shape generally depends on the source of blur. Some x-ray system components, such as intensifying screens and image intensifier tubes,

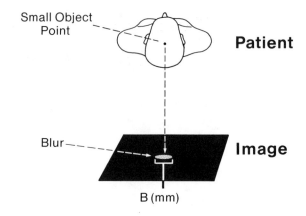

Small Object Point

Patient

Blur

Image

B (mm)

Figure 18-1 The Blur of an Individual Object Point

Blur Shapes

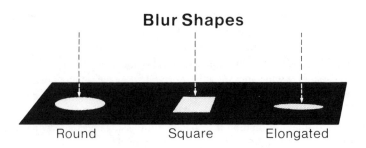

Round   Square   Elongated

Figure 18-2 Blur Shapes Encountered in Medical Imaging

generally produce round blur patterns. Most imaging methods that produce digital images (digital subtraction angiography (DSA), CT, MRI, etc.) produce square blur patterns that correspond to the dimensions of the image pixel or tissue voxel. Motion during the imaging process typically produces an elongated blur pattern. X-ray tube focal spots produce a variety of blur shapes.

In addition to a size and shape, the blur produced by a specific factor has a specific intensity distribution. This characteristic is related to the manner in which the point image is spread, or distributed, within the blur area. Two blur distribution patterns are illustrated in Figure 18-3. The actual distribution of the image intensity within the blur area is often illustrated by means of an intensity profile. Some sources of blur uniformly distribute the object-point image intensity within the blur area. This gives the blur pattern a precise dimension, as illustrated in Figure 18-3. Many sources of blur, however, do not uniformly distribute blur. Common examples are intensifying screens and defocused optical systems. A

Blur Distribution (Profiles)

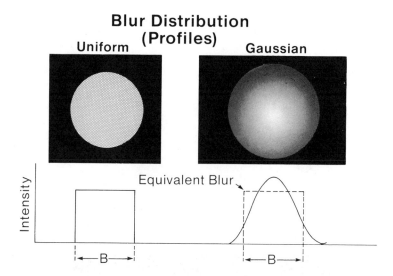

Figure 18-3 Blur Distribution Patterns

common distribution pattern is one with a relatively high intensity near the center with a gradual reduction of intensity toward the periphery. The profile of this type of distribution is often a Gaussian curve, as illustrated. The full dimension (diameter) of a Gaussian blur pattern is not used to express the amount of blur because it would tend to overstate the blur in relation to blur that is uniformly distributed. A more appropriate value is the dimension of a uniform distribution that would produce the same general image quality as the Gaussian distribution. This is designated the equivalent blur value. For example, the two blur patterns shown in Figure 18-3 have the same general effect on image quality even though the total dimension of the Gaussian distribution is larger.

VISIBILITY OF DETAIL

The most significant effect of blur in an imaging process is that it reduces the visibility of details such as small objects and structures. In every imaging process, blur places a definite limit on the amount of detail (object smallness) that can be visualized.

The direct effect of blur is to reduce the contrast of small objects and features, as illustrated in Figure 18-4. In effect, blur spreads the image of small objects into the surrounding background area. As the image spreads, the contrast and visibility are reduced.

The visibility of specific objects is very dependent on the relationship between object size and the blur value. If the blur value is less than the dimension of an

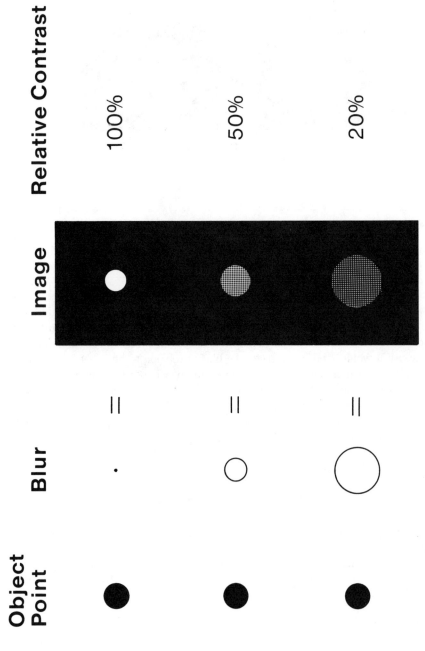

Figure 18-4 General Effect of Blur on Image Contrast

object, the reduced contrast will generally not affect visibility. When the amount of blur approaches the dimensions of the object, the blurring process can significantly reduce contrast. In some situations, especially in which small objects already have a low inherent contrast, the blur can significantly affect visibility. As a general rule, the blur value can be considered as an approximate detail-visibility threshold. In most situations, body structures much smaller than the blur value will not be visible.

The basic concept we need to emphasize is that the blur that is present as part of an imaging procedure reduces the contrast, and the resulting visibility, of small objects (detail) within the body. The extent to which the contrast is reduced depends on the relationship between the amount of blur and the size of the object, as illustrated in Figure 18-5. This diagram shows how the contrast of objects is affected by blur. The maximum value on the relative contrast scale (100%) represents the contrast of each object in the absence of blur; it does not mean that all objects, both small and large, have the same amount of inherent contrast. In projection x-ray imaging, small objects tend to produce much less contrast than large objects because of their increased penetration. The contrast and visibility of small objects are actually reduced by two factors: the increased x-ray penetration and the effects of blur, which we are considering here.

No medical imaging method produces images that are free of blur; the no-blur line is included in the illustration as a point of reference. In this particular example, the blur values are described only in the relative terms of low, medium, and high.

Let us now consider the effect of a small amount of blur on the imaging process. The contrast of the larger objects is not affected. The loss of contrast because of blur increases with decreasing object size (detail). The contrast is eventually reduced to zero at some point along the detail scale, and no smaller objects will be visible. For objects that produce relatively low contrast, even without blur, the threshold of visibility might occur at object sizes larger than the point at which blur produces zero contrast. The visibility threshold is related to, but not necessarily equal to, the object size at which blur produces zero relative contrast.

As blur is increased in the imaging process, the loss of contrast increases for all objects, and the visibility threshold moves to the left.

UNSHARPNESS

An image that shows much detail and distinct boundaries is often described as being sharp. The presence of blur produces unsharpness. Image unsharpness, as the term is commonly used, and blur refer to the same general image characteristic. In a more exact sense, however, image unsharpness is one of several visual effects produced by the basic process of blurring.

Unsharpness is especially noticeable at the boundaries and edges within an image.

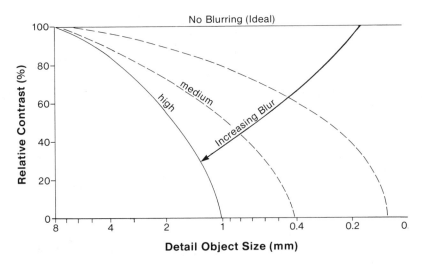

Figure 18-5 Effect of Blur on the Contrast of Objects of Different Size

In the early days of radiography, the term *penumbra* was often used to describe the unsharpness, or blur, produced by x-ray tube focal spots. Penumbra is primarily an astronomical name for the unsharp shadow boundaries created by the moon because of its finite size. Because a number of different sources of blur in x-ray imaging produce the same visual effects and are not true penumbras, use of the term should be discouraged.

RESOLUTION

Resolution describes the ability of an imaging system to distinguish or separate (ie, resolve) objects that are close together. The resolving capability of a particular imaging process is determined by the amount of blur. When blur is present, the images of individual objects begin to run together until the separate objects are no longer distinguishable. For objects to be resolved, their separation distance must be increased in proportion to the amount of blur present.

The resolving ability, or resolution, of an imaging system is relatively easy to measure and is often used to evaluate system blur. Figure 18-6 shows one type of test object used for this purpose; it consists of parallel lead strips separated by a distance equal to the width of the strips. The common practice is to describe the line width and separation distance in terms of line pairs (lp) per unit distance (millimeters or centimeters). One line pair consists of one lead strip and one adjacent separation space. The number of line pairs per millimeter is actually an expression of spatial frequency. As the lines get smaller and closer together, the spatial frequency (line pairs per millimeter) increases. A typical test pattern

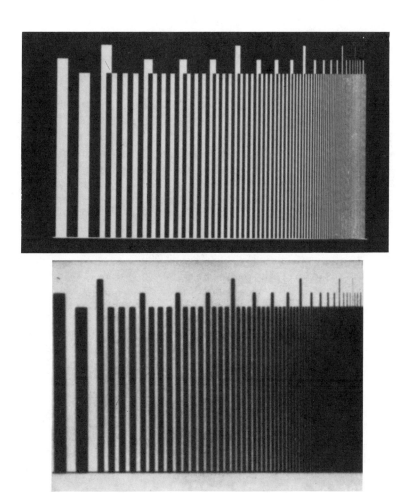

Figure 18-6 A Test Pattern Used to Measure the Resolution of an X-Ray Imaging System

contains areas with different spatial frequencies. An imaging system is evaluated by imaging the test object and observing the highest spatial frequency (or minimum separation) at which the separation of the lines is visible.

Figure 18-7 illustrates the effect of blur on resolution. When no blur is present, all of the line-pair groups can be resolved. As blur is increased, however, resolution is decreased, and only the lines with larger separation distances are visible.

Figure 18-8 compares how the contrast within the various line-pair groups is reduced by various levels of blur. Note the similarity between this illustration and Figure 18-5. Increasing spatial frequency corresponds to increasing image detail and reducing object size. Curves like those shown in Figure 18-8 are generally

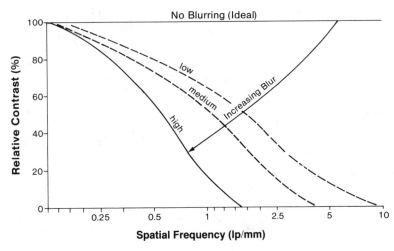

Figure 18-7 Effect of Blur on Resolution

designated contrast transfer functions (CTF). They show the ability of an imaging system to transfer contrast of objects of different sizes in the presence of blur.

The shape of the curve depends, to some extent, on the major source and distribution of blur within the system, as shown in Figure 18-9. For example, the

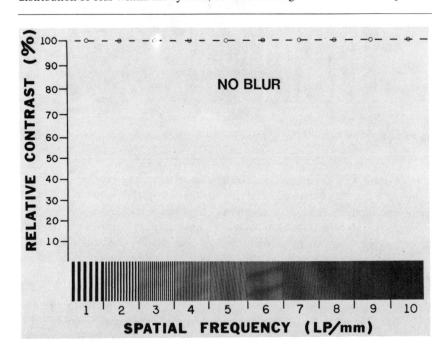

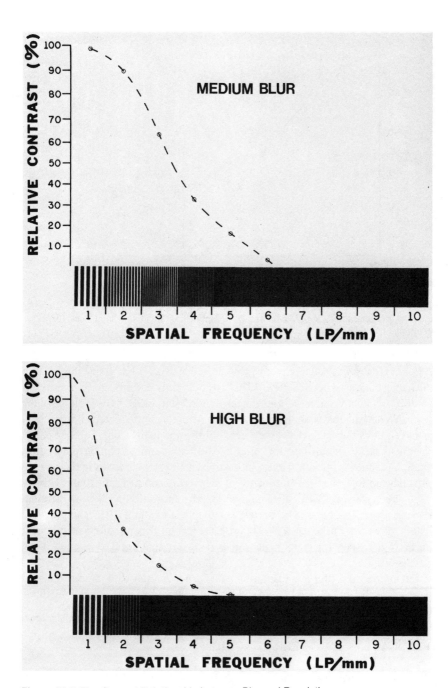

Figure 18-8 The General Relationship between Blur and Resolution

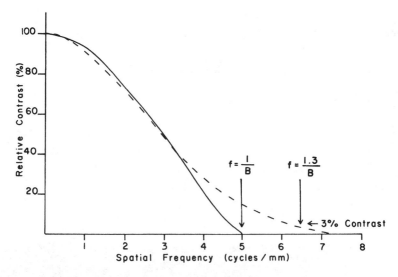

Figure 18-9 The Contrast Transfer Function Associated with Two Types of Blur. The Solid Line (——) is Characteristic of Motion and Focal Spot Blur. The Dotted line (----) is Generally Characteristic of Receptor Blur.

typical CTF curve associated with focal spot blur usually has a specific point at which the contrast becomes zero. This is commonly referred to as the disappearance frequency and represents the resolution limit, or resolving ability, of the system. When the major source of blur is the receptor, ie, the intensifying screen or image intensifier tube, the curve might not show a distinct zero-contrast point. Criteria must be established for defining the maximum resolution point. It is common practice to specify the resolution of such a system in terms of the spacing frequency, in line pairs per millimeter, at which the contrast falls to a relatively low value, typically 3%. When comparing the resolution values of different systems, this practice should be taken into consideration. For example, if a manufacturer arbitrarily uses a 3% contrast, the resolution values for its equipment will be higher than for equipment from a company that uses 10%, even if the systems are identical.

The approximate blur and resolution values encountered with various imaging methods are shown in Figure 18-10, which illustrates why some imaging methods are much better than others in visualizing anatomical detail.

MODULATION TRANSFER FUNCTION

The modulation transfer function (MTF) is a graphical description of the blur, or resolution characteristics, of an imaging system or its individual components. In

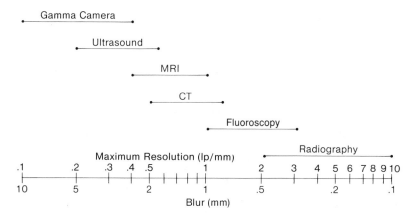

Figure 18-10 Comparison of Blur and Resolution Values for the Different Imaging Methods

many respects, the MTF is similar to the CTF shown in Figure 18-9. The difference is that the CTF describes a system's ability to image line pairs, whereas the MTF describes its ability to image sine-wave shapes, or spatial frequencies. Rather than lines and spaces, as in the CTF test object, a true MTF test object has peaks and valleys. Actually, the MTF is seldom determined by using such a test object, but the idea is useful in understanding the concept of MTF. One peak and valley make up 1 cycle of the object. Such a test object is characterized by its spatial frequency, which is the number of cycles (peaks and valleys) per millimeter of length. In other words, an MTF test object has a certain number of peaks and valleys (cycles) per millimeter, whereas a CTF test object has a certain number of lines and spaces (line pairs) per millimeter. The ability of a system to image the various spatial frequencies is related to the amount of blur present.

A large flat object of relatively uniform thickness contains low frequency components. At the edge of such an object, however, high frequency components are created by the sudden change in thickness. Generally speaking, small objects of a given cross-sectional shape have higher frequency components than larger objects.

In order to form an unblurred image of the object, the x-ray imaging system must be able to produce sufficient contrast for all spatial frequencies contained in the object. If some of the frequency components are lost in the imaging process, the image will not be a true representation of the object. For example, if the high frequency components are not present in the image, the image will be blurred. The spatial frequency content of the image that reaches the film is determined by the frequency content of the object being imaged and the MTF of the imaging system. This is illustrated in Figure 18-11. The image content at a specific frequency is found by multiplying the object content by the MTF. For example, in Figure

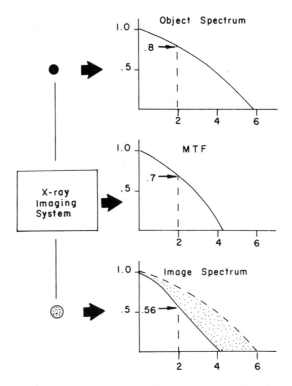

Figure 18-11 The Relationship of an Image Spatial Frequency Spectrum to the Object Spectrum and the MTF of the Imaging System

18-11, the object contains 0.8 (80%) at a frequency of 2 cycles per mm. The MTF at this frequency is 0.7. Multiplying these two quantities shows that the image will contain only 0.56 (56%) at this frequency. The shaded area is the portion of the object's spatial frequency spectrum that is lost because of the MTF of the imaging system. Any frequency components of the object that are above the resolution limit of the system are completely lost. In effect, the MTF of the imaging system can cut out the higher frequency components associated with an object, and the image will be made up only of lower frequency components. Since low frequency components are associated with large objects with gradual changes in thickness, as opposed to sharp edges, the image will be blurred.

A property of MTFs that is not possessed by CTFs is their ability to be cascaded. Consider an imaging system in which the sources of blur are the focal spot and receptor. The blur characteristics of each of these can be described by an MTF curve, as shown in Figure 18-12. The MTF of the total system is found by multiplying the two MTF values at each frequency. For example, if at 2 cycles per

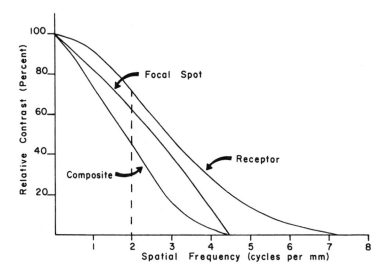

Figure 18-12 The Composite MTF

mm the MTF for the focal spot is 62%, and for the receptor is 72%, the total system will have an MTF value of 44%. It should be observed that a system cannot have frequency components that are higher than the resolution limit of either the receptor or the focal spot. This is equivalent to saying that the total system blur cannot be less than the blur from either of the two sources. If the MTFs of the different blur sources (focal spot, motion, or receptor) are significantly different, the one with the lowest limiting frequency (the largest blur) will generally determine the MTF of the total system. In other words, if one source is producing significantly larger blur than the other sources, the total system blur will be essentially equal to the largest blur value.

Chapter 19

Radiographic Detail

INTRODUCTION AND OVERVIEW

Of all medical imaging systems, radiography has the ability to produce images with the greatest detail. All radiographs, however, contain some blur. The three basic sources of radiographic blurring and loss of detail are indicated in Figure 19-1 and are (1) the focal spot, (2) motion during film exposure, and (3) the receptor. Most receptor blur is produced by the spreading of light within the intensifying screen, as described in Chapter 14. Light crossover between the two film emulsions can add to receptor blur. If the intensifying screen and film surfaces do not make good contact, additional blurring is produced.

The amount of blur in radiographs is generally in the range of 0.15 mm to approximately 1 mm. The blur value for a specific radiographic procedure depends on a combination of factors including focal spot size, type of intensifying screen, location of the object being imaged, and exposure time (if motion is present). The general objective is not to produce a radiograph with the greatest possible detail but to produce one with adequate detail within the confines of x-ray tube heating and patient exposure.

We begin by considering the characteristics of the three basic blur sources, and then show how they combine to affect image quality.

OBJECT LOCATION AND MAGNIFICATION

Before proceeding with a discussion of the various types of blur, it is necessary to establish the relationship of several distances within the imaging system. Figure 19-2 shows the three basic distances. The focal-spot-to-receptor distance, FRD, is always the sum of the focal-spot-to-object distance, FOD, and the object-to-receptor distance, ORD. With respect to image formation and image quality, the significant values are not the actual distances, but certain distance ratios.

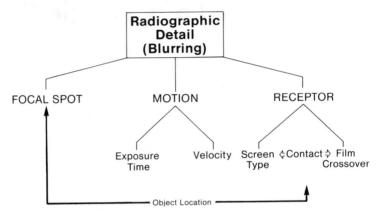

Figure 19-1 The Sources of Blur in Radiographs

In the formation of an x-ray image, the image will always be larger than the object if the object is separated from the receptor. The amount of enlargement, or magnification, is equal to the FRD:FOD ratio. Magnification, m, is increased either by increasing the FRD or bringing the object closer to the x-ray tube, which decreases the FOD.

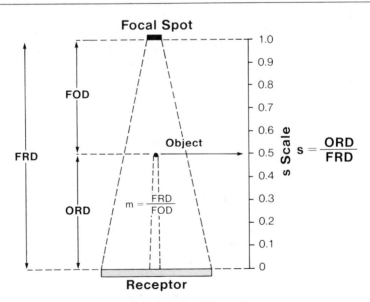

Figure 19-2 Distance Relationships in Radiographic Imaging

Another useful relationship is the ORD:FRD ratio. This quantity, s, is used to specify the distance between the object and receptor (ORD) in relation to the total distance between focal spot and receptor (FRD). It is helpful to think of a scale running from the receptor to the focal spot: The receptor would be at the zero-end, and the focal spot at the other end, which has a value of 1. The position of the object being radiographed can be specified with respect to this scale; for example, if it is located at s = 0.2 on the scale, the ORD is 20% of the FRD. For certain types of blurring, the blur value is dependent on s, rather than on the actual distance between object and receptor.

When blur is given a specific value, the location within the imaging system must be specified. Blur values are generally specified for either the receptor input surface (plane) or the location of the object being radiographed. If an x-ray system has a blur value of 0.3 mm when measured in the object plane, and a magnification factor of 1.2, the image at the receptor location will have a blur value of 0.3 × 1.2 or 0.36 mm. Conversely, if an imaging system has a blur value specified at the receptor, the amount of blur with respect to the object size is found by dividing by the magnification factor. In all cases, as shown in Figure 19-3, the relationship between the blur with respect to the size of the object, and as measured at the receptor surface, is just the magnification, m.

The visibility of detail within a radiograph is determined by the relationship of the blur to the size of the objects being imaged. As blur values begin to exceed object dimensions, contrast and visibility are greatly diminished. Therefore, the

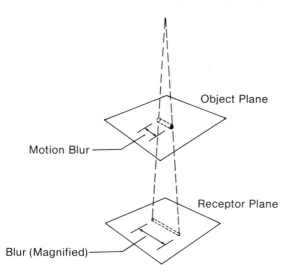

Figure 19-3 Magnification of Blur

most appropriate location for evaluating blur is at the location of the object where the blur values have meaning with respect to image detail. Another major reason for evaluating blur at the location of the object, rather than at the receptor, is that the relationship of blur values to all contributing factors is a simple linear relationship, as described below.

MOTION BLUR

Blurring will occur if the object being imaged moves during the exposure. The amount of blur in the object plane is equal to the distance moved during the exposure. As shown in Figure 19-3, the blur value at the receptor is larger and is in proportion to the magnification factor, m. The effect of motion on each point within the object is to reduce contrast and spread the image over a larger area, as indicated. If motion of body parts cannot be temporarily halted, motion blur can be minimized by reducing exposure time.

A misconception regarding motion blur is that it is increased by magnification. Although it is true that the blur at the receptor surface is increased, image quality generally depends on the amount of blur with respect to the object size. This value is not affected by magnification.

FOCAL SPOT BLUR

All x-ray tube focal spots have a finite size, and this contributes to image blur. Consider the example shown in Figure 19-4. X-ray photons passing through each point of the object from the focal spot diverge and form a blurred image of the object point. The blur value with respect to the object size (in the object plane) is given by

$$Bf = F \times s$$

where F is the dimension of the focal spot. Note that the value of focal spot blur, for a given focal size, is directly related to the position of the object on the s scale. If the object is in direct contact with the receptor (s = 0), focal-spot blur vanishes. As the object is moved away from the receptor, the blur increases in direct proportion to the value of s. The significance of this is illustrated in Figure 19-5. When the object is moved away from the receptor, both the image and blur are magnified, but the blur increases faster than the size of the image. Therefore, the blur value is increased in proportion to the object size, causing a deterioration in image quality.

Figure 19-5 shows the relationship of focal-spot blur to object size as it is affected by object location(s). The amount of blur relative to the size of the object

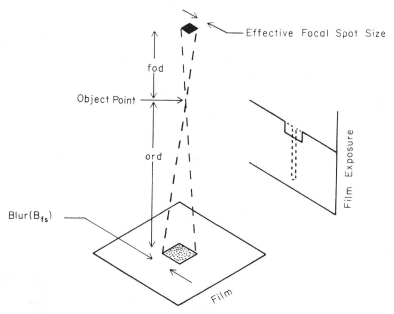

Figure 19-4 Focal Spot Blur

in the object plane increases in proportion to the relative distance(s) between the object and the receptor. The maximum blur occurs at the focal spot where the blur value becomes equal to the actual size of the spot.

The effect of focal spot size on the visibility of a specific object depends on three factors: (1) the size of the object, (2) the size of the focal spot, and (3) the location of the object.

Focal Spot Size

The most significant characteristic of a focal spot is its size. Most x-ray tubes have labels that specify the size of the focal spot. The size specified by the manufacturer on the label is generally referred to as the nominal size. The dimension that determines the blur characteristics of the focal spot is the effective blur size. The relationship between these two sizes is illustrated in Figure 19-6.

A distinction must be made between the focal spot dimension, which determines its blur characteristics, and the focal spot size, as specified by the tube manufacturer. Because of several factors, the generally stated size of a focal spot and its blur-producing size are significantly different. Blur is related to the equivalent size of a focal spot, rather than to its actual dimensions. The equivalent size is defined as the size of a rectangular focal spot with uniform x-ray emission over its surface that will produce the same blur as the focal spot in question.

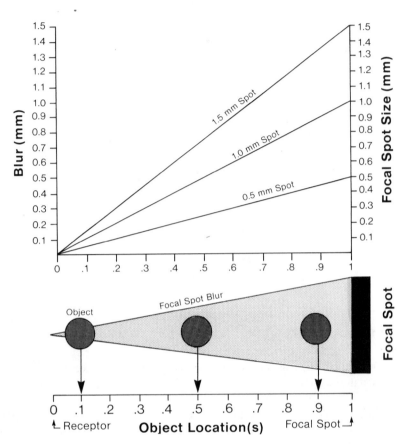

Figure 19-5 Relationship of Focal Spot Blur to Focal Spot Size and Object Location

Manufacturer's Tolerance

It is a general practice to allow a discrepancy between the manufacturer's stated nominal size and the actual measured size of focal spots. In almost all cases, the allowed tolerance is such that the stated nominal size is less than the measured size. The allowed tolerance generally depends on the size of the focal spot but is as large as 50% for the smaller focal spot sizes. For example, a focal spot that has a measured size of 0.9 mm could be labeled as a 0.6-mm focal spot because it falls within the accepted tolerance values.

Blooming

A common characteristic of many focal spots is that they undergo a change in size with changes in MA and KV_p. This effect is known as blooming. If the size of

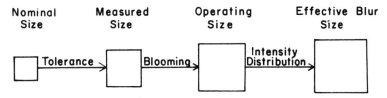

Figure 19-6 Different Focal Spot Sizes

a focal spot is measured at a relatively low tube current, the size during operation at higher tube current values can be significantly larger. The amount of blooming with an increase in tube current varies from tube to tube. In some tubes, the blooming of the focal spot in one direction is more than in the other. Blooming is generally greater for small focal spots.

KV_p generally has less effect on focal spot size than current. Some focal spots undergo a slight reduction in size with increased KV_p.

Intensity Distribution

Most focal spots do not have a uniform distribution of radiation over their entire area. A non-uniform distribution of x-ray intensity causes a focal spot to have an effective blur size different from its actual physical size. The variation in x-ray emission can be represented by an intensity profile, as shown in Figure 19-7. The focal spot with a rectangular intensity distribution (center) has an effective blur size identical with the dimensions of the spot. A focal spot with a double peak distribution (top) has an effective blur size significantly larger than the actual dimension of the spot. This double-peak distribution is characteristic of many focal spots produced by a line focus cathode.

The intensity distribution shown at the bottom of the illustration has a Gaussian shape. A focal spot with this type of intensity distribution has an effective blur size less than its actual physical size. Gaussian-shaped focal spots are highly desirable because they have a relatively low effective blur size in comparison to their heat capacity. A focal spot with an approximate Gaussian distribution can be produced in line focus tubes by applying a bias voltage between the cathode elements.

Anode Angle

The size of the focal spot is usually specified with reference to the center of the x-ray beam area, or field. Because of the angle of the anode surface, the effective focal spot size changes with position in the field: It becomes smaller for points toward the anode end and larger toward the cathode end of the field. The variation in effective focal spot size with position within the field is more significant in tubes with small anode angles.

Equivalent
Size

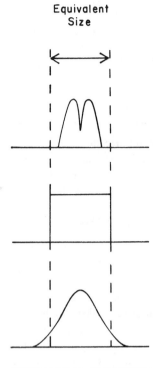

Figure 19-7 Three Focal-Spot Intensity Distributions with Approximately the Same Effective Blur Size

Measurement of Focal Spot Sizes

Two methods are used to determine the size of focal spots. The principles of the two methods are entirely different and generally produce different dimensions for the same focal spot. The pin-hole camera can be used to determine the actual dimensions of a focal spot, whereas the star test pattern is used to determine the effective blur size.

Pin-Hole Camera

The principle of the pin-hole camera is illustrated in Figure 19-8. The pin-hole camera consists of a very small hole in a sheet of metal, such as gold or lead. The pin-hole is positioned between the focal spot and a film receptor, as shown. When the x-ray tube is energized, an image of the focal spot is projected onto the film. The size of the focal spot can be determined by measuring the size of the image and applying a correction factor if there is any geometric magnification present. If the pin-hole is located at the midpoint between the focal spot and film, no correction factor will be required.

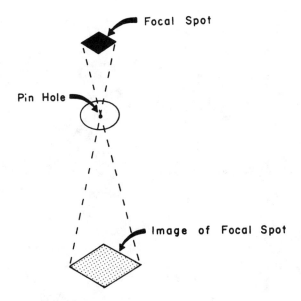

Figure 19-8 Pin-Hole Method of Determining Focal Spot Size

Star Test Pattern

The effective blur size of a focal spot can be measured by using a test object that measures blur or resolution. The most common object used for this purpose has alternating lines and spaces arranged in a star pattern, as shown in Figure 19-9. The first step in determining focal spot size is to make a radiograph with the test object located at approximately the midpoint between the focal spot and receptor. An image is obtained in which there is a zone of blurring at some distance from the center of the object. The distance between the blur zones is measured and used to calculate the size of the focal spot by using the following formula:

$$F = \frac{\pi \, \Theta \, D}{180(M - 1)}$$

where F is the effective focal spot size, D is the diameter of the blur circle illustrated in Figure 19-9, M is the magnification factor, and Θ is the angle of one test-pattern segment.

RECEPTOR BLUR

If the receptor input surface that absorbs the x-ray beam has significant thickness, blur will be introduced at this point. Blurring of this type generally occurs in

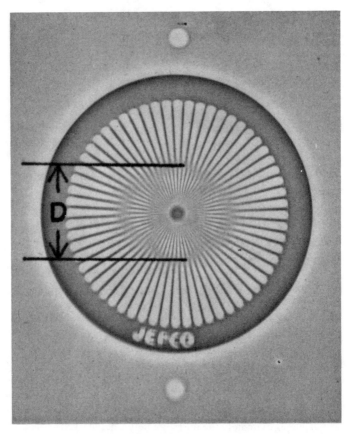

Figure 19-9 The Image of a Star Test Pattern Used to Determine Focal Spot Size

intensifying screens and in the input phosphor layers of image intensifiers. Blur production was illustrated in Figure 14-5. X-ray photons that pass through a point within the object are absorbed by the phosphor layer and converted into light. The light created along the x-ray "path" spreads into the surrounding portion of the phosphor layer. When the light emerges from the screen it covers an area that is larger than the object point. In other words, the x-rays that pass through each point within an object form an image that is blurred into the surrounding area.

Because this type of blur is caused by the spreading, or "diffusing," of light, the blur profile generally has a shape different from that of motion blur. In most cases, the blur profile is "bell-shaped" or Gaussian in nature. Because it is somewhat difficult to specify an exact blur dimension, receptor blur is more appropriately described in terms of an effective blur value. The amount of blur is primarily dependent on the thickness of the phosphor layer.

Intensifying screens generally have effective blur values in the range of 0.15 mm to 0.6 mm. The approximate breakdown for the basic screen types is as follows:

- mammographic, 0.15–0.2 mm
- detail, 0.2–0.35 mm
- medium speed, 0.5–0.6 mm
- high speed, 0.6–0.7 mm.

Since there must be a compromise between image detail and patient exposure, the objective is not always to use intensifying screens that produce maximum detail but to select screens that provide adequate detail with the lowest possible exposure.

In a given imaging system, the receptor blur value with respect to the size of the object can be decreased by introducing magnification. This is illustrated in Figure 19-10, in which a small object is being imaged. The presence of receptor

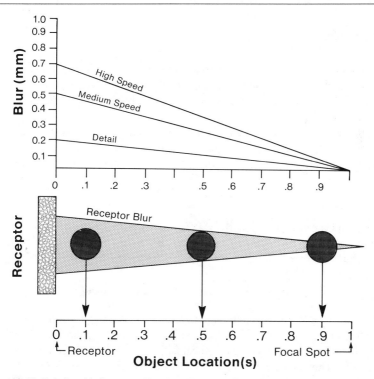

Figure 19-10 Relationship between Receptor Blur and Object Location for Three Types of Intensifying Screens

blur produces a zone of unsharpness around the object. The actual blur dimension at the receptor surface is fixed by the receptor characteristics and is unaffected by magnification. When magnification is relatively small, the blur is large in comparison to the object. When magnification is increased, the relative blur-to-image size is decreased. What actually happens is that magnification causes the image of a specific object to be enlarged at the receptor. This changes the relationship between the amount of blur and the size of the object image because the blur value at the receptor remains fixed. However, the amount of receptor blur projected back to the location of the object is reduced by magnification. Receptor blur in the object plane, Br, is related to the position of the object, s, by

$$Br = Bro\ (1 - s)$$

where Bro is the equivalent blur value of the receptor measured at the receptor surface. Although magnification can be used to reduce receptor blur with respect to object size, it must be approached with caution. Since focal spot blur increases with magnification, the two blur sources must be considered together.

COMPOSITE BLUR

The total blur in an image is a composite of the three different types of blur: (1) motion, (2) receptor, and (3) focal spot. In some situations one source of blur might predominate. When this occurs, the total blur is essentially equal to the largest blur value.

In order to determine the total, or composite, blur in a system, it is necessary to combine the three blur values. Although the exact relationship may vary, depending on conditions, it is generally accepted that the total value is given by

$$Bt = \sqrt{Br^2 + Bf^2 + Bm^2}.$$

For example, if receptor blur, Br, is 0.3 mm; focal spot blur, Bf, is 0.2 mm; and motion blur, Bm, is 0.2 mm; the total blur, Bt, would be found by substituting in the equation above as follows:

$$Bt = \sqrt{0.3^2 + 0.2^2 + 0.2^2} = 0.41 \text{ mm}.$$

It was shown earlier that blur from two sources, the receptor and the focal spot, depends on the position of the object with respect to the s scale. As an object is moved away from the receptor, focal spot blur increases and receptor blur decreases. This means that the position of the object must be taken into account when considering the blur characteristics of a specific x-ray system. For most systems, there is an object position on the s scale that produces the minimum blur.

Moving the object in either direction, toward or away from the receptor, increases the blur.

The relationship between blur and object position is easy to visualize by using a blur nomograph, as shown in Figure 19-11. The nomograph has three scales: (1) blur, (2) focal spot size, and (3) the position of the object, or s scale. The lines representing the blur from the three sources are drawn on the diagram according to the following simple rules:

The line representing receptor blur is drawn between a point on the blur scale that represents the equivalent blur of the particular receptor being used and a point located at a value of 1 on the s scale.

The line representing focal spot blur is drawn between the zero (0) point on the s scale and a point on the focal spot scale that corresponds to the size of the focal spot.

The line for motion blur is drawn horizontally and intersects the blur scale at a value equal to the distance the object moved during the exposure interval. The significance of the horizontal line for motion blur is that its value relative to the size of an object does not change with magnification. In most applications, the actual value for motion blur is difficult to estimate. It is included in this illustration primarily for the sake of completeness.

The three lines represent the blur of an object from the three blur sources. The composite, or total blur, is found for any point on the s scale by combining the three blur values, using the equation given above. It is of special significance that

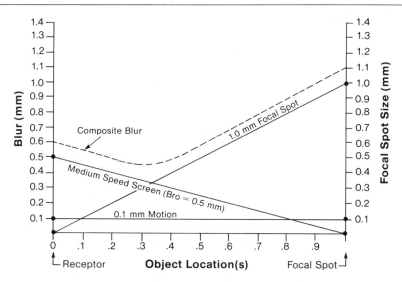

Figure 19-11 A Nomogram Used to Determine Radiographic Blur at Different Object Locations

the total system blur usually has a minimum value at a point on the s scale. An exception is when the major source of blur is motion, in which case the total blur is essentially the same at any point along the s scale. However, when most of the blur arises from either the receptor or the focal spot, a minimum point is usually present. The position of the minimum blur point along the s scale depends on the characteristics of the receptor and the focal spot. If the receptor has a relatively low characteristic blur value, the minimum point will be located in the lower portion of the s scale, which represents a position close to the receptor surface. Either increasing receptor blur or decreasing focal spot size shifts the minimum blur point to higher values on the s scale. Inspection of the diagram leads to two significant observations:

1. When an object is located near the receptor surface (low s scale value), the total blur is essentially a function of the receptor.
2. As an object is moved away from the receptor surface (high s scale value), the focal spot becomes the major determining factor in overall system blur.

Figure 19-12 shows the composite blur for a radiographic system using high-speed screens and a 0.5-mm focal spot. With this combination, the intensifying screen is the most significant blur source. Notice that the blur decreases with magnification over the useful range of object locations.

Figure 19-13 illustrates the blur produced when using detail screens and a 1-mm focal spot. With this combination, the focal spot is the predominant blur source for most object locations.

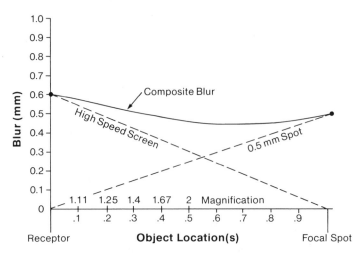

Figure 19-12 Blur Produced by High Speed Screens and a 0.5-mm Focal Spot

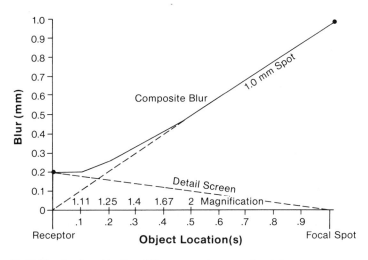

Figure 19-13 Blur Produced by Detail Screens and a 1-mm Focal Spot

These two examples show how either the receptor or the focal spot can be the predominant source of blur in a specific radiographic system. The dominating blur source is determined by the relationship of receptor blur to focal spot size and the location of the object; these are the factors that must be considered when setting up a radiographic system.

Chapter 20

Fluoroscopic Imaging Systems

INTRODUCTION AND OVERVIEW

The fluoroscope produces an instantaneous and continuous image that is especially useful for guiding a procedure, searching through a body section, or observing a dynamic function. Fluoroscopic examinations began soon after the discovery of x-radiation. Since that time, however, the fluoroscopic imaging system has undergone several major changes that have improved image quality, reduced patient exposure, and provided much more flexibility and ease of use.

The receptor for the first-generation fluoroscope was a flat fluorescent screen, which intercepted the x-ray beam as it emerged from the patient's body. The x-ray beam carrying the invisible image was absorbed by the fluorescent material and converted into a light image. In fact, it is the fluorescent screen receptor that gives the name "fluoroscopy" to the procedure.

Under normal operating conditions, the image had a relatively low brightness level. Because of the low light intensity, it was usually necessary to conduct examinations in a darkened room with the eyes dark-adapted by wearing red goggles or remaining in the dark for approximately 20 minutes. The contrast sensitivity and visibility of detail were significantly less than what can be achieved with contemporary fluoroscopic systems.

The first major advancement was the introduction of the image intensifier tube. The intensifier tube produces a much brighter image than the fluorescent screen, and its images can be viewed in a lighted room. The quality of the image produced by the intensifier tube was generally an improvement over the fluoroscopic screen image. An examination was performed by viewing the image from the intensifier tube through a system of mirrors. The viewing was generally limited to one person unless a special attachment was used.

The next step in the evolution of the fluoroscope was the introduction of a video (TV) system to transfer the image from the output of the image intensifier tube to a large screen.

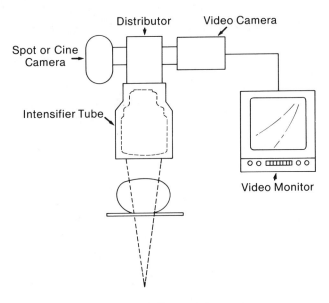

Figure 20-1 Components of a Fluoroscopic Receptor System

The receptor system of a contemporary fluoroscope is shown in Figure 20-1. It consists of an image intensifier tube, an optical image distribution system, and a closed-circuit video system containing a camera, monitor, and associated electronics. A spot film or cine camera is often included as part of the receptor system.

INTENSIFIER TUBES

In any x-ray imaging process, it is necessary to convert the invisible x-ray image into a visible image. There are two major reasons for this conversion: A light image can be visualized by the human eye, and film is generally more sensitive to light than it is to x-radiation. We have already seen that certain fluorescent materials are used in intensifying screens to convert the x-rays into light images. Although intensifying screens are used in a wide range of radiographic applications, the brightness of the light produced by the screen is relatively low. The brightness is sufficient to expose film placed in direct contact with the screen, but the light output is generally too low for direct visualization, photographing with a camera (cine or spot film), or viewing with a television camera. In many applications, a device is needed that will convert the x-ray into light and intensify, or increase the brightness of, the light in the process. The image intensifier tube is such a device.

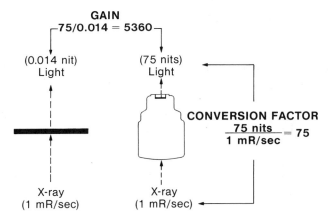

Figure 20-2 Gain Characteristics of an Image Intensifier Tube

Before considering the details of intensifier tube function, let us compare its overall function to that of a fluorescent screen, shown in Figure 20-2. The tube is exposed to the x-ray beam, and light is emitted from the other end. One of the important characteristics of a specific intensifier tube is its ability to produce a bright light image.

Gain

Gain is one factor used to describe the ability of a tube to produce a bright image. As illustrated in Figure 20-2, the gain value of a specific tube is the ratio of its light brightness to that of a reference fluorescent screen receiving the same x-ray exposure. Contemporary intensifier tubes have gains of 5,000 or more.

Conversion Factor

A factor that is easier to measure, especially in the clinical setting, is the conversion factor. The conversion factor of a specific tube is the ratio of the output light brightness to the input x-ray exposure rate. Gain and conversion factor are merely two terms used to describe the same general characteristic of an intensifier tube: its ability to convert an x-ray exposure into a bright image. The approximate relationship between the gain value and the conversion factor value is

$$\text{Gain} = 70 \times \text{Conversion factor.}$$

The brightness of the light from the intensifier tube is several thousand times brighter than from a fluorescent screen. This is achieved in two ways.

A fluorescent screen is a passive device that converts a portion of the absorbed x-ray energy into light energy. On the other hand, an image intensifier tube is an active device that adds energy to the process. This additional energy enters the tube in the form of electrical energy from a high-voltage energy source.

The second factor that contributes to the increase in image brightness, or intensity, is the minification of the image as it passes through the tube. The output light image from an intensifier tube appears on a small screen with a diameter of approximately 1 in. The input field of view of the intensifier tube generally has a diameter in the range of 4 in. to 14 in. The maximum input image size is determined by the size of the tube. Tubes can be adjusted to receive input images smaller than the tube diameter. The amount of minification gain is the ratio of the areas of the input image to the output image.

The method by which electrical energy is used to intensify the image is illustrated in Figure 20-3. The intensifier tube body is essentially an evacuated glass bottle. The large area forming the bottom of the bottle is the input screen, and the small area that forms the "cap" on the bottle is the output screen.

The input surface, or screen, of the intensifier tube is in two layers. The first layer encountered by the x-ray beam is a fluorescent material, typically cesium iodide. In direct contact with the fluorescent screen is a layer of material that functions as a photocathode.

The x-ray photons entering the tube are absorbed by the fluorescent input screen. A portion of the absorbed energy is converted into light. Since light photons contain much less energy than x-ray photons, one x-ray photon can

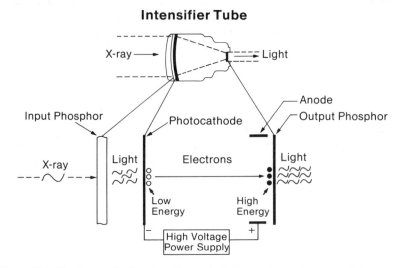

Figure 20-3 The Events that Produce Electronic Gain in an Image Intensifier Tube

produce a light flash consisting of many light photons. The light photons are, in turn, absorbed by the photocathode layer by the photoelectric process, which results in the emission of electrons into the tube. At this point, the electrons possess very little kinetic energy.

The intensifier tube is connected to an electrical energy source (power supply) that applies a relatively high voltage between the cathode surface and an anode located near the output end of the tube. The electrical energy accelerates the cluster of electrons toward the output end of the tube where they strike the output screen. The output screen absorbs the electron energy and converts it into a relatively bright flash of light.

In a simple fluorescent screen, the x-ray energy is converted directly into light energy. In the intensifier tube three steps are added to the process. These are:

1. Transferring energy from light to electrons in the photocathode
2. Adding electrical energy to the electrons
3. Converting electron energy back to light within the output screen.

These additional steps are necessary to add energy, or intensify the image. It is not possible to increase the energy of photons. It is possible, however, to increase the energy of electrons. The result of this process is that an x-ray photon can produce a much brighter light at the output of an intensifier tube than in a fluorescent screen.

Along the length of the tube is a series of electrodes that focus the electron image onto the output screen. The voltage applied to the focusing electrodes can be switched to change the size of the input image, or field of view, as shown in Figure 20-4. The maximum field of view is determined by the diameter of the tube.

In most tubes, the input image area can be electrically reduced. When the tube is switched from one mode to another, the factors that change include field of view, image quality, and receptor sensitivity (exposure). The tube should be operated in the large field mode when maximum field of view is the primary consideration. In this mode, the tube has the highest gain and requires the lowest exposure because the minification gain is proportional to the area of the input image. The small field mode is used primarily to enhance image quality. As an image passes through an intensifier tube, its quality is usually reduced.

Contrast

We know that the contrast in an image delivered to the film is reduced by both object penetration and scattered radiation. When image intensifier tubes are used, there is an additional loss of contrast because of events taking place within the tube. Some of the radiation that penetrates the input screen can be absorbed by the output screen and can produce an effect similar to scattered radiation. Also, some

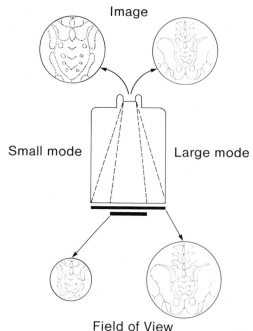

Figure 20-4 A Dual-Mode (FOV) Image Intensifier Tube

of the light produced in the output screen travels back to the photocathode and causes electrons to be emitted. These electrons are accelerated to the output screen where they contribute additional exposure to the image area and further reduce contrast. The contrast reduction in modern intensifier tubes is generally in the range of 5 to 15%.

Blur

There are several potential sources of blur within the system. The spreading of light in the input and output screens of the image intensifier tube produces blur as it does in intensifying screens. In many image intensifier tubes, both screens are significant sources of blur. Actually, the blur in the output screen is quite small and becomes significant only when it is referred back to the input screen. The minification of the image within the tube has the effect of magnifying the blur of most image intensifier tubes so that blur increases with the size of the input image. With dual-mode tubes, the larger field generally produces more blur than the smaller field. In most tubes, the blur varies over the image area; it is generally the smallest near the center of the field and increases toward the periphery.

Blur is also produced by improper focusing of the electrons in the tube. Most intensifier systems have controls that can adjust the electron focus.

Noise

The problem of quantum noise in intensified systems is discussed in Chapter 21. If it were not for the limitations of quantum noise, modern intensifier systems could operate at much lower input exposure values.

VIDEO SYSTEMS

The primary function of a video system is to transfer an image from one location to another. During the transfer process, certain image characteristics, such as size, brightness, and contrast, can be changed. However, as an image passes through a video system, there can be a loss of quality, especially in the form of blur and loss of detail visibility.

Video Principles

The two major components of a video system are the camera and the monitor, or receiver. Conventional broadcast television systems transmit the image from the camera to the receiver by means of radio frequency (RF) radiation. In a closed circuit system, the image is transmitted between the two devices by means of electrical conductors or cables. However, other than for the means of image transmission, the basic principles of the two systems are essentially the same.

A basic video system is illustrated in Figure 20-5, which shows the major functional components contained in the camera and the monitor. The ''heart'' of each is an electronic tube that converts the image into an electrical signal or vice versa.

The function of the camera tube is to convert the light image into an electronic signal. Broadcast television systems use camera tubes known as image orthicons. Fluoroscopic systems generally use either vidicon or plumbicon tubes; they are smaller and less complex than image orthicons. They also require brighter input images, but this is not a problem in fluoroscopy. The significant difference between the vidicon and plumbicon is one of image persistence, or lag.

The typical camera tube is cylindrical with a diameter of approximately 25 mm and a length of 15 cm. The image to be transmitted is projected onto the input screen of the tube by a lens like that in a conventional film camera. The other end of the tube contains a heated cathode and other electrodes that form an electron gun. The electron gun shoots a small beam of electrons down the length of the evacuated tube. The electron beam strikes the rear of the screen surface on which the input image is projected.

Electrical signals are applied to the camera tube, which causes the electron beam to be swept over the surface of the input screen. One signal moves the beam

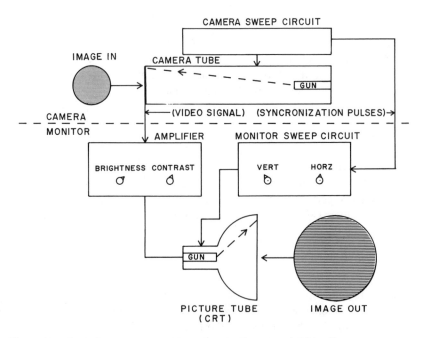

Figure 20-5 Basic Components and Function of a Fluoroscopic Video System

in a horizontal direction, and the other signal moves it vertically. The two signals are synchronized so that they work together to move the beam in a specific pattern. Although the input screen is round, the area covered by the scanning electron beam is generally rectangular. The beam begins in the upper left-hand corner and moves across the screen horizontally, as shown in Figure 20-6. In the conventional American 525-line video system, lines are scanned at the rate of 15,750 per second. When the beam reaches the right-hand side, it is quickly "snapped back" to the left and deflected downward by approximately one beam width. It then sweeps across to form a second scan line. This process is repeated until the beam reaches the bottom of the screen, which usually requires 1/60th of a second. After reaching the bottom, the beam returns to the top and resumes the scanning process. This time, however, the scan lines are slightly displaced with respect to the first set so that they fall between the lines created in the first scan field. This is known as interlacing.

Interlacing is used to prevent flicker in the picture. If all lines were scanned consecutively, it would take twice as long (1/30th of a second) for the beam to reach the bottom of the screen. This delay would be detectable by the human eye and would appear as flicker. With interlacing, the face of the screen is scanned in two sets of lines, or fields. The pattern of scan lines produced in a video system is

INTERLACED SCAN

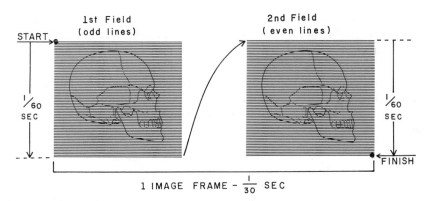

Figure 20-6 An Interlaced Scan Format

known as raster. The conventional video system is generally set to contain 525 lines. The raster, however, contains approximately 485 lines. The remaining lines are lost during the return of the electron beam to the left side of the screen. In a 525-line system, 30 complete raster frames (60 fields) are formed per second.

The screen of the camera tube is made of a material with light-sensitive electrical properties. Several types of tubes are used, but the general concept of tube function can be described as follows.

The electrical conductivity of the screen surface depends on its illumination. When an image is projected onto the screen, the conductivity varies from point to point. A dark area is essentially nonconductive, and a brightly illuminated area is the most conductive. As the electron beam sweeps over the surface, it encounters areas with various levels of conductivity, which depend on the brightness at each point. When the beam strikes a bright spot, it is "conducted through" and creates a relatively high signal voltage at the output terminal of the tube. As the spot moves across the screen, it creates a signal that represents the brightness of the image at each point along its path.

The heart of the receiver, or monitor, is the picture tube. The picture tube differs from the camera tube in size and shape. One end of the tube is the screen on which the video image is displayed. Like the camera tube, the picture tube has an electron gun located in the end opposite to the screen. The electron gun produces a beam of electrons that strike the rear of the screen in the picture tube. The electron beam scans the surface of the picture tube screen just as it scans the camera tube screen. In fact, the scanning in the two tubes is synchronized by a signal transmitted from the camera to the monitor. If the scanning becomes unsynchronized, the image will roll in the vertical direction or become distorted horizontally. The horizontal and vertical controls on a video monitor are used to adjust the scan rates so that they are identical with those of the camera and can maintain synchronization.

When the electron beam in the picture tube strikes the screen, it produces a bright spot. The brightness of the spot is determined by the number of electrons in the beam, which is controlled by the signal from the camera tube. In other words, the brightness of a spot on the picture tube screen is determined by the brightness of the corresponding point on the camera tube screen. As the two electron beams scan the two screens, the image is transferred from the camera tube to the picture tube. In the 525-line system, complete images are transferred at the rate of 30 per second.

Contrast

In the typical video system, image contrast can be changed by adjusting a control located in the monitor. The contrast control changes the amplification of the video signal. The brightness of each point within the image on the picture tube screen is determined by the voltage of the video signal associated with the point. The contrast of an image on the screen is the brightness difference between two points, such as background and object area, and is determined by the voltage difference in the video signal for the two areas. When a video signal is amplified, the voltage difference between two points is increased. This, in turn, produces a larger difference in brightness, or more contrast. At first, it might appear that amplification of the video signals not only increases contrast, but also produces a brighter image. Most circuits are designed, however, so that changing the contrast control does not appreciably change the average signal level. The average video signal level is changed by adjusting the brightness control.

Although the contrast and brightness controls are essentially separate and independent, they must generally be adjusted together for optimum image quality. The typical picture tube has a maximum brightness level that cannot be exceeded, regardless of the value of the incoming video signal. If the average signal level is pushed toward this upper limit by turning up the brightness control, contrast will generally decrease. This is because the bright (white) areas have reached a limiting value, and the darker areas are increasing in brightness. Since the bright areas cannot increase above the maximum limit, the contrast between the two areas is reduced.

Blur

One generally undesirable characteristic of a video imaging system is that it introduces blur into the image. One source produces blur in the vertical direction, and the other in the horizontal. Although the blur values can be different for the

Image on
Camera Tube

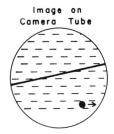

Image on
Picture Tube

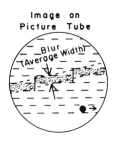

Figure 20-7 Vertical Blur Produced by Scan Lines

two directions, the overall image quality is usually best when they are approximately equal.

Vertical Blur

Vertical blur is caused by the finite size of the electron beam and the scan lines. The effect of vertical blur is illustrated in Figure 20-7. If a small-line-type object is oriented at a slight angle to the scan lines, the images of the object will appear to be wider because of blur. At any instant, the width of a line in the image cannot be less than the width of one scan line. An object is normally not perfectly aligned with a single scan line. Therefore, the width of the image of the line is slightly larger than the width of a single scan line. The approximate relationship between blur (image line width), Bv, and scan line width, w, is given by

$$Bv = 1.4 \, w.$$

The width of a scan line, w, is, in turn, related to the vertical field of view (FOV) and the number of actual scan lines. These factors can be incorporated into the relationship above to give the following:

$$Bv = 1.4 \, FOV/n$$

where FOV is the vertical dimension of the image, and n is the number of useful scan lines within that dimension. For an image containing a given number of scan lines, vertical blur is directly proportional to the dimension of the image, or FOV. Where within the system is the image dimension determined? Should it be on the monitor screen, at the camera tube, or at some other point? The appropriate location for determining image size is in the plane through the object being imaged, as illustrated in Figure 20-8.

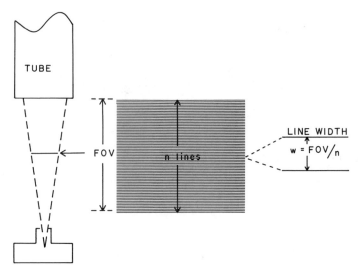

Figure 20-8 The Factors that Affect Line Width and Vertical Detail in a Video Image

The blur value determined by using this image dimension is properly scaled to the size of the object and can be easily compared to blur values for the focal spot and receptor. In the plane of the object, the image diameter, FOV, is equal to the FOV of the image at the input to the image intensifier divided by the geometric magnification factor, m. Substitution of this expression for image size gives an expression for image blur that is related to three specific factors:

$$Bv = 1.4 \text{ FOV (image tube)}/nm.$$

Special attention is called to the fact that video blur is directly proportional to the FOV at the input to the image intensifier tube, as illustrated in Figure 20-9. A small FOV produces better detail. For example, assume that a system has 485 useful lines and a magnification factor, m, of 1.2. For a 15-cm (6-in.) input image size, the blur is 0.36 mm. If the image size is switched to 23 cm (9 in.), the blur will increase to 0.55 mm. When the size of the image at the input of the image intensifier is increased, the video lines are spread over a larger object area. Since the number of lines is not changed, the width of the lines must increase. Since blur is directly related to line width, it is obvious that it must increase with an increase in image size.

Blur can be decreased by increasing the number of lines used to form the video image. Figure 20-10 illustrates two of the most common video formats used in fluoroscopy. Most are classified as 525-line systems. In special applications that require more image detail, 1,050-line systems are used.

SMALL FIELD OF VIEW   LARGE FIELD OF VIEW

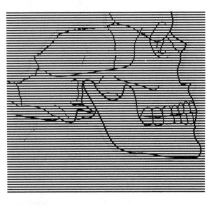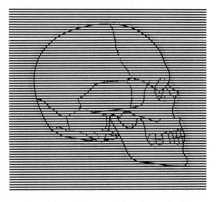

Figure 20-9 Improvement in Image Detail Using a Small Field of View

525 LINES   1050 LINES

Figure 20-10 Improvement in Image Detail by Increasing the Number of Scan Lines

Horizontal Blur

Blur in the horizontal direction is determined by the response time of the electronic circuitry through which the video signal passes in going from the camera to the picture tube. The response time of a video circuit is generally specified in terms of a frequency bandwidth. The bandwidth is in the units of megahertz (MHz). In most cases, the bandwidth can be readily changed by the circuit designer and is usually the factor used to adjust the horizontal blur value. In most systems, the horizontal blur is adjusted to be approximately equal to the vertical blur. There is probably no advantage in having significantly more or less blur in one direction than the other.

Noise

The two types of noise in a fluoroscopic system are electronic and quantum. Electronic noise produces "snow," which is familiar to most television viewers. It is usually significant only when the video signals are extremely weak. Since signal strength is not a problem in the typical closed circuit video system, the presence of significant "snow" or electronic noise usually indicates problems within the video system.

Quantum noise depends on the number of photons used to form the image. The number of photons involved in image formation is directly related to the receptor input exposure. The input exposure, for a specific image brightness, can be adjusted by changing the automatic brightness control circuit reference level, as discussed in Chapter 21. An input exposure rate of approximately 0.025 mR/sec (1.5 mR/min) is usually required to reduce quantum noise to an acceptable level in fluoroscopy.

The noise level is related to the total number of photons used to form an image, not the rate. The human eye has an effective "collection" time of approximately 0.2 seconds. In some video systems, the time during which photons are collected to form an image is longer because of the persistence, or lag, inherent in the camera tube. Vidicon tubes generally have more lag than plumbicons. Because of this, they average photons over a longer period of time and produce less quantum noise for the same input exposure rate.

THE OPTICAL SYSTEM AND CAMERAS

An optical system is used to transfer the image from the output screen of the intensifier tube to the input screen of the video camera tube or to the film in the spot or cine camera. The components of the total optical system are contained in the image distributor and the individual cameras, as shown in Figure 20-11, and are lenses, apertures, and mirrors. Before we consider the operation of the optical system, we will review the basic characteristics of two of these components, lenses and apertures.

Lens

A lens is the basic element that can transfer an image from one location to another. The curvature of the lens focuses the light that passes through the lens.

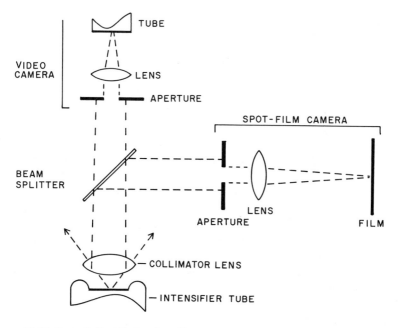

Figure 20-11 Basic Optical System for a Fluoroscope

A fundamental characteristic of a lens is its focal length, which expresses its focusing power. The focal length is the distance between the lens and the point at which all parallel light rays that enter the lens are brought together, or focused. The focal length is determined by the curvature of the lens and is typically expressed in millimeters. The focal length of eye-glasses is expressed in the units of diopters, which is the reciprocal of the actual focal length in meters. For example, a 2-diopter lens has a focal length of 50 cm.

The focal length of a lens is a major factor in determining the size of an image projected onto a film or screen.

Aperture

Another important characteristic of a lens is its size (diameter, or aperture). This determines the amount of light that is captured by the lens. This, in turn, affects the efficiency of light transfer through the optical system and the exposure to film in the camera. Actually, the factor that determines the efficiency of a lens is the ratio of its size to its focal length, which is generally expressed in terms of the f number, which is

f number = focal length of lens/diameter of lens.

It should be noted that the f number is inversely related to the diameter of the lens. In other words, as the size of the lens is increased, the value of the f number is decreased. The efficiency of a lens is given by

$$\text{Efficiency} = 1/4 \, f^2.$$

Certain f number values are commonly used and correspond to the different multiples of two of the lens areas. This relationship between f number and relative lens area is shown in Table 20-1.

The difference between any two adjacent standard f numbers is referred to as one stop. A change of one stop corresponds to changing the relative area, or efficiency, of the lens (and film exposure) by a factor of two.

In many applications, it is desirable to adjust the aperture size, or light-gathering efficiency, of a lens. This is accomplished by covering a portion of the lens with a circular mask with a hole in the center. In conventional photographic cameras, the aperture can usually be adjusted to different sizes. In many radiographic systems, the size of the aperture is changed by replacing one mask (aperture) with another.

Image Distributor

When intensifying screens are used in radiography, the light is transferred directly to the film because the film is in direct contact with the screen. This results in a film image that is the same size as the image from the intensifying screen. The output image from the typical intensifying tube, however, is only about 20 mm in diameter and must be enlarged before it is applied to the film. In order to be enlarged, the film must be separated from the output screen. The transfer of the image from the image intensifier output to the film surface is the main function of the optical system. If only one camera is to be used, it will be a relatively simple

Table 20-1 Standard f Number Values and Relative Lens Areas

f number	Relative lens area (efficiency)
16	1
11	2
8	4
5.6	8
4	16
2.8	32
2.0	64
1.4	128
1.0	256

process to mount the camera so that it views the image from the intensifier tube. With many fluoroscopic systems, however, it is desirable to transfer the image to spot film or cine cameras in addition to the video camera. This is the function of the part of the optical system known as the image distributor.

Collimator Lens

The first component of the optical system encountered by the light from the intensifier output screen is the collimator lens. Its function is to collect the light from the output screen and focus it into a beam of parallel light rays, as shown in Figure 20-11. The parallel rays are produced by positioning the lens so that the image intensifier screen is located near the focal point of the lens. One of the fundamental characteristics of a converging lens is that light originating at its focal point forms a beam of parallel rays after passing through the lens. Light originating from points at distances other than the focal length from the lens forms into either a diverging or converging beam after passing through the lens. The formation of the image into a parallel beam makes it possible to distribute the image to two or more devices, such as a spot film camera and a video camera, for fluoroscopy.

Mirrors

The next element in the path of the light is a beam splitter. A splitter is usually a mirror that is only partially reflective. A portion of the light is reflected by the mirror to one camera. The remaining light passes through the mirror to a second camera. In some systems, the mirror is attached to a rotating mechanism so that it can be shifted from one camera to another. The mirrors are generally designed to divide the light unevenly between two devices. For example, a 70-30 mirror sends 70% of the light to a film camera and 30% to a video camera to form the fluoroscopic image.

Vignetting

A potential problem with a two-lens optical system is vignetting. Vignetting is the loss of film exposure around the periphery of the image. Light that leaves a point near the center of the intensifier output screen passes through the collimator lens and forms a beam that is parallel to the axis running through the two lenses. Light that originates from points near the periphery of the image also passes through the collimator lens but is projected in a beam that is not parallel to the axis. In order for a camera lens to capture light from the periphery of the image, it must be located in an area where the beams overlap. Vignetting usually occurs when the camera lens is mounted too far from the collimator, or the camera lens is too large to be contained in the overlap area. Since the effective diameter of the camera lens is often determined by the size of the aperture, changing the aperture setting to a larger value (smaller f number) might introduce vignetting.

Camera

After passing through the aperture, a second lens focuses the light onto the surface of the film to form the final image. This lens is part of the camera and serves the same function as a conventional camera lens. The most significant characteristic of this lens is its focal length.

Image Size and Framing

The amount of enlargement, or magnification, in the image between the image intensifier output and the film is given by:

Magnification (m) = focal length of camera lens/focal length of collimator lens.

The camera lens must be selected to give the desired image size on the film, as shown in Figure 20-12. Four film sizes are generally used in intensified radiography: 35 mm, 70 mm, 90 mm, and 105 mm. These are the dimensions of the film. The size of the image area is somewhat less because of sprocket holes and borders. For example, 35-mm film typically has an image area of 25 mm × 18 mm. The image at the intensifier output screen is circular, but all films have either square or rectangular image areas. Because of this, it is impossible to get exact coverage on the film.

For a given film size, it is possible to obtain different degrees of coverage, or framing. With underframing, all of the image appears on the film but is circular; the corners of the film area are not exposed. On the other hand, with overframing, all of the film is used, but some portions of the image are lost.

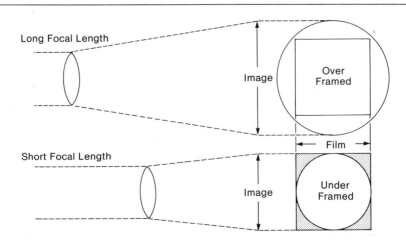

Figure 20-12 Relationship of Image and Film Size for Different Degrees of Framing

Unless the optical system is properly focused, it will also be a source of image blur. Both the collimator and camera lens can be out of focus. Proper focusing of the collimator lens requires special equipment and should be attempted only by qualified personnel.

Film Exposure

Only a fraction of the light emitted by the image intensifier reaches the film. The reasons for this are that the optical system does not capture all of the light, and a significant portion of the light is absorbed by the lenses and mirrors within the system or is stopped by the aperture. Only a fraction of light captured by the collimator lens and passed through the aperture reaches the film because of absorption in the lens. This fraction is typically about 0.8. If the light that reaches the film is spread over an area that is larger than the output screen, the intensity, but not the total number of light photons, will be reduced.

RECEPTOR SENSITIVITY

Fluoroscopy

The sensitivity during fluoroscopic operations is set by the equipment engineer through an adjustment of the video camera sensitivity or the video camera aperture. The sensitivity and exposure also change with the field of view (mode), as described above. The fluoroscope is most sensitive when operated with the maximum field of view. Increasing field of view increases sensitivity and decreases required exposure. Because the x-ray beam then covers more of the patient's body, however, the total radiation energy to the patient is not significantly reduced.

Some fluoroscopic systems have a control that allows the operator to change the sensitivity. This is used to control the level of quantum noise in the fluoroscopic image. The low sensitivity (low noise) settings are used to improve visibility in certain demanding procedures, such as angioplasty.

Radiography

The overall sensitivity of an intensified radiography receptor system depends on three major factors: (1) the gain or conversion factor of the image tube, (2) the efficiency of the optical system, and (3) the sensitivity of the film. The input exposure increases as the square of the magnification, which is, in effect, the film image size. If all other factors remain unchanged, four times as much x-ray exposure will be required if the film size is doubled. This is because doubling the size (diameter) of the film increases the image area by a factor of 4.

Image size usually changes twice in an intensified system. The image is reduced, or minified, in the image intensifier and then magnified in the optical system. Minification increases image intensity, whereas magnification produces a decrease. Much of the gain in the image intensifier tube obtained from minification will be lost if the image is remagnified on the film. In fact, if the film size is the same as the input phosphor size, these two factors will cancel each other.

Within a given system, the receptor sensitivity can usually be changed by adjusting the aperture. If the film is changed to one with a different sensitivity, the aperture can be used to compensate for the change and to maintain the same receptor sensitivity, if desired. The aperture is also used to compensate for image intensifier tubes with different conversion factors.

The two factors used by the equipment engineer to set the sensitivity level are the film sensitivity and the aperture of the camera lens. The gain (conversion factor) of the intensifier tube has a major effect on overall receptor sensitivity. The only way the gain of the specific tube can be changed is by changing the field of view, or mode of a multi-mode tube. Tube gain, and therefore receptor sensitivity, is proportional to the area of the field of view. Therefore, a tube operating in a large field mode is more sensitive and requires less radiation exposure than when it is operated in the small field mode. The sensitivity is usually set in relationship to the size of the film being used. In general, maximum sensitivity (minimum exposure) is obtained with the smallest film size.

Chapter 21

Image Noise

INTRODUCTION AND OVERVIEW

It is generally desirable for film density, or image brightness, to be uniform except where it changes to form an image. There are factors, however, that tend to produce variation in film density even when no image detail is present. This variation is usually random and has no particular pattern. In many cases, it reduces image quality and is especially significant when the objects being imaged are small and have relatively low contrast. This random variation in film density, or image brightness, is designated *noise*.

All medical images contain some visual noise. The presence of noise gives an image a mottled, grainy, textured, or snowy appearance. Figure 21-1 compares two images with different levels of noise. Image noise comes from a variety of sources, as we will soon discover. No imaging method is free of noise, but noise is much more prevalent in certain types of imaging procedures than in others.

Nuclear images are generally the most noisy. Noise is also significant in MRI, CT, and ultrasound imaging. In comparison to these, radiography produces images with the least noise. Fluoroscopic images are slightly more noisy than radiographic images, for reasons explained later. Conventional photography produces relatively noise-free images except where the grain of the film becomes visible.

In this chapter we consider some of the general characteristics of image noise along with the specific factors in radiography and fluoroscopy that affect noise.

EFFECT ON VISIBILITY

Although noise gives an image a generally undesirable appearance, the most significant factor is that noise can cover and reduce the visibility of certain features within the image. The loss of visibility is especially significant for low-contrast

Figure 21-1 Comparison of Radiographic Images with High and Low Noise Levels

objects. The general effect of noise on object visibility was described in Chapter 1 and illustrated in Figure 1-7. The visibility threshold, especially for low-contrast objects, is very noise dependent. In principle, when we reduce image noise, the "curtain" is raised somewhat, and more of the low-contrast objects within the body become visible.

If the noise level can be adjusted for a specific imaging procedure, then why not reduce it to its lowest possible level for maximum visibility? Although it is true that we can usually change imaging factors to reduce noise, we must always compromise. In x-ray imaging, the primary compromise is with patient exposure; in MRI and nuclear imaging, the primary compromise is with imaging time. There are also compromises between noise and other image characteristics, such as contrast and blur. In principle, the user of each imaging method must determine the acceptable level of noise for a specific procedure and then select imaging factors that will achieve it with minimum exposure, imaging time, or effect on other image quality characteristics.

QUANTUM NOISE

X-ray photons impinge on a surface in a random pattern. No force can cause them to be evenly distributed over the surface. One area of the receptor surface might receive more photons than another area, even when both are exposed to the same average x-ray intensity.

In all imaging procedures using x-ray or gamma photons, most of the image noise is produced by the random manner in which the photons are distributed within the image. This is generally designated *quantum noise*. Recall that each individual photon is a quantum (specific quantity) of energy. It is the quantum structure of an x-ray beam that creates quantum noise.

Let us use Figure 21-2 to refresh our concept of the quantum nature of radiation to see how it produces image noise. Here we see the part of an x-ray beam that forms the exposure to one small area within an image. Remember that an x-ray beam is a shower of individual photons. Because the photons are independent, they are randomly distributed within an image area somewhat like the first few drops of rain falling on the ground. At some points there might be clusters of several photons (drops) and, also, areas where only a few photons are collected. This uneven distribution of photons shows up in the image as noise. The amount of noise is determined by the variation in photon concentration from point to point within a small image area.

Fortunately we can control, to some extent, the photon fluctuation and the resulting image noise. Figure 21-2 shows two 1-mm square image areas that are subdivided into nine smaller square areas. The difference between the two areas is the concentration of photons (radiation exposure) falling within the area. The first has an average of 100 photons per small square, and the second a concentration of 1,000 photons per small square. For a typical diagnostic x-ray beam, this is equivalent to receptor exposures of approximately 3.6 μR and 36 μR, respectively.

Notice that in the first large area none of the smaller areas has exactly 100 photons. In this situation, the number of photons per area ranges from a low of 89 photons to a high of 114 photons. We will not, however, use these two extreme values as a measure of photon fluctuation. Because most of the small areas have photon concentrations much closer to the average value, it is more appropriate to express the photon variation in terms of the standard deviation. The standard deviation is a quantity often used in statistical analysis (see Chapter 31) to express the amount of spread, or variation, among quantities. The value of the standard deviation is somewhat like the "average" amount of deviation, or variation, among the small areas. One of the characteristics of photon distribution is that the amount of fluctuation (standard deviation value) is related to the average photon concentration, or exposure level. The square root of the average number of photons per area provides a close estimate for the value of the standard deviation.

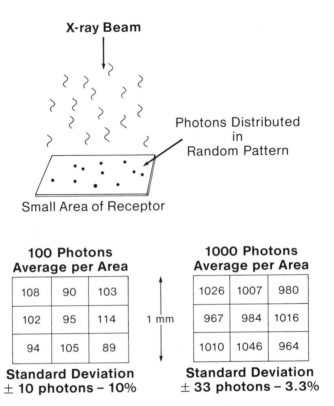

Figure 21-2 The Concept of Quantum Noise

In this example the standard deviation has a value of ten photons per area. Since this is 10% of the average value, the quantum noise (photon fluctuation) at this exposure has a value of 10%.

Let us now consider the image area on the right, which received an average of 1,000 photons per area. In this example, we also find that none of the small areas received exactly 1,000 photons. In this case, the photon concentrations range from 964 photons to 1,046 photons per area. Taking the square root of the average photon concentration (1,000) gives a standard deviation value of 33.3 photons. It appears we have an even higher photon fluctuation, or noise, than in the other area. However, when we express the standard deviation as a percentage of the average photon concentration, we find that the noise level has actually dropped to 3.3%.

We have just observed what is perhaps the most important characteristic of quantum noise: It can be reduced by increasing the concentration of photons (ie, exposure) used to form an image. More specifically, quantum noise is inversely proportional to the square root of the exposure to the receptor.

The relationship between image noise and required exposure is one of the issues that must be considered by persons setting up specific x-ray procedures. In most situations, patient exposure can be reduced, but at the expense of increased quantum noise and, possibly, reduced visibility. It is also possible, in most situations, to decrease image noise, but a higher exposure would be required. Most x-ray procedures are conducted at a point of reasonable compromise between these two very important factors.

RECEPTOR SENSITIVITY

The photon concentration, or exposure, that is required to form an image is determined by the sensitivity of the receptor. The sensitivities of the receptors used in x-ray projection imaging (radiography and fluoroscopy) vary over a considerable range, as shown in Figure 21-3. This chart shows the approximate values used for specific imaging applications.

Screen-Film Radiography

The sensitivity of a radiographic receptor (cassette) is determined by characteristics of the screen and the film and the way they are matched. The factors that affect receptor sensitivity do not necessarily alter the quantum noise characteristics of the receptor. The major factors that affect radiographic receptor sensitivity are film sensitivity, screen conversion efficiency, and screen absorption efficiency. The quantum noise level is determined by the concentration of photons actually absorbed by the receptor, rather than the concentration of photons

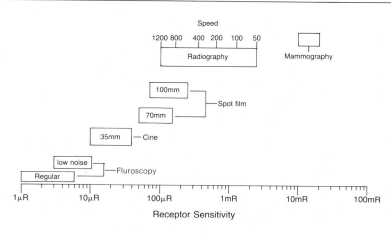

Figure 21-3 Receptor Sensitivity Values Used in X-Ray Imaging

delivered to it. Increasing receptor sensitivity by changing any factor that decreases the number of photons actually absorbed will increase the quantum noise.

The receptor exposure required to form an image (receptor sensitivity) can be changed by modifying several factors, as indicated in Figure 21-4. Film sensitivity, which is shown to the right in the illustration, determines the amount of light required to produce the desired film density. If film sensitivity is increased to reduce the amount of light required, this, in turn, will reduce the number of x-ray photons that must be absorbed in the screen. The result would be an image with increased quantum noise. Recall that the effective sensitivity of a particular film and screen combination depends on the matching of the spectral sensitivity characteristics of the film to the spectral characteristics of the light produced by the screen. When the two characteristics are closely matched, maximum sensitivity and maximum quantum noise are produced. In radiography, changing the film sensitivity (ie, changing type of film) is the most direct way to adjust the quantum noise level in images. Quantum noise is usually the factor that limits the use of highly sensitive film in radiography.

Conversion efficiency is the characteristic of an intensifying screen that is, in effect, the fraction of absorbed x-ray energy actually converted into light. The conversion efficiency value for a particular screen is determined by its composition and design. It cannot be changed by the user. In principle, a high conversion efficiency increases receptor sensitivity and reduces patient exposure. Unfortu-

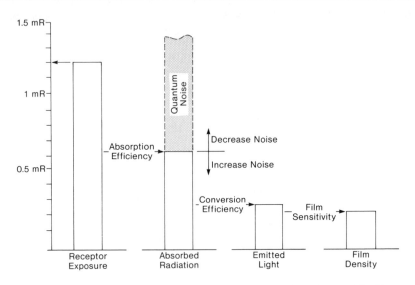

Figure 21-4 Relationship of Radiation Quantities Within an Intensifying Screen-Film Receptor

nately, an increase in conversion efficiency decreases the quantity of x-radiation that must be absorbed in the screen, and this, in turn, increases quantum noise. Therefore, a high conversion efficiency is not always a desirable characteristic for intensifying screens. It should be adjusted by the manufacturer to a value that produces a proper balance between receptor sensitivity and quantum noise.

The only way to increase radiographic receptor sensitivity without increasing quantum noise is to increase the absorption efficiency. An increase in absorption efficiency does not change the amount of radiation that must be absorbed to produce an image. It does, however, reduce the required incident exposure since a greater proportion of the radiation is absorbed.

Recall that several factors determine absorption efficiency; namely, screen composition, screen thickness, and photon energy spectrum. The relationship between radiographic receptor sensitivity and quantum noise can be summarized as follows. The amount of quantum noise in a properly exposed image is directly related to the amount of x-ray energy actually absorbed in the intensifying screen. Changing factors, such as type of screen material, screen thickness, and KV_p (photon energy spectrum), that affect absorption efficiency will alter the overall receptor sensitivity in relation to the quantum noise level. On the other hand, changing film sensitivity, spectral matching, and the conversion efficiency of the intensifying screen generally changes quantum noise and receptor sensitivity.

Two screen-film combinations with the same sensitivity are shown in Figure 21-5. One system uses a relatively thick high-speed screen and a film with conventional sensitivity. The other system uses a thinner detail-speed screen and a more sensitive film. The images produced by these two systems differ in two respects. The system using the thicker screen has more blur but less quantum noise than the system using the more sensitive film. The reduction in noise comes from the increases in absorption efficiency and blur.

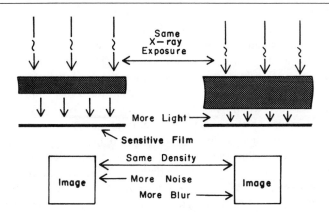

Figure 21-5 Comparison of Image Quality Between Two Screen-Film Combinations

Intensified Radiography

Quantum noise is sometimes more significant in intensified radiography (cine and spot films) than in screen-film radiography because of generally higher receptor sensitivity values (ie, lower receptor exposures). With such systems, the quantum noise level can be adjusted.

Absorption efficiency of image intensifier tubes has gradually improved over the years. Like intensifying screens, absorption efficiency depends on the composition of the input screen, its thickness, and the photon energy spectrum. However, a manufacturer generally does not offer choices. Most modern intensifier tubes have input screens designed to provide a reasonable compromise between absorption efficiency (sensitivity) and image blur.

The variations in intensifier tube–receptor system sensitivity are related to characteristics of the intensifier tube, the optical system, and the film. The gain (conversion factor) of an image intensifier tube cannot be adjusted by the user except by changing the input field of view (mode).

Changing the size of the optical aperture is the most common method of adjusting the receptor sensitivity and quantum noise level. This adjustment can usually be made in the clinical facility by a service engineer. The other factors associated with the optical system that affect overall receptor sensitivity, such as magnification (film size) and light transmission through the lens and distributor components, are not generally adjustable by the user and cannot be used to modify the quantum noise level.

The sensitivity of the film has a direct effect on the overall receptor system sensitivity. If the film is changed to one with a greater sensitivity, images can be produced with less x-radiation, but the amount of quantum noise will be increased. However, the aperture size can be decreased to compensate for the increase in film sensitivity and prevent an increase in noise.

Whenever film sensitivity or the aperture is changed, the AEC system must be readjusted to produce a properly exposed film.

The basic x-ray system illustrated in Figure 21-6 is used to illustrate how the input exposure to the image intensifier can be adjusted to obtain a specified quantum noise level. In most systems, the input to the AEC circuit is a light sensor that monitors the output of the image intensifier. The intensifier output luminance, or exposure (luminance multiplied by time), is electronically compared with a preestablished reference level. The output signal from the control circuit adjusts the x-ray machine exposure factors until the desired luminance, or exposure, is obtained. In most spot film and some cine systems, the KV_p and MA are preset, and the AEC circuit adjusts the exposure time to achieve proper film exposure. In some cine systems, the AEC circuit adjusts the KV_p, MA, or both, and the exposure time is preset. In some systems, the control circuit can adjust all three exposure factors. Generally, the time is changed within certain limits. If the

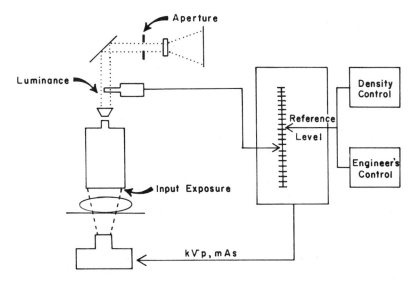

Figure 21-6 Factors that Determine the Input Exposure (and Quantum Noise) of an Intensified Radiography System

desired exposure is not obtained when time reaches a limit, either KV_p or MA will be changed.

The reference level for the luminance output of the intensifier is generally adjusted by two controls: the operator's control, which is used to adjust film density, and the engineer's control, which is used to set the approximate intensifier light output. This second control is usually located within the equipment and is not accessible to the equipment operator. The operator's control is essentially a fine adjustment of the engineer's control. For a given setting of the reference level, the AEC circuit produces a fixed value of intensifier input exposure. The readjustment of this reference level by means of the engineer's control is used to alter the input exposure and control quantum noise.

The reference level cannot be changed without making other adjustments, or film exposure will be incorrect. The relationship of film density to light output from the image intensifier is determined by the film sensitivity and the size of the aperture within the optical system. The aperture and reference level are usually adjusted together to obtain the desired film exposure and image intensifier input exposure.

Assume that a cine system is producing properly exposed films, but the quantum noise is considered to be too high. A measurement of the input exposure shows that it is 10 μR per frame. It might be desirable to increase this to at least 25 μR to reduce quantum noise. This can be achieved by changing the output light reference level to a higher value by means of the engineer's control. It is then necessary to reduce the size of the aperture to prevent the film from being overexposed.

In considering the image intensifier input exposure, the relationship between the size of the image intensifier input and film must be considered. In most systems, the size of the image on the film is less than the size of the image at the image intensifier input. When minification is present, an image can be formed with a given noise level by using less radiation. The significant factor is the concentration of x-ray photons with respect to a given film area.

Many imaging systems use intensifier tubes with selectable input image sizes, or fields of view, as illustrated in Figure 21-7 in which three image intensifier inputs, or modes, are compared with a 100-mm film. Intensifier input exposure values that give approximately the same quantum noise on the film are also indicated. The relationship among the exposure values is determined by the ratios of the respective areas. In all three cases, the number of photons forming the image is the same. This is because the total photon number is related to the product of the exposure and the image area.

When an image intensifier can be operated with different input image sizes, there is a different sensitivity value for each size. Sensitivity changes because the gain of the intensifier tube is proportional to the area of the input.

Fluoroscopy

The same basic principles apply to a fluoroscopic imaging system except that the sensitivity of the video camera, rather than the film, is a determining factor. The sensitivity of a video camera is generally not fixed but can be varied through adjustments in the internal amplification, or gain. The quantum noise level for a fluoroscope is generally set to an acceptable level by adjusting either the video camera or aperture, or both.

The receptor sensitivity of a conventional fluoroscope is typically in the range of 1 μR to 10 μR per image frame. This relatively low exposure produces images with considerable quantum noise. In normal fluoroscopic viewing, however, we do not see one image frame at a time but an average of several frames, as discussed below.

Some fluoroscopic systems can be switched into a low-noise mode, which will improve the visibility of low-contrast detail. In the low-noise mode, the receptor sensitivity is reduced, and more exposure is required to form the image.

It is possible to develop receptor systems that would have greater sensitivity and would require less exposure than those currently used in x-ray imaging. But, there is no known way to overcome the fundamental limitation of quantum noise. The receptor must absorb an adequate concentration of x-ray photons to reduce noise to an acceptable level.

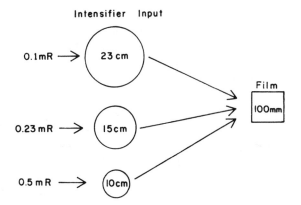

Figure 21-7 Relationship of Intensifier Tube Input Diameters to Film Size and Exposure Values Required to Produce the Same Image Quality

GRAIN AND STRUCTURE NOISE

Although the quantum structure of the x-ray beam is the most significant noise source in most x-ray imaging applications, the structure of the film, intensifying screens, or intensifier tube screens can introduce noise into images.

An image recorded on film is composed of many opaque silver halide crystals, or grains. The grains in radiographic film are quite small and are not generally visible when the film is viewed in the conventional manner. The grainy structure sometimes becomes visible when an image recorded on film is optically enlarged, as when projected onto a screen. Whenever it is visible, film grain is a form of image noise.

Film-grain noise is generally a more significant problem in photography than in radiography, especially in enlargements from images recorded on film with a relatively high sensitivity (speed).

Image-intensifying screens and the screens of intensifier tubes are actually layers of small crystals. An image is formed by the production of light (fluorescence) within each crystal. The crystal structure of screens introduces a slight variation in light production from point to point within an image. This structure noise is relatively insignificant in most radiographic applications.

ELECTRONIC NOISE

Video images often contain noise that comes from various electronic sources. Video image noise is often referred to as snow. Some of the electronic components that make up a video system can be sources of electronic noise. The noise is in the form of random electrical currents often produced by thermal activity within the device. Other electrical devices, such as motors and fluorescent lights, and even natural phenomena within the atmosphere generate electrical noise that can be picked up by video systems.

The presence of noise in a video system becomes especially noticeable when the image signal is weak. Most video receivers have an automatic gain (amplification) circuit that increases the amount of amplification in the presence of a weak signal. This amplifies the noise and causes it to become quite apparent within the image. This effect can be easily observed by tuning a TV (video) receiver to a vacant channel or a channel with a weak signal. The presence of excessive electronic noise in a fluoroscopic image is often the result of a weak video signal because of system failure or misadjustment.

EFFECT OF CONTRAST ON NOISE

The noise in an image becomes more visible if the overall contrast transfer of the imaging system is increased. This must be considered when using image displays with adjustable contrast, such as some video monitors used in fluoroscopy, and the viewing window in CT, MRI, and other forms of digital images. High contrast film increases the visibility of noise.

EFFECT OF BLUR ON NOISE

The visibility of image noise can often be reduced by blurring because noise has a rather finely detailed structure. The blurring of an image tends to blend each image point with its surrounding area; the effect is to smooth out the random structure of the noise and make it less visible.

The use of image blurring to reduce the visibility of noise often involves a compromise because the blurring can reduce the visibility of useful image detail.

High-sensitivity (speed) intensifying screens generally produce images showing less quantum noise than detail screens because they produce more image blur. The problem is that no screen gives both maximum noise suppression and visibility of detail.

A blurring process is sometimes used in digital image processing to reduce image noise, as described in Chapter 22.

IMAGE INTEGRATION

Integration is the process of averaging a series of images over a period of time. Since most types of image noise have a random distribution with respect to time, the integration of images can be quite effective in smoothing an image and reducing its noise content. Integration is, in principle, blurring an image with respect to time, rather than with respect to space or area. The basic limitation of using this process is the effect of patient motion during the time interval.

Integration requires the ability to store or remember images, at least for a short period of time. Several devices are used for image integration in medical imaging.

Human Vision

The human eye (retina) responds to average light intensity over a period of approximately 0.2 seconds. This integration, or averaging, is especially helpful when viewing fluoroscopic images.

The conventional fluoroscopic display is a series of individual video images. Each image is displayed for one thirtieth of a second. Because a relatively low receptor exposure (less than 5 μR) is used to form each individual image, the images are relatively noisy. However, since the eye does not ''see'' each individual image, but an average of several images, the visibility of the noise is reduced. In effect, the eye is integrating, or averaging, approximately six video images at any particular time. The noise actually visible to the human eye is not determined by the receptor exposure for individual fluoroscopic images but by the total exposure for the series of integrated images.

Video Camera Tubes

Certain types of video camera tubes have an inherent lag, or slow response, to changes in an image. This lag is especially significant in vidicon tubes. The effect of the lag is to average, or integrate, the noise fluctuations and produce a smoother image. The major disadvantage in using this type of tube for fluoroscopy is that moving objects tend to leave a temporary trail in the image.

Digital Processing

When a series of images is acquired and stored in a digital memory, the images can be averaged to reduce the noise content. This process is frequently used in DSA and MRI.

IMAGE SUBTRACTION

There are several applications in which one image is subtracted from another. A specific example is DSA. A basic problem with any image subtraction procedure is that the noise level in the resulting image is higher than in either of the two original images. This occurs because of the random distribution of the noise within each image.

Relatively high exposures are used to create the original images in DSA. This partially compensates for the increase in noise produced by the subtraction process.

Chapter 22

Digital Imaging Systems and Image Processing

INTRODUCTION AND OVERVIEW

Digital computers are now an integral part of medical imaging. In some applications, such as CT and MRI, general-purpose digital computers are part of the system. In other applications, such as digital radiography and ultrasound imaging, special-purpose digital processors (computers) are built into the equipment. Nuclear imaging systems use both general-purpose and specialized computer systems. The computer, or digital processor, performs a variety of functions including

- image acquisition control
- image reconstruction
- image storage and retrieval
- image processing
- image analysis.

DIGITAL IMAGES

Images must be in a digital form to be processed by a computer. A digital image consists of a matrix in which each element, or pixel, is represented by a numerical value, as shown in Figure 22-1.

Matrix Size

The matrix size (number of rows and columns) for a particular image generally depends on the specific application and capabilities of the system that creates the image. The most common format is a square, although it is possible to have

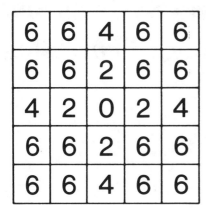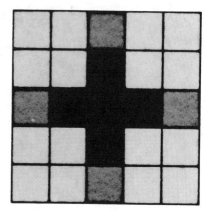

Figure 22-1 A 16-Pixel Digital Image

rectangular digital images. The number of rows and columns in an image matrix is usually a multiple of the number 2 because of the binary characteristics of digital systems. Matrix sizes encountered in medical imaging include 64 × 64, 128 × 128, 256 × 256, 512 × 512, and 1,024 × 1,024. The number of pixels contained in an image is the product of the number of rows and columns. For the square matrix, the number of pixels is proportional to the square of the matrix size. When a matrix dimension is increased by a factor of 2 (eg, from 256 to 512), the number of pixels increases by a factor of 4.

The selection of a matrix size has two important consequences. A large matrix, ie, 512 or 1,024, has smaller pixels, which produce better image detail. But the larger matrix requires more numbers to represent each image and, thus, requires more storage capacity and processing time.

Pixel Values

Devices that process and store digital images operate with binary numbers rather than decimal numbers. The difference is that digits in a binary number always express multiples of the base number 2, whereas digits in a decimal express multiples of the base number 10. A basic knowledge of the binary number format is especially helpful in understanding the storage requirements for digital images.

When a computer, or digital processor, writes a number in memory, it does so by filling in, or marking, specific spaces. This is somewhat analogous to what humans do when they fill out forms where a space is designated for each digit (or letter of the alphabet). Let us use Figure 22-2 to develop this analogy. Consider the decimal number first. Each digit in a decimal number represents a multiple of 10. The specific multiple value is determined by the position, or order, of the digit

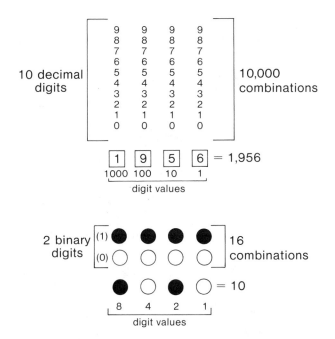

Figure 22-2 Comparison of Binary and Decimal Numbers

within the total number. When humans fill in a decimal number, they do so by writing 1 of 10 different numbers (0–9). The total value of the number is determined by the digit selected and the position in which it is entered. For example, the digit 3 entered into the space to the extreme right has the value of 3, whereas if it is entered into the third space from the right, it has a value of 300. The value of a number is simply the sum of its individual digit values.

In the binary number format, each digit position is indicated by a circle. Notice that the value of each digit position is a multiple of the number 2. When a computer fills in a binary number, it has a choice of only two values, 0 and 1. A 0 is indicated by leaving the position blank, and a 1 is indicated by placing a mark in the position. Each space represents one binary digit, or bit. A bit can have only two different values, whereas a decimal digit can have 10 different values.

Most digital devices work with groups of bits. A group of 8 bits is often used, and it is known as a byte. Within a byte, each blank, or unmarked bit, has a value of 0. Each marked bit has a value determined by its position within the byte. When the bit on the extreme right is marked, it has a value of 1; the bit on the extreme left would have a value of 128, etc. The total value of a byte is the sum of the values for the marked bits.

One byte can represent 256 different values. A byte with all blank bits (all bits equal to 0) has a value of 0. The other extreme is when all bits are marked, which gives a total value of 255. There are 254 other combinations that can be formed with marked and unmarked bits.

The number of different values a binary number can represent is much less than with a decimal number of the same number of digits. This is because a binary digit can have only one of two possible values, whereas a decimal digit can have one of ten different values. We have just seen that an 8-bit binary number, or 1 byte, can have only 256 different values. By comparison, a three-digit decimal number can have 1,000 different values, 0 to 999.

Our primary interest in binary numbers, bits and bytes, is that they are used to represent the pixels in digital images. Different byte configurations represent different shades of gray in the pixels. Figure 22-3 shows the general relationship of byte configurations, pixel values, and shades of gray.

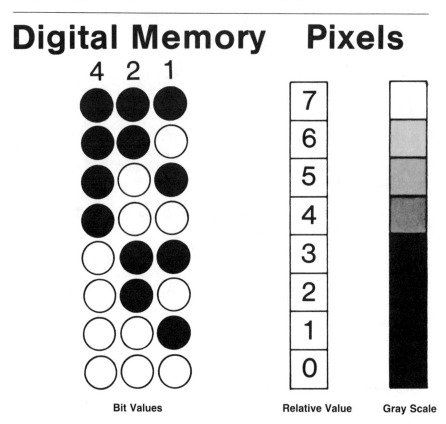

Digital Memory Pixels

Bit Values **Relative Value** **Gray Scale**

Figure 22-3 Relationship between Pixel Values and Image Gray Scale

Image Conversion

Since digital images are not formed directly, like conventional radiographs, they must be created by a conversion process. In CT, MRI, and emission tomography, the digital images are mathematically reconstructed from data collected during the scanning, or acquisition phase. In ultrasound and nuclear imaging, digital images are formed by processing the signals from the transducer, or gamma camera. The digital images in digital radiography and fluoroscopy are generally created by converting a video image into a digital format.

The transformation is performed by an electronic device generally known as an analog to digital (A to D) converter. The converter divides each line of video image into a row of pixels; measures the signal level, or brightness, for each pixel; and converts the value into a digital number, which is then stored in memory.

Nuclear Image Acquisition

In many nuclear medicine procedures, the computer has an important role in the acquisition of the image. The computer is inserted between the gamma camera and the display device and, in most applications, controls the acquisition, or flow, of data from the gamma camera. The acquired data is stored in the computer memory for later processing and display. The processing is usually of two types: the processing of an image to improve its quality and the processing, or abstraction, of quantitative information from the stored data. The computer also controls the manner in which images and data are displayed.

The two major functions of the computer during the acquisition phase are to collect data only during specific time intervals and to arrange the data into specific formats for storage.

The formatting of the data during the acquisition phase is often referred to as the mode of acquisition. The two most common formats (modes) are the frame (or matrix) and the list. The selection between these two modes depends on the type of processing to be performed.

Frame Mode

In the frame, or matrix, mode, the image area is divided into an array of pixels, as shown in Figure 22-4. Typically, the computer can be instructed to divide an image into pixels of different sizes. The selection of a specific matrix format depends, to some extent, on the type of study being conducted.

The formatting of an image into discrete pixels is, in effect, a blurring process. The image of a small object point can be no smaller than one pixel. Therefore, when it is necessary to visualize small objects, or to determine the size and shape of structures with a reasonable degree of precision, small pixel sizes must be used.

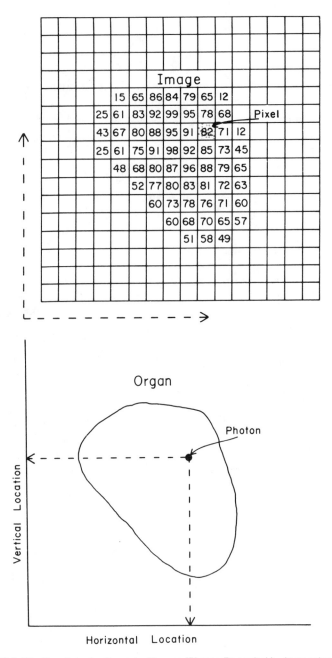

Figure 22-4 The Creation of a Numerical Image (Photon Recorded by Increasing the Count Value in the Corresponding Pixel)

If, on the other hand, the study is concerned with the build-up and elimination of activity in relatively large areas, large pixels can be used to advantage.

In the matrix mode, each pixel is represented by a specific location (address) in the computer memory. Recall that when each photon is detected by the gamma camera, an electrical signal (set of pulses) is created that represents its location within the image area. These signals are processed by the computer to determine the pixel in which the photon is located. It then goes to the corresponding memory location for that pixel and adds one count to the number stored there. In effect, each memory location is like a scoreboard that is continuously updated during the acquisition of data. The final number in the location represents the number of photons that originated within the corresponding pixel.

Let us consider the specific example illustrated in Figure 22-4. If a photon originates from a specific point in an organ, its vertical and horizontal coordinates will be sent to the computer. The computer then uses this information to identify the specific pixel that corresponds to the photon location. The computer goes to the memory location (address) that corresponds to the specific pixel and increases the stored count value by 1 unit. The image stored in the computer memory is in a numerical form. This is desirable because it can then be readily processed and analyzed.

Many studies require a series of images, as illustrated in Figure 22-5. To achieve this, the computer collects and stores counts for a series of specified time intervals. These data are stored as separate images, or frames.

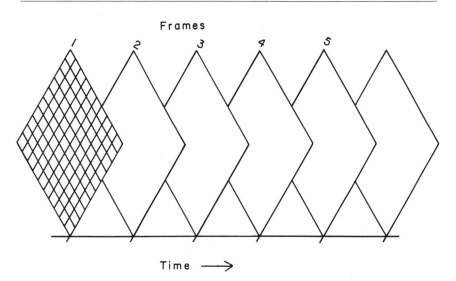

Figure 22-5 A Series of Images (Frames) as Recorded in the Matrix Mode

In some studies, it is desirable to have data collected only during specific phases of a physiological function, such as the cardiac cycle. This is achieved by obtaining a signal from the patient's body, in this case, an electrocardiogram (ECG), and using it to gate the acquisition process. For example, frames can be created to correspond to the different segments of the cardiac cycle, as illustrated in Figure 22-6. In this type of acquisition, the count data can be collected over several cardiac cycles. The counts in each interval are added together to form a series of images that are actually composites of several cycles.

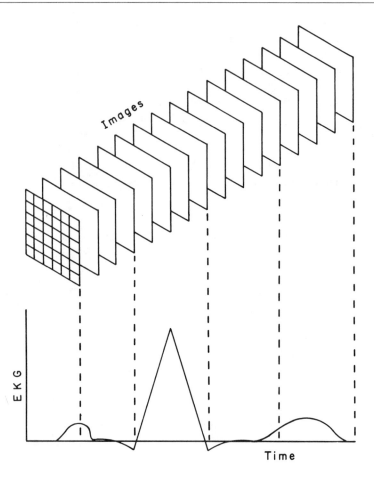

Figure 22-6 Relationship between a Series of Images and the ECG Signal as Created in a Gated Study

List Mode

In the list mode of data acquisition, the data are arranged in memory according to the sequence in which the photons are detected by the camera. Each time a photon is detected, a pair of numbers representing its vertical and horizontal location is stored in the computer memory, as illustrated in Figure 22-7. In addition to the position information, time marks and gate signals from the patient are also stored.

The major advantage in storing data in the list mode is that it can later be arranged in a variety of formats at the user's discretion. It is also usually faster. A disadvantage of the list mode is that it generally requires a larger computer memory because a memory location is required for each photon; in the frame mode, a memory location is required for each pixel (which can accommodate many photons).

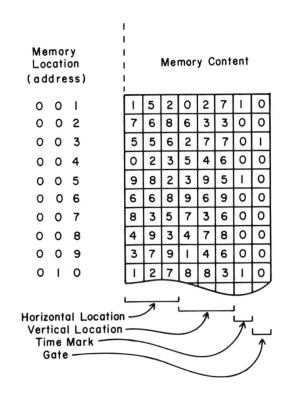

Figure 22-7 The Storage of Count Data in the List Mode

IMAGE PROCESSING

When image data are stored in computer memory, they are available for various kinds of processing. The processing is usually for the purpose of either altering a characteristic of the image or obtaining quantitative data from an image or series of images.

Noise Reduction

In some studies, the image can be processed to reduce the noise produced by the statistical fluctuation in photon concentration, as discussed in Chapter 21. The apparent noise can be reduced by blending the value for an individual pixel with the values for adjacent pixels. Several mathematical approaches can be used for this, but a specific one, the nine-point smoothing process, is illustrated in Figure 22-8. In this procedure, the computer calculates a new image from the old. The value for each new pixel is a weighted average value of the old pixel and the eight pixels surrounding it.

We can calculate a new value for each pixel shown in Figure 22-8. First, the original value is multiplied by 4. The values for the four pixels located on the four sides of the pixel being processed are multiplied by 2, and the values in the corner pixels are multiplied by 1. The results of these multiplications are then added, and the total is divided by 16 to give a weighted average. This process is repeated for each pixel within the image area. When this process is applied to the image section shown in Figure 22-8, the noise (1 standard deviation) is decreased from 10% to 1.8%. Image smoothing to reduce noise is generally a blurring process that reduces the sharpness and visibility of small structures.

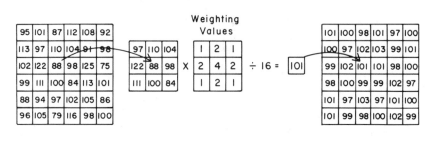

Noise $(1\sigma) = 10\%$ Noise $(1\sigma) = 1.8\%$

Figure 22-8 The Reduction of Image Noise by the Use of the Nine-Point Smoothing Process

Contrast Modification

Image contrast is related to the difference in the values among pixels. Contrast can be modified by multiplying the values by an appropriate factor and subtracting a value, as illustrated in Figure 22-9. Generally, the computer can be instructed to multiply the image by different factors.

The relationship between an original and modified image is shown by means of a graph in Figure 22-10. This graph shows the relationship between the new and old pixel values. The dotted line represents the relationship between two identical images, or when the multiplication factor is 1. If the pixel values of the original image are multiplied by a factor greater than 1, contrast will be increased. If they are multiplied by a factor less than 1 (a fraction), contrast will be reduced. Note that contrast is related to the slope of the lines in Figure 22-10. This graph is somewhat analogous to the characteristic curve for film.

Now let us consider in more detail the specific example shown in Figure 22-9. The original image has an average value of 100 per pixel in the background area, and 75 per pixel in the center of the object area. This gives a contrast between the object and background of 25, or 25%. An image with enhanced contrast is obtained by multiplying each of the values by a factor of 2 and subtracting 100. In the new image, the background has an average value of 100 per pixel, and the object area an average of 50 per pixel. This yields a contrast between the two areas of 50 (50%), or double the original contrast.

The illustration in Figure 22-9 shows no noise in order to emphasize the change in contrast. Noise is, however, always present in an actual image, and enhancing contrast in this manner increases noise. Therefore, it does not improve the image contrast-to-noise ratio.

One form of contrast enhancement is background subtraction. To achieve this, the computer will be instructed to set the new image pixel values at zero if the old image pixel values are below a specific threshold value.

Image Subtraction

Digital images can be readily subtracted to show a difference, or change, between images. Although this form of processing can be applied to any type of digital image, the most common procedure is DSA.

The basic principle of DSA is illustrated in Figure 22-11. The first image is acquired before the injection of contrast medium. This image (the mask) contains all anatomical structures normally revealed in an x-ray image. The second image is acquired after the contrast medium is injected into the vessel being imaged. If a dilute concentration of contrast medium is used, the vessels will have very little contrast in comparison to many other structures, especially bone. If the second

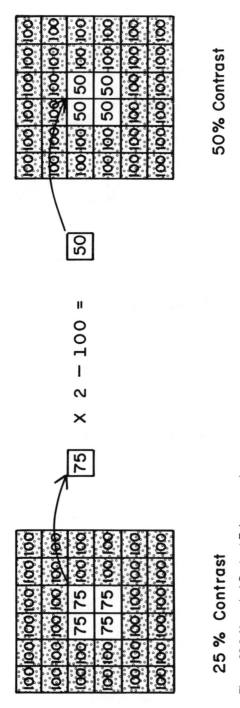

25 % Contrast

$\times 2 - 100 =$

50% Contrast

Figure 22-9 Numerical Contrast Enhancement

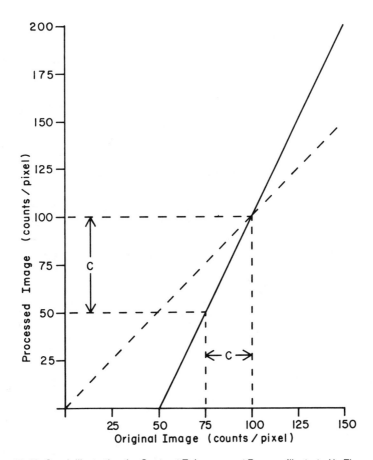

Figure 22-10 Graph Illustrating the Contrast Enhancement Process Illustrated in Figure 22-9

image is subtracted from the first under ideal conditions, an image showing only the vessel containing the contrast medium will be obtained.

Image subtraction is used to increase contrast sensitivity, with respect to conventional angiographic procedures, so that vascular structures with lower concentrations of contrast medium can be imaged. The improvement in contrast sensitivity is, however, often accompanied by an increase in image noise and artifacts.

As discussed in Chapter 21, image subtraction always increases image noise. In DSA the two original images are usually acquired with relatively high exposure levels to minimize quantum noise.

The primary source of artifacts in DSA is patient motion during the interval between the two images. If the anatomical structures are not in the same position for the two images, the subtraction process will produce an image of the move-

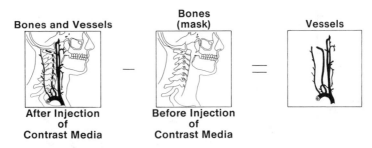

Figure 22-11 The Basic Principles of Digital Subtraction Angiography

ment, or displacement. This appears in the image as an artifact. Several methods can be used to reduce the effect of motion artifacts. Some imaging systems have a reregistration capability that allows the user to shift one image with respect to the other in an effort to compensate for the motion. Another procedure is to acquire a series of mask images, and then try different combinations to find one that produces the least artifact.

QUANTITATIVE DATA PROCESSING AND ANALYSIS

Profiles

The ability to compare a characteristic, such as density or activity of various areas within an image, is often improved by generating a profile. Typically, the computer is instructed to select a specific row of pixels and to create a graphic display of the pixel values.

Regions of Interest

Computers can be instructed to outline a region of interest (ROI) in an image. Then data such as the total counts or the average density within the region can be obtained.

A useful function for many dynamic nuclear studies is to produce a graphic display of the activity within the ROI as a function of elapsed time. Time-activity curves are useful for observing the quantitative build-up and elimination of activity within a specific body region or organ.

DISPLAY CONTROL

Digital images are not suitable for direct viewing. In most applications, the digital image is converted into a video image, which can then be observed or

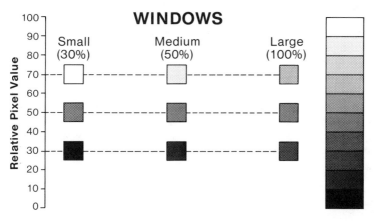

Figure 22-12 The Use of a Window for Viewing Digital Images

recorded on film. This conversion is performed by an electronic device: a digital to analog (video) converter. Most systems for viewing digitized images allow the observer to select the range of pixel values that will be converted into the full gray scale, or brightness range. This function is known as windowing. The two selectable variables associated with the window are its width, or range of pixel values, and its position along the pixel value scale. The windowing concept is illustrated in Figure 22-12.

When the window is set with specific variables, all pixels with values greater than the upper window limit are displayed as white, all pixels below the lower window limit are displayed as black, and pixel values between the two limits are spread over the full scale of gray. In principle, the window setting functions as a contrast control. Decreasing window width increases image contrast.

Some systems use a color display. In such a system, the computer translates pixel values into specific colors.

Chapter 23

Computed Tomography Image Formation

INTRODUCTION AND OVERVIEW

Computed tomography differs from conventional projection x-ray imaging in several respects. A major difference is the way in which the image is formed. The formation of the CT image is a multi-step process.

Image production begins with the scanning phase, as shown in Figure 23-1. During this phase, a thin fan-shaped x-ray beam is projected through the edges of the body section (slice) being imaged. The radiation that penetrates the section is measured by an array of detectors. The detectors do not ''see'' a complete image of the body section, only a profile from one direction. The profile data are measurements of the x-ray penetration along each ray extending from the x-ray tube to the individual detectors. In order to produce enough information to create a full image, the x-ray beam is rotated, or scanned, around the body section to produce views from many angles. Typically, several hundred views are taken, and the profile data for each view are stored in the computer memory. The total number of penetration measurements made during a scan is the product of the number of views and the number of rays within each view. The total scanning time for one slice can range from approximately 1 to 15 seconds, depending on the design of the scanner mechanism and the selection of scanning variables by the operator. In general, the quality of the image can be improved by using longer scanning times.

The second phase of image production is known as image reconstruction, as illustrated in Figure 23-2. This is performed by the digital computer, which is part of the CT system. Image reconstruction is a mathematical procedure that converts the scan data for the individual views into a numerical, or digital, image. The image is structured in an array of individual picture elements, or pixels. Each pixel is represented by a numerical value, or CT number. The specific value for each pixel is related to the density of tissue in the corresponding volume element, or voxel. Reconstruction usually takes several seconds, depending on the complexity

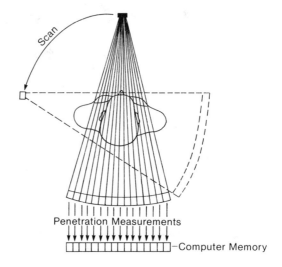

Penetration Measurements
Computer Memory

Figure 23-1 The Scanning Phase of CT Image Formation

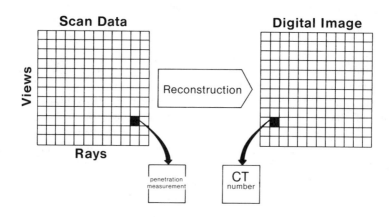

Scan Data

Views

Rays

Digital Image

Reconstruction

penetration measurement

CT number

Figure 23-2 The Reconstruction of a CT Image from Scan Data

of the image and the capabilities of the computer. The digital image is then stored in the computer memory.

The final phase is the conversion of the digital image into a video display so that it can be viewed directly or recorded on film. This phase is performed by electronic components that function as a digital-to-analog (video) converter. The relationship between the pixel CT number values and the shades of gray, or brightness, in the displayed image is determined by the window levels selected by the operator, as shown in Figure 23-3. Through the manipulation of the upper and lower window levels, it is possible to adjust the brightness and contrast of the displayed image. The window setting determines the range of CT numbers that are spread over the entire image gray scale.

In this chapter we consider the basic construction and operation of a CT scanner. In the next chapter we consider, in more detail, the image quality characteristics of CT imaging.

THE X-RAY SYSTEM

The x-ray beam in a CT system must have an appropriate shape, intensity distribution, and the ability to be rotated around the patient's body.

Tube and Gantry

The x-ray tube is mounted on a circular gantry assembly, which rotates it around the patient's body. Supplying electrical power to the tube while it is rotating is

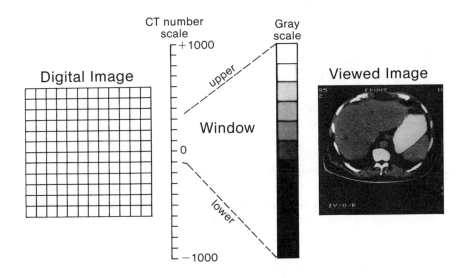

Figure 23-3 The Conversion of a Digital Image into a Gray Scale Image

awkward. Most scanners use cables that wrap around the gantry while it is rotating. This design allows only a few rotations; the gantry must then be stopped and rotated in the other direction to uncoil the cables. Another design uses sliding electrical contacts, or slip rings, that permit continuous high-speed rotation.

Collimation

The x-ray tube assembly contains collimating devices that determine the physical size and shape of the x-ray beam. One set of collimators determines the angular span of the beam, and another set determines its thickness. This latter set can usually be adjusted to vary slice thickness.

With current technology it is not possible to create an x-ray beam with sharply defined edges. This is because of the finite size of the x-ray tube focal spot, which results in a penumbra, or "partial shadow," along the beam edges, as shown in Figure 23-4. The radiation has the greatest intensity at the center of the slice and reduced intensity near the edges. Some radiation exposes the tissue adjacent to the slice being imaged.

Filtration

The x-ray tube assembly also contains metal filters through which the x-ray beam passes. CT x-ray beams are filtered for two purposes.

Beam Hardening

Beam hardening refers to the process of increasing the average photon energy, ie, hardening, that occurs when the lower-energy photons are absorbed as the beam passes through any material. This will normally occur when an x-ray beam passes through the human body if the beam contains a wide range of photon energies. In CT imaging, this hardening of the beam creates an image artifact because the peripheral tissue is exposed to a lower average photon energy than the inner portion of the slice. This can be minimized by hardening the beam with the filter material before it enters the body. This filtration reduces patient exposure by selectively removing the low-energy, low-penetrating part of the x-ray beam spectrum.

Compensation

A filter with a non-uniform thickness is often placed in the x-ray beam to compensate for the non-uniform thickness of the human body. This type of filter is

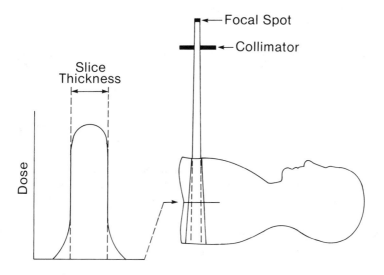

Figure 23-4 A Profile Showing the Distribution of Radiation Dose through a Slice

thicker near the edges and is sometimes referred to as a bow-tie filter. When it is used, the thick center section of the body is exposed to a higher radiation intensity than the thinner sections near the edges. The use of this type of compensation filter generally reduces patient exposure while maintaining a specified level of image quality.

Power Supply

The generator, or power supply, for a CT system is typically a constant potential type that can produce relatively high KV and MA values for a sustained period of time.

DETECTORS

In a CT system, the radiation receptor is an array of many small detectors. Several types of detectors are in use today. The way in which they are mounted within the gantry assembly can vary from one scanner type to another.

Function

The function of a detector element is to absorb the radiation it intercepts, and then to produce an electrical signal proportional to the radiation intensity. In principle, each detector measures the radiation that penetrates the body section in the direction of the detector.

Construction

Several materials are used for CT detectors. Solid-state detectors are made of solid scintillation crystals that convert the x-ray energy into light. The light is then converted into an electrical signal by either a photodiode or photomultiplier (PM) tube. In another design, each detector is a small chamber filled with a high pressure gas, typically xenon. The radiation absorbed within the chamber ionizes the gas, which, in turn, changes its electrical conductivity.

Two of the most important characteristics of an individual detector are its size and its efficiency for absorbing radiation. The most significant dimension is its width in the plane of the x-ray beam. This dimension is the detector aperture. Small detectors are necessary to achieve high detail in CT images.

The efficiency of a detector is the percentage of radiation in its "space" that it actually absorbs. Two factors affect detector efficiency, as shown in Figure 23-5. The geometric efficiency is determined by the ratio of the individual detector aperture to the total space associated with each detector. This space includes the detector itself and the inactive collimator or the interspace between it and the next detector. Radiation that enters the interspace is not absorbed by the detector and does not contribute to image formation. The ideal situation would be a large detector area in comparison to the dimensions of the interspace.

The other component of detector efficiency is determined by the percentage of radiation entering the detector that is absorbed. This depends on detector thickness and, to some extent, on the energy of the x-ray photons. The total detector efficiency is the product of the geometric and absorption efficiency values. High detector efficiency is desirable because it reduces patient dose for a specific level of image quality.

Sensitivity Profile

In the ideal situation, each detector would be uniformly sensitive to all radiation passing through the body section being imaged and would be insensitive to radiation coming from outside the slice. This would permit the imaging of well-defined slices with good detail. The slice thickness that is within the view of each detector is determined by the position of the collimating elements. The typical

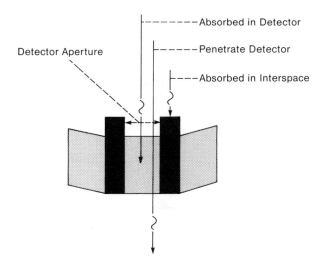

Detector Aperture

Absorbed in Detector

Penetrate Detector

Absorbed in Interspace

Figure 23-5 Factors that Determine Detector Efficiency

collimator geometry produces a variation in detector sensitivity along the axis passing through the body section. A typical detector sensitivity profile is shown in Figure 23-6. The significance of this is that a CT image can contain features produced by objects outside the nominal slice.

Detector Configurations

The way in which the detectors are arranged and moved during the scanning process has changed during the evolution of the CT scanner and is different among scanners used today. It is common practice to designate various detector configurations as either first, second, third, or fourth generation. The generation designations correspond to the order in which the various configurations were developed. Performance was improved in going from the first to the second and then on to the third and fourth generations. The concept of generation with respect to the third and fourth types, however, must be used with caution. They represent two different approaches to detector design. Each has its own operating characteristics, but one is not inherently superior to the other.

First and Second Types

The first two detector configurations are discussed for the sake of historical reference. The first CT scanner used a single detector element that was moved,

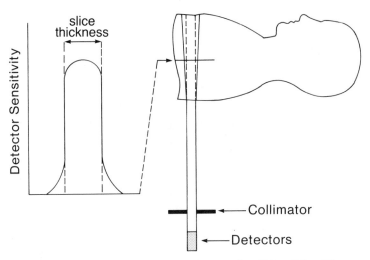

Figure 23-6 A Profile Showing the Variation in Detector Sensitivity within a Slice

along with the x-ray tube, in a straight line across the patient's body to form one view. The entire x-ray tube and detector assembly was then rotated approximately 1° and scanned across the body to form the second view. This combination of translate-rotate motions was continued until the number of views was adequate. Typical scanning time was approximately 4 minutes. The scanning time was reduced with the development of the second type of detector configuration, which used multiple detectors and reduced the number of rotations required to achieve a full scan. The second type also used a combined translate-rotate motion.

Third Type

The third type of detector configuration is shown in Figure 23-7. An array of individual detector elements that is just large enough to form one view is mounted on the gantry so that it rotates along with the x-ray tube. This is often referred to as a rotating detector configuration.

Fourth Type

The fourth type of detector configuration is a ring of detector elements that completely encircles the patient's body, as shown in Figure 23-8. The detectors are stationary and do not rotate. This arrangement has many more detector elements than the third type, but they are not all in use at the same time. Different segments of the detector array are exposed as the x-ray tube rotates. The functional difference between the third and fourth types is the way in which the individual views are created.

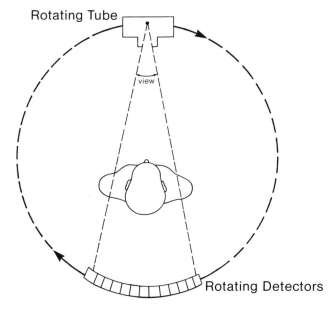

Figure 23-7 A Type 3, or Rotate-Rotate, Scanner

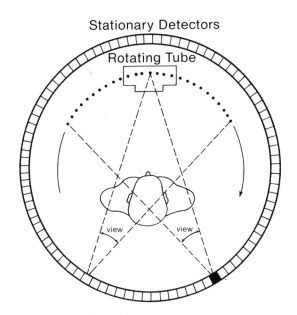

Figure 23-8 A Type 4, or Stationary-Rotate, Scanner

COMPUTER

The digital computer, which is a major component of a CT system, performs several functions.

Control

After the operator selects the appropriate scanning factors and initiates the scan, the procedure progresses under the control of the computer. The computer coordinates and times the sequence of events that occur during the scan, which includes turning the x-ray beam and detectors on and off at the appropriate time, transferring data, and monitoring the system operation.

Processing

The digital computer is directly involved in the formation of CT image through processing of the profile data to reconstruct the image. This function is made up of many steps that are written into the computer program. The reconstruction of one CT image requires millions of mathematical operations by the computer; the sequence of the mathematical operations makes up the reconstruction algorithm.

Storage and Retrieval

A third major function of the computer in the CT system is the transfer, storage, and retrieval of images and data. Data and images that are being processed are temporarily stored in the computer's electronic memory. Since this memory has a rather limited capacity, most of the images within the system are stored on magnetic disk. They can be recalled from the disk for processing or display very quickly. The disk also has a limited capacity, although it is much larger than the electronic memory. The long-term, or archival, storage of images requires the transfer to a storage medium that can be removed from the computer and stored independently. Magnetic tape and floppy disk are used for this purpose.

DISPLAY UNIT AND CAMERA

The two other units that make up a CT system are the display unit (viewing console) and the camera, which records the images onto film. Most CT systems use a multi-format camera.

The viewing unit is the interface between the CT system and the physician or operator. The image display is a CRT or video monitor. Before the digital images are transferred to the viewing unit by the computer, they are converted from a digital to a video form.

The viewer can communicate with the computer through a keyboard, joystick, or tracker ball. This allows the viewer to select specific images for display, control brightness and contrast, implement display functions such as zoom and rotation, and analyze region of interest (ROI).

SCANNING

The scanning process is the first step in the formation of a CT image. During the scanning phase, the data are collected that will be used as a basis for reconstructing the image. The scanning process consists of rotating the x-ray beam around the patient's body and making measurements of the penetration through the body from various directions. One scan will result in hundreds of thousands of individual penetration measurements, or samples.

Rays

A ray is the portion of an x-ray beam that is projected onto an individual detector, as shown in Figure 23-9. Typically, a ray passes through the body slice as shown. The radiation within the ray is absorbed by the tissue in the pathway. The rate of absorption at each point along the way is determined by the value of the linear attenuation coefficient. For the purpose of this discussion, let us divide the tissue into a line of individual blocks. Each block of tissue has an attenuation coefficient value that depends on the type of tissue and the energy of the photons within the x-ray beam. In principle, each block of tissue attenuates the x-ray beam by an amount equal to the value of the attenuation coefficient. The total attenuation (or penetration) along a ray is related to the sum of the individual attenuation coefficients of points along the ray.

The projection of one ray through a body section produces a measurement of the total attenuation, or penetration, along its path; the measurement represents the sum of the individual attenuation coefficient values for each voxel of tissue within the ray. With a single measurement, there is no way to determine the individual voxel attenuation coefficient values. However, by projecting many rays through a body section, making measurements for each, and then reconstructing the image, the attenuation coefficient value for each voxel within the slice can be calculated.

Views

A view consists of a collection of rays that share a common point. The common point can be either a focal spot location or an individual detector, depending on the specific detector configuration.

Third Type

In systems with the third type of detector configuration (Figure 23-7), a view is created by exposing all of the detectors from one focal spot location. All of the rays

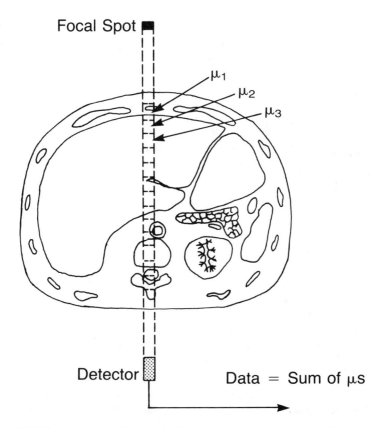

Figure 23-9 The Attenuation (Penetration) Measurement Made by an Individual Ray

within the view are projected simultaneously. The time required to create one view is relatively short and is controlled by turning either the x-ray tube or the detectors on and off. Additional views are created as the x-ray tube (focal spot) and detector array rotate around the body.

Fourth Type

In views created by CT scanners with the fourth type of detector configuration (Figure 23-8), one detector is common to all rays within one view. Individual rays are created as the focal spot moves along its circular path. The rays are not projected simultaneously, as in the third type, but are produced sequentially as the x-ray tube moves along.

During each scan, many views are being developed at the same time. This is possible because the x-ray beam exposes many detectors simultaneously. For example, when the focal spot is in a specific position, it can project the first ray of one view, the second ray of another view, and the third ray of yet another view, etc.

Measurements and Samples

The total number of measurements, or data samples, obtained during one scan is the product of the number of views and the number of rays per view. The actual number varies from one type of scanner to another; it also depends on the selection of scanning factors by the operator. In principle, increasing the number of measurements improves image quality but often increases scanning time. The number of measurements per scan is typically within the range of 500,000 to 1.5 million.

A typical scan is created by rotating the x-ray beam through an angle of 360°. Some systems can be set to scan through a smaller angle, to reduce time, or to scan through angles larger than 360°, to increase the number of measurements and image quality. The number of measurements per scan is generally not set directly by the operator but is affected by the examination type (or mode) and the scanning time.

IMAGE RECONSTRUCTION

CT image reconstruction is the process of transforming the x-ray penetration measurements into a digital image of the body section. It is a mathematical process performed by the computer using one of several mathematical methods of image reconstruction.

Image Format

The image is reconstructed in the form of an array of individual picture elements, or pixels. The number of pixels making up the image is typically in the range of 64 × 64 pixels to 512 × 512 pixels. The matrix size (number of pixels per image) is selected by the operator before the scan procedure. Pixel size has a significant effect on image quality and must be selected to fulfill the needs of the specific clinical procedure.

Each pixel in the image corresponds to a volume element, or voxel, of tissue in the body section being imaged. The size of the individual tissue voxel has a significant effect on image quality. Three examination variables affect the size of a voxel, as shown in Figure 23-10: (1) matrix size, (2) field of view, and (3) slice thickness. The slice thickness corresponds to the depth of a voxel. The dimension of a voxel area is the field of view divided by the matrix size. For example, a 25.4-cm (10-in.) field of view with a 256 matrix produces tissue voxels with

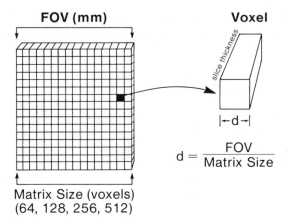

Figure 23-10 The Relationship of Voxel Size to FOV, Matrix Size, and Slice Thickness

dimensions (length and width) of 1 mm. Changing either the field of view or the matrix size alters the dimensions of the individual voxels.

CT Numbers

In the reconstructed image, each pixel is represented by a numerical value related to the linear attenuation coefficient value of the tissue in each voxel, as shown in Figure 23-11. In principle, the reconstruction process first calculates the

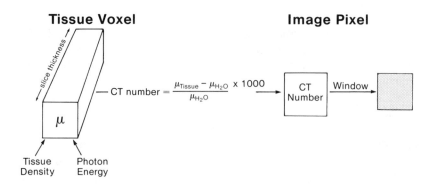

Figure 23-11 The Relationship of Pixel (CT) Number and Tissue Voxel Attenuation Coefficient Value (μ)

attenuation coefficient value for each voxel and then transforms it into an appropriate image pixel value. The pixel values are generally designated CT numbers.

Most systems express CT numbers in Hounsfield units. The relationship between a CT number and the corresponding attenuation coefficient value is given by

$$CT\ number = ((\mu_{Tissue} - \mu_{H_2O})/\mu_{H_2O}) \times 1,000.$$

Water is used as a reference material for determining CT numbers. By definition, water has a CT number value of 0. Materials that have attenuation coefficient values greater than that of water have positive CT number values, and materials with coefficient values less than that of water have negative CT numbers. CT scanners generally operate at relatively high KVs when Compton interactions predominate in the soft tissue. The linear attenuation coefficient values for Compton interactions are primarily determined by material density. Therefore, at least in the soft tissues, the CT numbers are closely related to tissue density. Tissue with a density less than that of water (specific gravity less than 1) generally has negative CT number values. Positive CT number values indicate a tissue density greater than that of water.

The same tissue will not produce the same CT numbers if scanned with different machines because of differences in x-ray beam energy (KV and filtration) and system calibration procedures. CT numbers obtained with the same scanner can

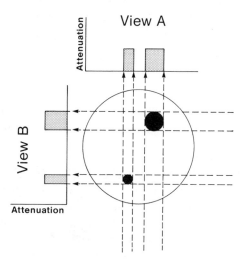

Figure 23-12 Two Views of a Body Section Used to Illustrate Back Projection

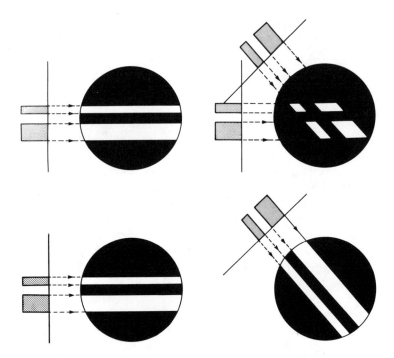

Figure 23-13 The Concept of Back Projection Image Reconstruction

vary from one time to another and if the location of the specific tissue is changed within the imaged area. If CT numbers are to be used for analytical purposes such as the determination of bone density, it is usually necessary to scan a set of reference materials along with the patient.

Back Projection

Although several mathematical methods can be used to reconstruct CT images, one method, filtered back projection, is used almost exclusively. In principle, the reconstruction of an image by the back projection method is the inverse of the scanning process. During the scanning of a body section, the x-ray beam is projected through the section from different directions to create different views, as shown in Figure 23-12. Since the x-ray beam is projected through the sides of the body section, a view "sees" only a composite attenuation profile rather than the individual anatomical structures within the slice. This illustration shows only two of the several hundred views usually made in an actual scan.

It will be possible to reconstruct an image of the body section if a number of the individual profiles are projected back onto an image area. The general concept of

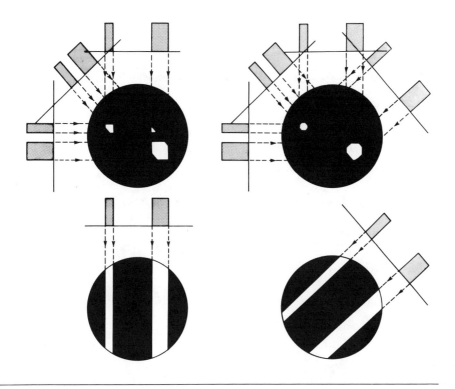

back projection is illustrated in Figure 23-13. The bottom row shows the back projection of four views onto an image surface. Each view profile contains only enough information to project lines, or bands, through the image. However, if the individual views are superimposed, as shown from left to right in the top row, the image will be recreated, or reconstructed.

In this example, we used only four views to reconstruct a relatively simple image. Several hundred views are normally required to reconstruct the more complex and detailed image of a body section.

Chapter 24

Computed Tomography Image Quality

INTRODUCTION AND OVERVIEW

The CT image is distinctly different from the conventional radiograph. The best use of CT imaging and accurate interpretation will be easier to achieve if one has a good understanding of CT image quality characteristics and how they can be altered to fit specific clinical needs.

Before initiating a scan, the operator must adjust values for a relatively large number of imaging factors. The factors for a typical CT system are shown in Figure 24-1; most will have a direct effect on one or more image quality characteristics. In many instances, changing a factor to improve one image characteristic will adversely affect some other characteristic. Therefore, the issue is not which factors give the "best" image, but which values produce maximum visibility of specific anatomic or pathologic features. For example, a selection of imaging factors to produce maximum visibility of detail generally lowers visibility of subtle differences in soft tissue. Image quality must also be balanced against patient exposure, x-ray tube heating, and imaging time.

In this chapter, we consider the characteristics of CT image quality and show how they are related to the various imaging factors.

In comparison with radiography, CT imaging generally has a higher contrast sensitivity and produces less visibility of detail, more noise, and more artifacts.

CONTRAST SENSITIVITY

Computed tomography has one image quality characteristic that is superior to conventional radiography: a high contrast sensitivity that makes it possible to visualize low-contrast structures and objects, especially within soft tissue. Several factors associated with the formation of CT images contribute to its high-contrast sensitivity.

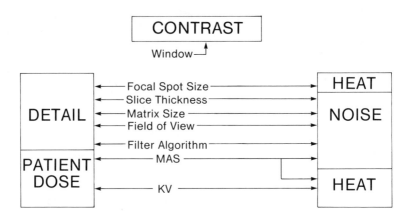

Figure 24-1 Operator-Selected Factors that Affect CT Image Quality

Tomography

In tomographic imaging, each anatomical feature is displayed directly and is not superimposed on other objects. This makes it possible to enhance the contrast in the areas of interest without interference from high-contrast bony structures.

Windowing

Another factor that contributes to the high-contrast sensitivity of CT imaging is its ability to window selected segments of the CT number scale, as illustrated in Figure 24-2. By adjusting the window levels, any segment of the CT number scale can be expanded to cover the entire gray scale range.

The window functions as a contrast control. In principle, tissue is divided into three categories according to window setting. Tissues with CT numbers lower than the lower window setting appear black in the image. Tissues with CT numbers greater than the upper window setting appear white. Tissues with CT numbers between the lower and upper levels appear as different shades of gray.

Image contrast is related to the difference between the upper and lower window levels. A small window produces high image contrast because small differences in tissue CT numbers are imaged with large differences in shades of gray. A large window setting produces an image with relatively low contrast, but visibility extends over a wider range of CT numbers.

The window function allows rather subtle differences in tissue CT numbers to be isolated from the full range and then displayed over the entire gray scale. This is a significant factor in achieving high-contrast sensitivity.

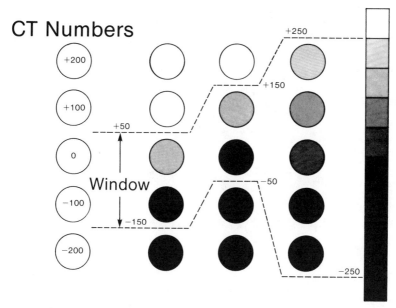

Figure 24-2 The Use of Windowing to Control Contrast in CT Imaging

Reduced Scattered Radiation

The relatively narrow x-ray beam used in CT produces much less scattered radiation than the much larger beams used in conventional radiography.

VISIBILITY OF DETAIL, BLUR, AND RESOLUTION

In CT imaging, several factors produce blurring of the image and a reduction in the visibility of detail. Some of the factors can usually be changed by the operator. CT blur values are usually in the range of 0.7 mm to 2.0 mm.

During scanning and image reconstruction, a series of factors contribute to the total (composite) blur, as illustrated in Figure 24-3.

Ray (Sample) Width

One of the most significant factors that blurs the CT image and limits visibility of detail is the width of the ray, also known as the sampling aperture. All anatomical detail within the width of a ray is blurred together during the measurement process.

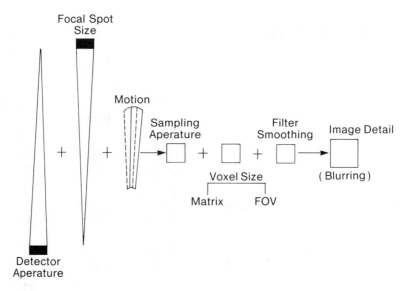

Figure 24-3 Factors that Produce Blurring and Loss of Detail in CT Imaging

Detector Aperture

The detector aperture is the effective size of each detector in the image plane and is one of the two major factors that determine ray width. A small detector aperture produces a narrow ray, less blur, and better image detail. Many scanners have adjustable collimating devices, which can be used to change the detector aperture. A small aperture setting produces maximum image detail. When a portion of the detector is covered, however, the geometric efficiency is reduced. An increase in radiation exposure to the patient is then required to produce the same image quality with respect to noise.

Focal Spot

Each ray is created by the x-ray tube focal spot. Two factors associated with the focal spot affect ray width: (1) the size of the focal spot and (2) movement during the interval of each measurement. Small focal spots create rays with narrow widths, which produce better image detail. However, the heat capacity of the focal spot area is often a limiting factor. Many scanners use x-ray tubes with dual focal spots; the small spot is used for maximum image detail and the large spot for maximum heat capacity.

The optimum imaging situation is generally one in which the focal spot size and detector aperture are approximately equal. If the objects being imaged are approximately the same distance from the focal spot and detector, no advantage is gained if the size of one greatly exceeds the size of the other. If the objects are closer to either the focal spot or detector, the closer device has more of an influence on the ray dimension.

Ray (Sample) Interval

Another factor that affects detail at the time the measurements are made is the distance, or interval, between adjacent rays. If the spacing between rays significantly exceeds the dimensions of small objects, or anatomical detail, the detail will not appear in the image. The rays must be sufficiently close during the scanning procedure to measure any anatomical detail that is to appear in the image. A relatively large interval between rays not only reduces image detail but causes aliasing artifacts.

Voxel and Pixel Size

The formation of an image into an array of pixels is, in itself, a blurring process. Since a specific pixel can have only one CT number value, there can be no detail within a pixel. In other words, all detail within the tissue voxel represented by a specific pixel is blurred together and assigned a single value. With respect to image quality, the significant dimension is not that of the pixel in the image but rather that of the corresponding voxel in the patient's body. Anatomical detail within a voxel cannot be imaged. Therefore, small voxels are needed when image detail is required.

Three factors determine voxel size: (1) field of view, (2) matrix size, and (3) slice thickness. In principle, voxel size can be changed by changing any one of these factors. Reducing voxel size generally, but not always, improves image detail. It will not significantly improve image detail if the voxel size is not the limiting factor, nor if the focal spot, detector, or other factors produce significantly more blur than the voxel.

The selection of the appropriate voxel size for a specific clinical procedure generally depends on the requirement for image detail. Noise increases as voxel size is decreased.

Reconstruction Filters

The scan data are typically passed through mathematical filter algorithms in the image reconstruction process. Most systems have several filters that can be selected by the operator. Functions performed by the filters include reducing artifacts, smoothing to reduce image noise, and enhancing edges. Since image smoothing is a blurring process, the use of this type of filter can limit visibility of detail.

Composite Blur

We have seen that several factors contribute to image blurring in CT. Many of them can be adjusted by the user. However, compromises must often be made between image detail and other factors. The following principles must be considered:

- Decreasing detector aperture decreases efficiency, leading to an increase in patient exposure or image noise.
- Decreasing focal spot size decreases x-ray tube heat capacity.
- Increasing matrix size increases image noise.
- Decreasing field of view increases image noise and can limit specific clinical applications.

Reducing blur by changing any one factor will not significantly improve image quality unless the factor is a significant source of blur with respect to the other factors. For example, using a small detector aperture will not improve image detail if the detail is limited by a large focal spot or large voxel. Figure 24-4 can be used to compare the image blur produced by individual factors; a scale of blur values is shown for the four most significant. The compromises associated with each factor are also indicated. Maximum image detail is obtained by reducing the blur values as much as possible.

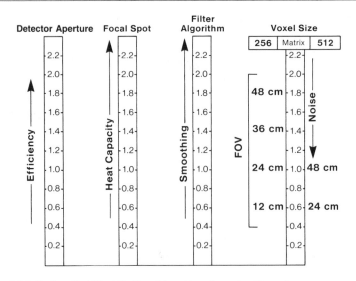

Figure 24-4 Factors that Must Be Considered in a Scanning Procedure

The best image procedure is generally one in which blur from all sources, except voxel size, is approximately the same. Voxel size can usually be adjusted to a smaller value than the other factors.

NOISE

Effect on Visibility

Image noise is significant in CT images since CT imaging is often used to visualize low-contrast tissue differences, which are especially sensitive to the presence of noise. The amount of noise in a CT image is a major factor in determining the effective contrast sensitivity (or contrast resolution) of an imaging procedure.

Noise in a CT image is a variation in CT number values from pixel to pixel and exists even when all pixels are associated with the same material. A section of a CT image of water is shown in Figure 24-5. Water has an average CT number value of

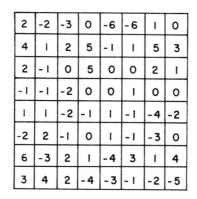

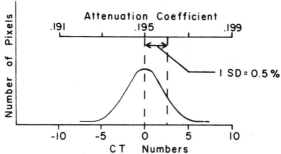

Figure 24-5 (A) Typical CT Numbers in an Image of a Volume of Water. (B) The Spread of Values (Standard Deviation) Is an Indication of the Amount of Image Noise.

0, but because of the presence of noise, individual pixels have a range of values as indicated. The variation in CT numbers (noise) can be expressed in terms of the standard deviation of the values. The graph in Figure 24-5 shows a typical distribution of CT numbers for water. The range of values represented by 1 standard deviation below and above the average value (0) is indicated. The value of the standard deviation can be expressed in CT numbers or as a percentage.

The amount of noise in a CT image can be determined by scanning a container of water and then using the viewing functions to display the standard deviation value for a specific region of interest (ROI).

Sources

In CT imaging, the predominant source of noise, in most cases, is the fluctuation of x-ray photon concentration, which we know as quantum noise.

Factors Affecting Noise

Several factors associated with a CT procedure affect the amount of image noise, and they can be changed, to some degree, by the operator. As each factor is changed to reduce noise, it either adversely affects another aspect of image quality or increases patient exposure. The amount of noise is inversely related to the total amount of radiation absorbed in each voxel; changing either the dimension of a voxel or the exposure produced by the x-ray beam alters the noise level.

Pixel Size

Noise can be decreased by increasing the dimensions of the pixel (voxel), but, as we have seen, this increases image blurring and reduces visibility of detail. This is one of the important compromises that must be made in selecting imaging factors.

Slice Thickness

Since slice thickness forms one dimension of the voxel, it affects image noise. Thin slices, which produce better detail and fewer partial-volume artifacts, produce higher noise levels. Again, a compromise must be made in selecting imaging factors.

Radiation Exposure

The amount of radiation used to create a CT image can usually be varied by changing either the MA or the scanning time. Changing either produces a proportional change in patient dose and the radiation absorbed in individual voxels.

Image noise can be decreased by increasing the quantity of radiation used (MAS), but the radiation dose absorbed by the tissue will also increase.

Window Setting

The visibility of noise in a CT image depends on the setting of the window used to view the image. Small windows, which enhance contrast, also increase the contrast and visibility of noise.

Filtration

Some of the mathematical filter algorithms used in the reconstruction process can reduce image noise by smoothing, or blurring, the image. The compromise that must be considered in using these filter functions is the reduction in image detail.

ARTIFACTS

Artifacts are significant problems in CT imaging. They come from a variety of sources but can usually be identified by their appearance. Typical artifact sources include

- patient motion (streaks)
- high-attenuation objects (streaks)
- aliasing (streaks)
- beam hardening (cupping)
- detector imbalance (rings)
- centering
- partial volume effect.

Chapter 25

Ultrasound Production
and Interactions

INTRODUCTION AND OVERVIEW

Sound is a physical phenomenon that transfers energy from one point to another. In this respect, it is similar to x-radiation. It differs from x-rays, however, in that sound can pass only through matter and not through a vacuum. This is because sound waves are actually vibrations passing through a material. If there is no material, nothing can vibrate and sound cannot exist.

One of the most significant characteristics of sound is its frequency, which is the rate at which the sound source and the material vibrate. The basic unit for specifying frequency is the hertz, which is one vibration, or cycle, per second. Pitch is a term commonly used as a synonym for frequency.

The human ear cannot hear or respond to all sound frequencies. The range of frequencies that can be heard by a normal young adult is from approximately 20 Hz to 20,000 Hz (20 kHz). Ultrasound has a frequency above this range. Frequencies in the range of 1 MHz (million cycles per second) to 15 MHz are used in diagnostic ultrasound. Ultrasound is used as a diagnostic tool because it can be focused into small, well-defined beams that can probe the human body.

The basic components of an ultrasound imaging system are shown in Figure 25-1. The source of the ultrasound pulses is the transducer, which is activated by electrical pulses from the pulse generator circuit. The ultrasound pulses, or beam, enter the body and are reflected from the various internal structures. The reflected pulses, or echoes, are picked up by the transducer and reconverted into electrical pulses. After appropriate amplification, the electrical pulses are used to form an image on the display device.

ULTRASOUND CHARACTERISTICS

Ultrasound has several physical characteristics that must be considered in order to use it properly in diagnostic applications.

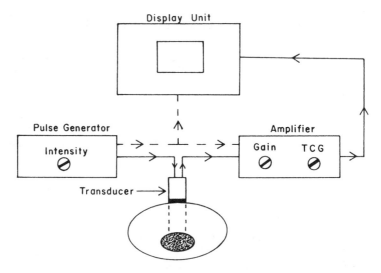

Figure 25-1 Basic Components of an Ultrasound Imaging System. The Solid Line and Arrows are the Pathway of Pulses. The Dotted Line is the Pathway of Synchronizing Signals.

Frequency

The basic principle of sound transmission is illustrated in Figure 25-2. For simplicity, the particles within the material are assumed to be arranged in rows. The source of sound is a vibrating object, such as the transducer crystal. Since the vibrating source in Figure 25-2 is in contact with the particles in the first row, they are caused to vibrate. Because they are in contact with particles in the second row,

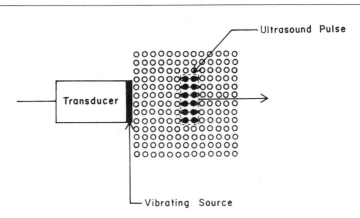

Figure 25-2 The Movement of an Ultrasound Pulse through Matter

these particles also begin to vibrate. This process continues, and the vibration, or sound, is passed along from one row of particles to another. The rate at which the particles vibrate back and forth is the frequency of the sound. The rate at which the vibrations move from row to row is the velocity of the sound.

The sound in most diagnostic ultrasound systems is emitted in pulses rather than a continuous stream of vibrations. At any instant, the vibrations are contained within a relatively small volume of the material. It is this volume of vibrating material that is referred to as the ultrasound pulse. As the vibrations are passed from one layer of material to another, the ultrasound pulse, but not the material, moves away from the source.

The diameter of the pulse is determined by the characteristics of the transducer. At the transducer surface, the diameter of the pulse is the same as the diameter of the vibrating crystal. As the pulse moves through the body, the diameter generally changes. This is determined by the focusing characteristics of the transducer and is discussed later.

As shown in Figure 25-3, the space through which the ultrasound pulse moves is generally referred to as the beam. In a diagnostic system, pulses are emitted at a rate of approximately 1,000 per second. The pulse rate (pulses per second) should not be confused with the frequency, which is the rate of vibration of the particles within the pulse.

The frequency of sound is determined by the source. For example, in a piano, the source of sound is a string that is caused to vibrate by striking it. Each string within the piano is adjusted, or tuned, to vibrate with a specific frequency. In diagnostic ultrasound equipment, the sound is generated by a device called a

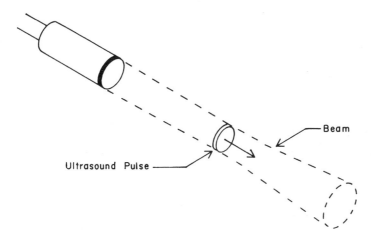

Figure 25-3 Relationship of the Ultrasound Pulse and Beam to the Transducer

transducer. The major element within the transducer is a crystal designed to vibrate with the desired frequency. A special property of the crystal material is that it is piezoelectrical. This means that the crystal will deform if electricity is applied to it. Therefore, if an electrical pulse is applied to the crystal it will have essentially the same effect as the striking of a piano string: the crystal will vibrate. If the transducer is activated by a single electrical pulse, the transducer will vibrate, or "ring," for a short period of time. This creates an ultrasound pulse as opposed to a continuous ultrasound wave. Most diagnostic procedures use pulsed ultrasound. The ultrasound pulse travels through the material in contact with the transducer and moves away from the transducer surface, as shown in Figure 25-2. A given transducer can vibrate with only one frequency, called its resonant frequency. Therefore, the only way to change ultrasound frequency is to change transducers. Certain frequencies are more appropriate for certain types of examination than others.

Velocity

The velocity with which sound travels through a medium is determined by the characteristics of the material and not the sound. There are several types of sound waves, depending on the direction of vibration with respect to the direction of movement of the pulse. In soft tissue and fluids, most of the vibration is in the same direction as that in which the sound moves. This type of vibration is designated longitudinal waves. Shear waves exist when the vibrations are at right angles to the direction of sound movement. The velocity of longitudinal sound waves in a liquid medium is given by

$$\text{Velocity} = E/\rho$$

where ρ is the density of the material, and E is a factor related to the elastic properties of the material. The velocities of sound through several materials of interest are given in Table 25-1.

Some solid materials, such as bone, transmit sound by means of shear waves.

Table 25-1 Approximate Velocity of Sound in Various Materials

Material	Velocity (m/sec)
Fat	1450
Water	1480
Soft tissue (average)	1540
Bone	4100

Wavelength

The distance sound travels during the period of one vibration is known as the wavelength, λ. It is related to the velocity, v, and frequency, f, by

$$\text{Wavelength} = \text{v/f.}$$

In other words, wavelength is simply the ratio of velocity to frequency. This means that the wavelength of ultrasound is determined by the characteristics of both the transducer (frequency) and the material through which the sound is passing (velocity). Although wavelength is not a unique property of a given ultrasound pulse, it is of some significance because the shape of an ultrasound beam is, to some extent, determined by the wavelength of the sound.

Amplitude

The distance through which the individual particles vibrate as the ultrasound pulse passes is the amplitude of the ultrasound pulse. Generally speaking, the amplitude is related to the energy content, or "loudness," of the ultrasound pulse. The amplitude of the pulse as it leaves the transducer is determined by how hard the crystal is "struck" by the electrical pulse. Most systems have a control on the pulse generator circuit that changes the size of the electrical pulse and the ultrasound pulse amplitude. We designate this the intensity control, although different names are used by various equipment manufacturers.

In diagnostic applications, it is usually necessary to know only the relative amplitude of ultrasound pulses. For example, it is necessary to know how much the amplitude, A, of a pulse decreases as it passes through a given thickness of tissue. The relative amplitude of two ultrasound pulses, or of one pulse after it has undergone an amplitude change, can be expressed by means of a ratio as follows:

$$\text{Relative amplitude (ratio)} = A_2/A_1.$$

There are advantages in expressing relative pulse amplitude in terms of the logarithm of the amplitude ratio. When this is done the relative amplitude is specified in the units of decibels (dB). The relative pulse amplitude, in decibels, is related to the actual amplitude ratio by

$$\text{Relative amplitude (dB)} = 20 \log (A_2/A_1).$$

When the amplitude ratio is greater than 1 (comparing a large pulse to a smaller one), the relative pulse amplitude has a positive decibel value; when the ratio is less than 1, the decibel value is negative. In other words, if the amplitude of a pulse is increased by some means, it will gain decibels, and if it is reduced, it will lose decibels.

Figure 25-4 compares decibel values to pulse amplitude ratios. The first two pulses differ in amplitude by 1 dB. In comparing the second pulse to the first, this corresponds to an amplitude ratio of 0.89, or a reduction of approximately 11%. If the pulse is reduced in amplitude by another 11%, it will be 2 dB smaller than the original pulse. If the pulse is once again reduced in amplitude by 11% (of 79%), it will have an amplitude ratio (with respect to the first pulse) of 0.71:1, or will be 3 dB smaller.

Perhaps the best way to establish a "feel" for the relationship between pulse amplitude expressed in decibels and in percentages is to notice that amplitudes that differ by a factor of 2 differ by 6 dB. A reduction in amplitude of 6 dB divides the amplitude by a factor of 2, or 50%. The doubling of a pulse amplitude increases it by 6 dB.

During its lifetime, an ultrasound pulse undergoes many reductions in amplitude. If the amount of each reduction is known in decibels, the total reduction can be found by simply adding all of the decibel losses. This is much easier than multiplying the various amplitude ratios, as illustrated in Figure 25-5. Here a pulse undergoes three reductions in amplitude. The relative amplitude of the pulse at any point can be found by adding the decibel losses. The advantage of doing this rather than multiplying the various ratios will become clear in later discussions.

In the following discussion of pulse amplitude, the reader is advised to think in terms of decibels without constantly trying to convert back and forth between decibels and amplitude ratios or percentages. It is much easier to use the decibel method for computing pulse amplitude changes.

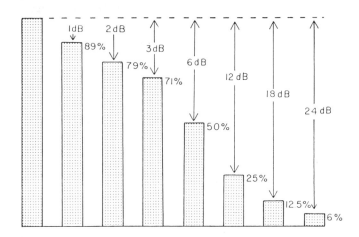

Figure 25-4 Pulse Amplitudes Expressed in Decibels and Percentages

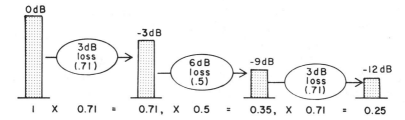

Figure 25-5 Final Pulse Amplitude Is Obtained by Adding Decibel Values

Intensity

Intensity is the amount of energy that passes through a specified area per second and is usually expressed in units of watts per square centimeter. The intensity of most diagnostic ultrasound beams at the transducer surface is on the order of a few milliwatts per square centimeter. Intensity is related to the amplitude of the individual pulses and the pulse rate. Since the pulse rate is fixed in most systems, the intensity of the beam is proportional to pulse amplitude when the amplitude is expressed in decibels.

INTERACTION OF ULTRASOUND WITH MATTER

As an ultrasound pulse passes through matter, such as the human body, it interacts with the matter in several different ways. Some of these interactions are necessary to form an ultrasound image, whereas others absorb much of the ultrasound energy and are generally undesirable in diagnostic examinations. The ability to conduct and interpret the results of an ultrasound examination depends on a thorough understanding of ultrasound interactions.

Attenuation

As the ultrasound pulse moves through matter, it continuously loses energy. This is generally referred to as attenuation. Several factors contribute to this reduction in energy. One of the most significant is the absorption of the ultrasound energy by the material, which converts it into heat. Ultrasound pulses lose energy continuously as they move through matter. This is unlike x-ray photons, which lose energy in "one-shot" photoelectric or Compton interactions. Scattering and refraction interactions remove some of the energy from the pulse and contribute to its overall attenuation.

The rate at which an ultrasound pulse is attenuated generally depends on two factors: (1) the material through which it is passing and (2) the frequency of the ultrasound. The attenuation rate is specified in terms of an attenuation coefficient in the units of decibels per centimeter. Since the attenuation in tissue increases with frequency, it is necessary to specify the frequency when an attenuation rate is given. The attenuation through a thickness of material, x, is given by

$$\text{Attenuation (dB)} = (\alpha)\,(f)\,(x)$$

where α is the attenuation coefficient (in decibels per centimeter at 1 MHz), and f is the ultrasound frequency, in megahertz. Approximate values of the attenuation coefficient for various materials of interest are given in Table 25-2.

From the attenuation coefficient values given in Table 25-2, it is apparent that there is a considerable variation in attenuation rate from material to material. The significance of these values is now considered. Of all the materials listed, water produces by far the least attenuation. This means that water is a very good conductor of ultrasound. Water within the body, such as in cysts and the bladder, forms "windows" through which underlying structures can be easily imaged. Most of the soft tissues of the body have attenuation coefficient values of approximately 1 dB per cm per MHz, with the exception of fat and muscle. Muscle has a range of values that depends on the direction of the ultrasound with respect to the muscle fibers. Lung has a much higher attenuation rate than either air or soft tissue. This is because the small pockets of air in the alveoli are very effective in scattering ultrasound energy. Because of this, the normal lung structure is extremely difficult to penetrate with ultrasound. Compared to the soft tissues of the body, bone has a relatively high attenuation rate. Bone, in effect, shields some parts of the body against easy access by ultrasound.

Table 25-2 Approximate Attenuation Coefficient Values for Various Materials

Material	Coefficient (dB/cm MHz)
Water	0.002
Fat	0.66
Soft tissue (average)	0.9
Muscle (average)	2.0
Air	12.0
Bone	20.0
Lung	40.0

Reflection

The reflection of ultrasound pulses by structures within the body is the interaction that creates the ultrasound image. The reflection of an ultrasound pulse occurs at the interface, or boundary, between two dissimilar materials. In order to form a reflection interface, the two materials must differ in terms of a physical characteristic known as acoustic impedance, Z. Although the traditional symbol for impedance, Z, is the same symbol used for atomic number, the two quantities are in no way related. Acoustic impedance is a characteristic of a material related to the density and elastic properties of the material. Since the velocity is related to the same material characteristics, a relationship exists between tissue impedance and ultrasound velocity. The relationship is such that the impedance, Z, is the product of the velocity, v, and the material density, ρ, which can be written as

$$\text{Impedance} = (\rho)\ (v).$$

At most interfaces within the body, only a portion of the ultrasound pulse is reflected. The pulse is divided into two pulses, and one pulse is reflected back toward the source and the other continues on into the other material, as shown in Figure 25-6. The quality of the ultrasound image depends on the strength of the reflection, or echo. This in turn depends on how much the two materials differ in terms of acoustic impedance. The amplitude ratio of the reflected to the incident pulse is related to the tissue impedance values by

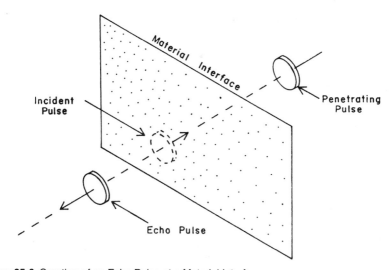

Figure 25-6 Creation of an Echo Pulse at a Material Interface

$$\text{Reflection loss (dB)} = 20 \log (Z_2 - Z_1)/(Z_2 + Z_1).$$

At most soft tissue interfaces, only a small fraction of the pulse is reflected. Therefore, the reflection process reduces the amplitude of the pulse that is reflected to the transducer. The reduction in pulse amplitude during reflection at several different interfaces is given in Table 25-3.

The amplitude of a pulse is reduced both by attenuation and reflection losses. Because of this, an echo returning to the transducer is much smaller than the original pulse produced by the transducer.

Table 25-3 Pulse Amplitude Loss Produced by a Reflection

Interface	Amplitude loss (dB)
Ideal reflector	0.0
Tissue-air	−0.01
Bone-soft tissue	−3.8
Fat-muscle	−20.0
Tissue-water	−26.0
Muscle-blood	−30.0

Chapter 26

Ultrasound Imaging

INTRODUCTION AND OVERVIEW

Most ultrasound images used for medical diagnostic purposes are formed by reflections, or echoes, from structural interfaces within the body. Reflected pulses, or echoes, are detected by the transducer, where they are converted into electrical pulses that are then amplified and displayed in an appropriate image format.

When an ultrasound pulse returns to the transducer, it brings with it two kinds of information, as illustrated in Figure 26-1. Its relative amplitude provides information as to the type of interface that produced the reflection. The time interval between when a pulse leaves and when it returns to the transducer is related to the distance between the transducer and the reflecting interface. These two pulse characteristics are used to form the ultrasound image. Other factors can alter the echo pulse and need to be taken into consideration when performing ultrasound examinations.

In most imaging situations, the ultrasound pulse passes through several different materials on its way to a reflection site (interface) and back to the transducer. As discussed previously, the velocity of the pulse depends on the characteristics of the material through which it is passing. Therefore, the velocity of the pulse actually changes as it passes from one material to another. The distance scale on most ultrasound equipment is calibrated for an ultrasound pulse velocity of 1,540 m/sec. This is assumed to be the average velocity of a pulse passing through most soft tissues. Distance errors because of variation in ultrasound velocity are relatively small, except in a material such as bone.

ECHO PULSE AMPLITUDE

When an echo pulse returns to the transducer, its amplitude is much less than when it left the transducer and began its journey into the body. The two factors that

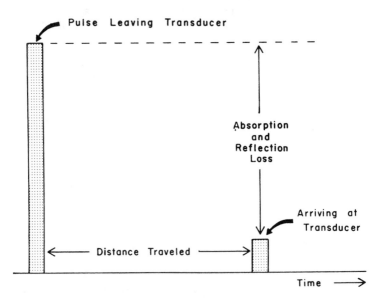

Figure 26-1 The Relative Amplitude and Time of Arrival of an Echo Pulse Provide the Information Necessary to Form an Ultrasound Image

account for this are the attenuation of the ultrasound pulse as it passes through the various materials and the reflection losses because of the splitting of the pulses at an interface.

The body section shown in Figure 26-2 is used to illustrate how attenuation and reflection reduce the amplitude of echo pulses. This body section does not represent a specific anatomical structure. The various materials were chosen to demonstrate several physical phenomena that are important in ultrasound imaging. The amplitude of the pulse is plotted with respect to distance into the body in Figure 26-3. Refer to both of these figures throughout the following discussion. The ultrasound frequency is 2.5 MHz.

As the pulse travels through the layer of fat, it is attenuated at the rate of 1.7 dB/cm (0.66 dB per cm per MHz × 2.5 MHz). This is represented by segment (a) in Figure 26-3. After traversing the 3-cm thickness of fat, the pulse amplitude is reduced by 5 dB (1.7 dB/cm × 3 cm). At the fat-muscle interface, the pulse is split by a reflection. The reflected pulse from a fat-muscle interface is reduced in amplitude by 20 dB, as indicated by segment (b). The reflected pulse returns through the same layer of fat where it undergoes an additional reduction in amplitude of 5 dB, as indicated by segment (c). The echo that returns to the transducer is 30 dB smaller than the original pulse.

The fat-muscle interface produces a relatively weak reflection. Therefore, most of the pulse energy passes through it into the muscle. As it moves through the

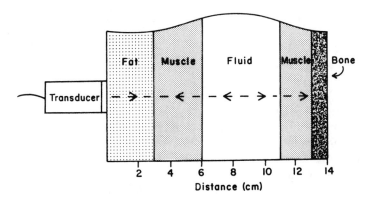

Figure 26-2 Body Section Containing Different Materials and Interfaces

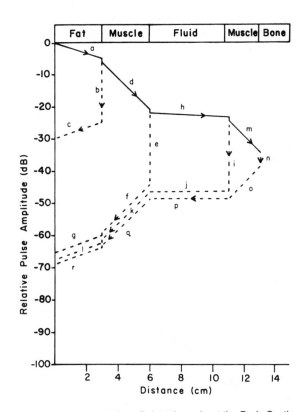

Figure 26-3 Pulse Amplitudes at Various Points throughout the Body Section

muscle, it is attenuated at the rate of 5 dB/cm for a total loss of 15 dB in the 3-cm muscle thickness. This is represented by segment (d). At the muscle-fluid interface, a reflected pulse is produced that is approximately 23 dB smaller, as indicated by segment (e). As the reflected pulse returns to the transducer through the muscle and fat layers, it undergoes additional attenuation, as indicated by segments (f) and (g). The echo from the muscle-fluid interface is 65 dB smaller than the original pulse.

At the muscle-fluid interface, most of the pulse energy passes on into the fluid. Since attenuation in fluid (water) is extremely small, the pulse amplitude is not significantly reduced in the fluid, as indicated by segment (h). A small part of this pulse is reflected at the second fluid-muscle interface and is returned to the transducer. The loss of amplitude for this reflected pulse is represented by segments (i), (j), (k), and (l).

The pulse energy that is not reflected continues on into the muscle where it undergoes additional attenuation, as represented by segment (m). At the muscle-bone interface, a relatively strong reflection occurs, and the echo is reduced by only 3.8 dB, as indicated by segment (n). This echo pulse returns to the transducer after undergoing the additional attenuation losses represented by segments (o), (p), (q), and (r). When it reaches the transducer, its amplitude is 69 dB smaller than the original pulse.

AMPLITUDE DISPLAY (A-MODE)

In the foregoing example, each ultrasound pulse sent out by the transducer resulted in four echoes. The returning echo pulses are intercepted by the transducer and converted into electrical pulses. The electrical pulses are passed through an amplifier, which increases their amplitude. The pulses from the amplifier go into an oscilloscope, which produces a visual display on a CRT. As pointed out earlier, the returning echo pulses picked up by the transducer differ in both amplitude and time of arrival after the initial pulse is sent out. The amplitude (A) display, or mode, displays these two characteristics. The "pulses" appear on the screen of the display. The amplitude of the echo pulses is represented by the height of the pulses on the display. The position of the display pulses along the horizontal scale is proportional to echo return time, which is interpreted as distance from the transducer.

The purpose of an A-mode display is to show the location and relative reflectivity of the various tissue interfaces. The relationship between the A-mode display and the structure of the body section is shown in Figure 26-4. In the ideal A-mode display, the amplitude of the displayed pulse would indicate the strength of the echo reflection. For example, in Figure 26-3 the echo pulse from the muscle-bone interface is much larger than the pulses from the fat-muscle and muscle-fluid

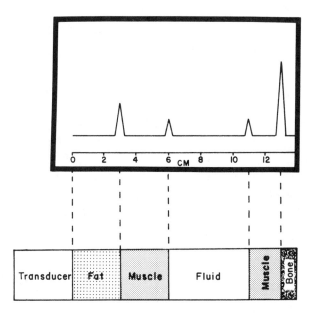

Figure 26-4 Relationship between A-mode Display and Body Structure

interfaces. This relationship between pulse amplitude and type of interface can provide useful diagnostic information.

Recall, however, that the amplitude of the pulses returning to the transducer depends not only on the strength of the reflections but also on the amount of attenuation along their path of travel. The attenuation losses can alter pulse amplitudes and make it difficult to determine the strength of a reflection from the size of a returning pulse. In Figure 26-3, the echo from the relatively weak fat-muscle interface returns to the transducer with a reduction in amplitude of only 30 dB. However, the much stronger echo from the muscle-bone interface is reduced in amplitude by 70 dB by the time it returns to the transducer. The reason the echo from the muscle-bone interface is smaller than the fat-muscle echo when it reaches the transducer is that it travels a much greater distance and undergoes much more attenuation. The amplitude of the echo pulses reaching the transducer is shown by the solid lines in Figure 26-5. The height of these should be compared to the height of the pulses in Figure 26-4. As stated previously, the echo pulse from the fat-muscle interface is much larger than from the muscle-bone interface because it undergoes less attenuation.

In order for the pulse amplitude to represent the strength of the reflection, it is necessary to remove the effects of attenuation on the pulse size. This can be done by amplifying the various pulses more or less in proportion to their attenuation losses. This, in turn, depends on the distance traveled by the ultrasound pulse and

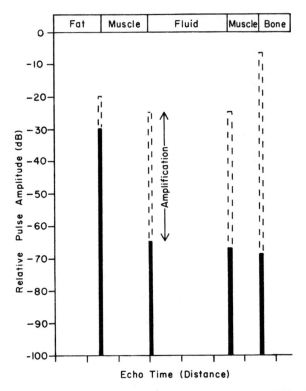

Figure 26-5 Amplitude of Echo Pulses without Amplification (———) and After Time-Controlled Amplification (- - -).

the attenuation coefficient values of the material through which it passes. The attenuation loss of a 2.5-MHz pulse that is reflected from various distances within the body section is shown in the bottom of Figure 26-6. For example, an echo from the fat-muscle interface undergoes a 10-dB attenuation: It loses 5 dB in traveling from the transducer to the interface and another 5 dB traveling from the interface back to the transducer. As would be expected, pulses reflected from deeper within the body undergo the most attenuation. For example, echoes from the muscle-bone interface decrease in amplitude by 60 dB because of attenuation.

It is desirable to amplify the returning echo pulses in proportion to their attenuation losses. This is achieved by having the amplifier gain increase with time after each pulse leaves the transducer. This is generally referred to as time-controlled gain, or TCG. Since the distance traveled by a pulse is proportional to its travel time, it gives a relationship between amplifier gain and distance to a reflection site. The fact that the rate of attenuation (decibels per centimeter) is not

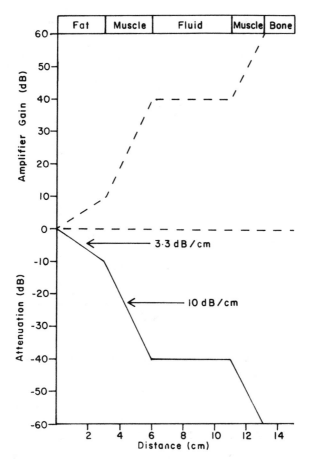

Figure 26-6 TCG Curve (Top) that Compensates for the Pulse Attenuation Described by the Bottom Curve

the same in all tissues must also be taken into account. When the pulse is passing through muscle, the gain must increase faster than when the pulse is passing through fat. The rate at which the amplifier gain changes with time (distance) is generally expressed in units of decibels per centimeter.

With most ultrasound equipment, TCG values can differ over various distances within the body. The relationship between amplifier gain and the distance to an echo site is usually described by means of a TCG curve, such as the one shown in the top of Figure 26-6. This particular TCG curve is one that would exactly compensate for the attenuation losses shown in the bottom half of the figure. In other words, the amplifier TCG curve that is a mirror image of the attenuation curve provides complete compensation for attenuation within the tissues.

When the echoes from the four interfaces are amplified in a time-controlled manner, their relative amplitudes are changed, as shown in Figure 26-5. The echo from the fat-muscle interface is amplified by only 10 dB. The echo from the muscle-fluid interfaces is amplified by 40 dB, and the muscle-bone echo is amplified by 60 dB. The increase in pulse size produced by the amplification is represented by the dotted lines in Figure 26-5. After passing through a properly adjusted TCG amplifier, the pulse amplitudes represent the strength of the various ultrasound reflections. Note that the amplified pulses in Figure 26-5 with respect to a 30-dB baseline have the same relative amplitudes as the pulses in the ideal display of Figure 26-4.

BRIGHTNESS (B-MODE)

Another useful type of ultrasound image is formed by using the amplitude of the various echo pulses to control the brightness of a spot on the display unit screen. This is called a B-mode display. A simple B-mode image is shown in Figure 26-7. If you compare it with the A-mode image shown in Figure 26-4, you will observe that the brightness (or film density) on the B-mode display corresponds to the amplitude of the echo pulses shown in the A-mode display. The brightness of the

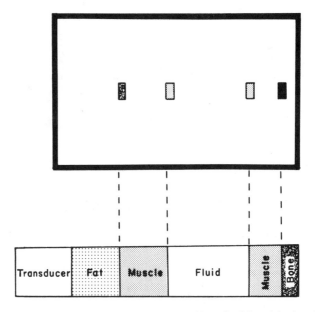

Figure 26-7 Relationship between a B-Mode Display (Gray Scale) and the Interfaces within a Body Section

spot is controlled by the amplitude of the echo pulse, as shown in Figure 26-7. The relationship between image point brightness and the amplitude of the echo pulse is determined by the characteristics and the control setting of the ultrasound system.

An important characteristic of an ultrasound system is its dynamic range. The dynamic range is the range of pulse amplitudes corresponding to the full brightness range of the viewing unit. The dynamic range of an ultrasound system is somewhat analogous to the latitude of an x-ray film.

If the transducer is not moved during the recording of an ultrasound image, only echoes from structures within the relatively small beam area will be recorded. This is the type of image illustrated in Figure 26-7. B-mode image is obtained by moving, or scanning, the ultrasound beam over the area of interest within the body. As the ultrasound beam is scanned through the area of interest, the image from each beam position is stored within the viewing unit.

SCAN METHODS

Several designs are used for transducers that scan the ultrasound beam.

Manual Scanners

A manual scanner is a single-element transducer mounted on an articulating arm. The operator manually moves the transducer over the surface of the patient's body to produce the scan. Several seconds are required for one complete image scan. The joints in the articulating arm assembly contain electrical sensors that measure the location and angulation of the ultrasound transducer. Signals from these sensors are used along with the echo-produced pulses to form the image.

Mechanical Scanners

With a mechanical scanner, the scanning motion is produced by a small motor within the transducer head. Several mechanical designs are used. Typically, the transducer element or a reflector is either oscillated or rotated to produce the scanning action.

Mechanical scanning transducers can scan at rates sufficiently high to produce real-time images capable of showing motion within the body.

Electronic Scanners

Electronic scanners use a transducer assembly that contains a phased array. The basic construction and function of a phased-array transducer is shown in Figure 26-8. It contains many small transducer elements that are mounted in an array. Each transducer element can be pulsed independently.

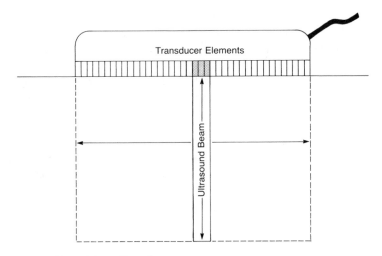

Figure 26-8 Phased-Array Transducer

A beam of ultrasound pulses is created by applying electrical pulses to a small group of transducer elements, as shown. When pulsed in this manner, the group of elements function together to produce a single ultrasound pulse. The beam can be scanned rapidly along the array by switching the electrical pulses to other groups of transducer elements.

An ultrasound beam can be angulated and focused by pulsing the elements within each group sequentially, rather than at the same time.

SCAN PATTERNS

Several scanning patterns are used to move the ultrasound beam over the body section being imaged. Four of the basic patterns are compared in Figure 26-9.

A linear scan pattern is produced by moving the beam so that all beams remain parallel. The imaged areas have the same width at all depths. General advantages of a linear scan are a wide field of view for anatomical regions close to the transducer and a uniform distribution of beam areas throughout the region. General disadvantages include a limited field of view for deeper regions and difficulty in intercostal imaging.

Sector scanning is performed by angulating the beam path from one transducer location. Imaging can be performed through an intercostal space. A general disadvantage is the small field of view for regions close to the transducer surface.

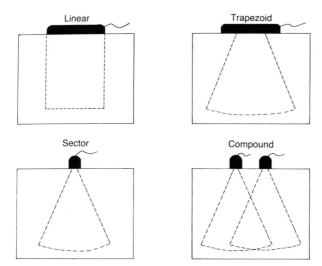

Figure 26-9 Four Basic Ultrasound Scan Patterns

A trapezoid pattern is, in principle, a combination of linear and sector scanning. The beam is both angulated and moved as in the linear scan.

Compound scanning is, in principle, sector scanning from several different transducer positions.

MOTION (M) MODE

In the motion (M) mode, the ultrasound system records the motion of internal body structures. In conventional M-mode systems, the transducer is stationary with respect to the body, and the echo pulses control the brightness of the display, as in B-mode operation. This display of image points is moved across the screen. Each echo site, in effect, leaves a track across the screen. A moving echo site produces a curved track. By using a properly calibrated distance scale, the amount of movement of the body structures can be readily determined.

DOPPLER IMAGING

The Doppler effect produces echoes with a frequency different from the original ultrasound pulse when the echoes are reflected from a moving object. This phenomenon can be used selectively to image moving substances such as blood and to produce displays showing flow velocities.

IMAGE QUALITY

The range of structures that can be visualized in an ultrasound image depends on the design characteristics of the particular system and the imaging variables selected by the operator.

Contrast Sensitivity

Contrast sensitivity in ultrasound imaging is primarily related to the system's ability to detect and display weak echoes. This characteristic is often referred to as sensitivity. It is most directly affected by the gain of the receiver amplifier. Increasing the gain has the effect of increasing the sensitivity and causing weaker echoes to become visible in the image.

Another aspect of contrast sensitivity is the ability to see (in the image) amplitude *differences* for echoes well above the threshold level. This depends on how the various echo amplitudes are translated into image brightness levels, or shades of gray. The imaging systems contain image processors that can be used to alter the relationship between image brightness and echo amplitude. Different processing functions can either enhance or suppress image contrast in different parts of the echo amplitude range.

Visibility of Detail

The major factor that limits visibility of detail in ultrasound imaging is the blurring associated with the size of the ultrasound pulse. The amount of blur is essentially the physical dimensions of the pulse. A pulse has two dimensions that must be considered.

Lateral Blur

Lateral blur, or resolution, is determined by the diameter of the ultrasound pulse, or beam, at the time it interacts with the object creating the echo. The width of the ultrasound beam is determined by certain characteristics of the transducer. The two basic types of transducers, with respect to beam shape, are the focused and unfocused, as shown in Figure 26-10.

The beam from an unfocused transducer is divided into two regions. The region nearest the transducer is designated the near field, or Fresnel zone. The other region is designated the far field, or Fraunhofer zone.

In the near field, the beam has a constant diameter that is determined by the diameter of the transducer. The length of the near field is related to the diameter, D, of the transducer and the wavelength, λ, of the ultrasound by

$$\text{Near field length} = D^2/4\lambda$$

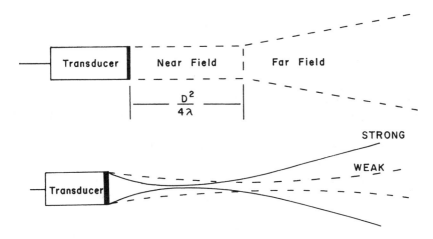

Figure 26-10 Beam Profiles Produced by Both Unfocused (a) and Focused (b) Transducers

Recall that the wavelength is inversely related to frequency. Therefore, for a given transducer size, the length of the near field is proportional to frequency. Another characteristic of the near field is that the intensity along the beam axis is not constant; it oscillates between maximum and zero several times between the transducer surface and the boundary between the near and far fields. This is because of the interference patterns created by the sound waves from the transducer surface. An intensity of zero at a point along the axis simply means that the sound vibrations are concentrated around the periphery of the beam. A picture of the ultrasound pulse in the region would look more like concentric rings or "donuts" than the disc that has been shown in various illustrations.

The major characteristic of the far field is that the beam diverges. This causes the ultrasound pulses to be larger in diameter but to have less intensity along the central axis. The approximate angle of divergence is related to the diameter of the transducer, D, and the wavelength by:

$$\text{Divergence angle (degrees)} = 70\lambda/D.$$

Because of the inverse relationship between wavelength and frequency, divergence is decreased by increasing frequency. The major advantage of using the higher ultrasound frequencies (shorter wavelengths) is that the beams are less divergent and generally produce less blur.

An acoustical lens can be attached to the transducer to produce a focused beam. Focusing can produce an ultrasound pulse with a diameter less than that of the transducer at some locations along the beam axis. The degree of focusing (strong or weak) is determined by the characteristics of the acoustic lens. A smaller beam can be produced by a strongly focused transducer, but the small pulse size is limited to a rather short distance along the beam axis.

Axial Blur

Axial, or depth, blur is determined by the length, or time duration, of the ultrasound pulse. This, in turn, is determined by the characteristics of the transducer and amplifier circuit.

Since smaller beams can be produced by increasing the ultrasound frequency, it is desirable to use the higher frequencies when imaging small structures where blur might become a significant problem. However, the attenuation is much greater at the higher frequencies. Therefore, a transducer (frequency) must be selected that will provide a reasonable compromise between attenuation and blur.

Noise

The predominant source of image noise comes from within the receiver and amplifier or is picked up as electrical interference from the environment or power lines. The noise becomes especially significant with high amplifier gain settings.

Artifacts

Artifacts are relatively common in ultrasound images. We now consider some of the most common.

Shadowing

Some objects produce shadows in ultrasound images. If the object has either high reflection or attenuation characteristics, very little pulse energy will pass through it. This artifact appears in the image as a streak of reduced intensity (shadow) behind the object and is often produced by bones and stones.

Enhancement

Enhancement is the opposite of shadowing. Certain objects, such as fluid-filled cysts and vascular structures, produce much less attenuation than adjacent tissue. This appears as a streak with increased intensity extending beyond the object.

Reverberation

Reverberation can occur if two or more reflecting structures are located at different points along the ultrasound beam. The artifact is produced because some of the pulses are reflected back and forth between the two objects. This causes a time delay before the echo pulse returns to the transducer. Because of this delay, the echo appears to have originated from a structure that is deeper within the body than it actually is. Therefore, the image shows the structure at several points along the beam path.

Chapter 27

Nuclear Magnetic Resonance Imaging

INTRODUCTION AND OVERVIEW

When certain materials are placed in a magnetic field, they take on a resonant characteristic. This means the materials can absorb and then reradiate electromagnetic radiation that has a specific frequency, as illustrated in Figure 27-1. The radiation is typically in the form of radio signals. The characteristics of the RF signals emitted by the material are determined by certain physical and chemical characteristics of the material. In the process of magnetic resonance imaging (MRI), the radio signals also carry information as to the spatial location of the tissue within the human body. The magnetic resonance (MR) image is an array of pixels showing the intensity of the RF signals originating from each tissue voxel within the body section.

The brightness of each pixel within the image is determined by the intensity of the RF signal emitted by the corresponding tissue voxel. The signal intensity from each voxel is determined by four characteristics of the tissue, as listed in Figure 27-1. The extent to which any one of the characteristics contributes to image brightness and contrast is determined by certain imaging factors selected by the operator. For example, it is possible to "weight" an image so that the RF signal is primarily determined by either nuclear density or concentration, longitudinal relaxation rate (T1) values, or transverse relaxation rate (T2) values. Selecting the imaging factors so as to control these variables is discussed later.

The tissue components that interact with the magnetic field and the RF energy are the individual nuclei. Therefore, this general phenomenon is known as nuclear magnetic resonance (NMR). It was discovered in 1946 by Felix Bloch and Edward Purcell and has been used extensively since that time for the in-vitro analysis of a wide range of chemical substances. NMR techniques can be used to measure a number of physical and chemical characteristics of materials. However, the predominant application has been the determination of molecular structure through the process of NMR spectroscopy.

381

Magnetic Resonance Imaging

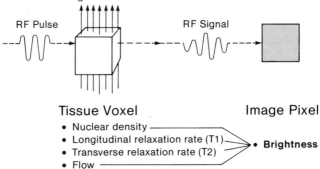

Figure 27-1 The Basic Principle of Magnetic Resonance Imaging

In the 1970s, several investigators, including Damadian and Lauterbur, developed systems that could perform in-vivo NMR analysis and display the results in tomographic images. By the early 1980s, nuclear magnetic imaging systems were being investigated for their diagnostic potential. The technology continues to advance and yield improvements in image quality and reduction in the time required to perform a diagnostic examination.

This chapter presents the basic concepts and principles of NMR and the application of these principles to the process of magnetic resonance imaging.

MAGNETIC NUCLEI

Materials that participate in the MR process must contain nuclei with specific magnetic properties. In order to interact with a magnetic field, the nuclei themselves must be small magnets and have a magnetic moment. The magnetic characteristic of an individual nucleus is determined by its neutron-proton composition. Only certain nuclides with an odd number of neutrons and protons are magnetic. Even though most chemical elements have one or more isotopes with magnetic nuclei, the number of magnetic isotopes that might be useful for either imaging or in-vivo spectroscopic analysis is somewhat limited. Among the nuclides that are magnetic and can participate in an NMR process, the amount of signal produced by each varies considerably.

The magnetic property of a nucleus has a specific direction known as the magnetic moment. In Figure 27-2, the direction of the magnetic moment is indicated by an arrow drawn through the nucleus.

Magnetic Nuclei

Nonmagnetic Nuclei

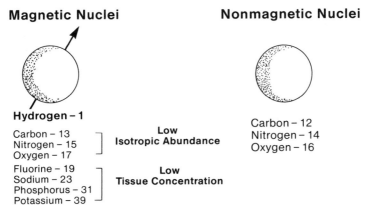

Hydrogen – 1

Carbon – 13
Nitrogen – 15   ] **Low Isotropic Abundance**
Oxygen – 17

Fluorine – 19
Sodium – 23   ] **Low Tissue Concentration**
Phosphorus – 31
Potassium – 39

Carbon – 12
Nitrogen – 14
Oxygen – 16

Figure 27-2 Isotopes that Have Magnetic Nuclei

The intensity of the RF signal emitted by tissue is probably the most significant factor in determining image quality and the time necessary to acquire an image. This important issue is considered in detail later. We now begin to introduce the factors that contribute to signal intensity.

During the imaging process, the body section is divided into an array of individual volume elements, or voxels. It is the signal intensity from each voxel that determines image quality. The signal is produced by the magnetic nuclei within each voxel. Therefore, signal intensity is, in general, proportional to the quantity of magnetic nuclei within an individual voxel. We now consider the factors that affect the number of nuclei within an individual voxel.

Tissue Concentration

The concentration of chemical elements in tissue covers a considerable range, depending on tissue type and factors such as metabolic or pathologic state. The concentrations of elements in tissue are in two groups. Four elements, hydrogen, carbon, nitrogen, and oxygen, typically make up at least 99% of the tissue mass. Other elements, such as sodium, phosphorus, potassium, and magnesium, are present in very low concentrations. Calcium is concentrated in bone or in localized deposits.

The most abundant isotopes of the four elements that account for more than 99% of tissue mass are:

- hydrogen-1
- carbon-12
- nitrogen-14
- oxygen-16.

Hydrogen is the only one of these four isotopes that has a magnetic nucleus. The nucleus of the hydrogen-1 atom is a single proton. Among all the chemical elements, hydrogen is unique in that it occurs in relatively high concentrations in most tissues, and the most abundant isotope (H-1) has a magnetic nucleus.

Within the group of elements with low tissue concentrations are several with magnetic nuclei. These include:

- fluorine-19
- sodium-23
- phosphorus-31
- potassium-39.

Isotopic Abundance

Most chemical elements have several isotopes. When a chemical element is found in a naturally occurring substance, such as tissue, most of the element is typically in the form of one isotope, with very low concentrations of the other isotopic forms. Unfortunately, some of the magnetic isotopes are the ones with a low abundance in the natural state. Examples are:

- carbon-13
- nitrogen-15
- oxygen-17.

Relative Sensitivity

The signal strength produced by an equal quantity of the various nuclei also varies over a considerable range. This inherent nuclear magnetic resonance (NMR) sensitivity is typically expressed relative to hydrogen-1, which produces the strongest signal of all of the nuclides. The relative sensitivity of some magnetic nuclides are:

- hydrogen-1, 1
- fluorine-19, 0.83
- sodium-23, 0.093
- phosphorus-31, 0.066.

Relative Signal Strength

The relative signal strength from the various chemical elements in tissue is determined by three factors: (1) tissue concentration of the element, (2) isotopic abundance, and (3) sensitivity of the specific nuclide.

In comparison to all other nuclides, hydrogen produces an extremely strong signal. This results from its high values for each of the three contributing factors. Of the three factors, only the concentration, or density, of the nuclei varies from point to point within an imaged section. The quantity is often referred to as spin-density and is the most fundamental tissue characteristic that determines the intensity of the RF signal from an individual voxel, and the resulting pixel brightness. In most imaging situations, pixel brightness is proportional to the density (concentration) of nuclei in the corresponding voxel, although additional factors modify this relationship.

THE IMAGING CYCLE

The formation of an MR image is not instantaneous, but occurs in steps. These steps include the application of RF energy pulses to the patient, creating gradients in the magnetic field, and detecting RF signals emitted by the tissue. These events are repeated within each imaging cycle. In order to acquire enough signals to form an entire image, the cycle must be repeated many times, as illustrated in Figure 27-3. The minimum number of cycles is determined by the size (number of columns and rows) of the matrix. The matrix size can be selected by the operator and usually has a dimension of 64, 128, or 256 voxels (pixels). The formation of a typical 256-matrix image requires a minimum of 256 imaging cycles.

In many clinical procedures, the individual cycles are often repeated and the signals averaged to improve image quality. The number of repetitions depends on the specific clinical requirements.

The duration of an imaging cycle is set by the operator and is designated TR (repetition time). Values typically range between 250 msec and 2,500 msec for conventional imaging methods. The total time required to acquire signals for one image (or one set of multi-slice or multi-echo images) is the product of three factors:

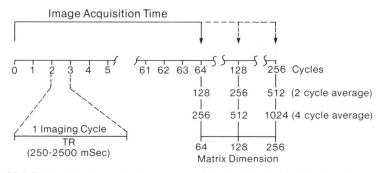

Figure 27-3 Factors that Determine the Number of Cycles Required to Create an Image

1. TR
2. matrix dimension (64, 128, 256, etc.)
3. number of cycles averaged together (1, 2, 4, etc.).

TR is a significant factor in image acquisition. It not only determines acquisition time, but also affects image contrast and image noise.

It is possible to create several types of MR images. The general image type is determined by the sequence of RF pulses and magnetic field gradients. Most clinical procedures use the spin-echo pulse sequence, which is applied during each cycle. The general discussion that follows describes spin-echo imaging. Some alternate imaging methods are introduced later.

MAGNETIC FIELDS

NMR occurs only when a magnetic nucleus is within a magnetic field. The magnetic field for in-vivo imaging and spectroscopy is typically created by a superconducting electrical coil surrounding the patient's body, as shown in Figure 27-4. At any point within a magnetic field, its two primary characteristics are *field direction* and *field strength*.

Field Direction

It will be easier to visualize a magnetic field if it is represented by a series of parallel lines, as shown in Figure 27-4. The arrow on each line indicates the direction of the field. On the surface of the earth, the direction of the magnetic field is specified with reference to the north and south poles. The north-south designa-

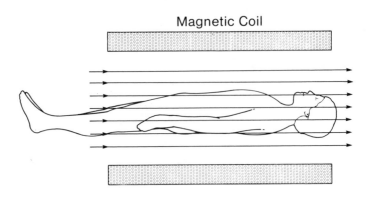

Magnetic Coil

Figure 27-4 General Direction of the Magnetic Field Used for Imaging

tion is generally not applied to magnetic fields used for imaging. The electromagnets used for imaging produce a magnetic field that runs through the bore parallel to the major patient axis. As the magnetic field leaves the bore, it spreads out and encircles the magnet. This part of the field is not shown in the illustration.

Field Strength

Each point within a magnetic field has a particular intensity, or strength. Field strength is expressed either in the units of tesla (T) or gauss (G). The relationship between the two units is that 1 T is equal to 10,000 G (or 10 kG). At the earth's surface, its magnetic field has a strength of less than 1 G. Magnetic field strengths in the range of 0.15 T to 1.5 T are used for imaging. The significance of field strength is considered as we explore the characteristics of MR images and image quality in the next chapter. In our pictorial representation of a magnetic field, the relative strength is indicated by the spacing, or concentration, of the lines.

MRI requires a magnetic field which is uniform, or homogeneous. Field homogeneity is affected by magnet design, adjustments, and environmental conditions. Imaging generally requires a homogeneity (field uniformity) on the order of a few parts per million (ppm) within the imaging area.

During an imaging procedure, the individual voxels are formed by a temporary distortion of the uniform field. This distortion is in the form of a variation in field strength across the imaging space and is known as a gradient. The use of the magnetic field gradient is considered later.

RADIO FREQUENCY ENERGY

During an imaging procedure, RF energy is exchanged between the imaging system and the patient's body, as shown in Figure 27-5. This exchange takes place through a set of coils located relatively close to the patient's body. The RF coil is the antenna that transmits energy to and receives energy from the tissue.

Pulses

RF energy is applied to the body in several short pulses during each imaging cycle. The strength of the pulses is described in terms of the angle through which they rotate tissue magnetization, as described below. Most imaging methods use both 90° and 180° pulses in each cycle.

Signals

At a specific time in each imaging cycle, the tissue is stimulated to emit an RF signal, which is picked up by the coil, analyzed, and used to form the image. The

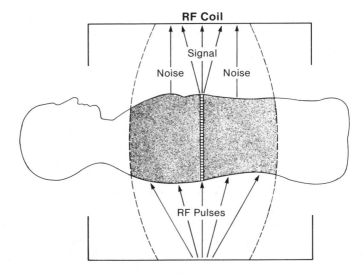

Figure 27-5 RF Coils and Energy Exchange with the Human Body

---

spin-echo technique is generally used to stimulate signal emission. Therefore, the signals from the patient's body are commonly referred to as echoes.

NUCLEAR MAGNETIC INTERACTIONS

The NMR process is a series of interactions involving the magnetic nuclei, a magnetic field, and RF energy pulses and signals.

Nuclear Alignment

Recall that a magnetic nucleus is characterized by a magnetic moment. The direction of the magnetic moment is represented by a small arrow passing through the nucleus. If we think of the nucleus as a small conventional magnet, then the magnetic moment arrow corresponds to the south pole–north pole direction of the magnet.

In the absence of a strong magnetic field, magnetic moments of nuclei are randomly oriented in space. Many nuclei in tissue are not in a rigid structure and are free to change direction. In fact, nuclei are constantly tumbling, or changing direction, because of thermal activity within the material.

When a material containing magnetic nuclei is placed in a magnetic field, the nuclei experience a torque that encourages them to align with the direction of the field. In the human body, however, thermal energy agitates the nuclei and keeps most of them from aligning parallel to the magnetic field. The number of nuclei that do align with the magnetic field is proportional to field strength. The magnetic fields used for imaging can align only a few of every million magnetic nuclei present.

Resonance

When a magnetic nucleus aligns with a magnetic field, it is not fixed; the nuclear magnetic moment precesses, or oscillates, about the axis of the magnetic field, as shown in Figure 27-6. The precessing motion is a physical phenomenon that results from an interaction between the magnetic field and the spinning momentum of the nucleus. Precession is often observed with a child's spinning top. A spinning top does not stand vertical for long, but begins to wobble, or precess. In this case, the precession is caused by an interaction between the earth's gravitational field and the spinning momentum of the top.

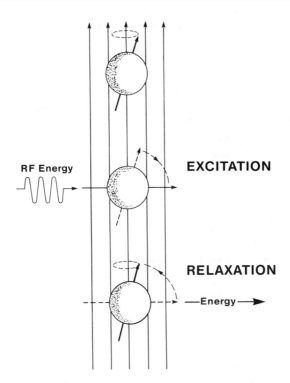

Figure 27-6 Interactions between RF Energy and Nuclei in a Magnetic Field

The significance of the nuclear precession is that it causes the nucleus to be extremely sensitive, or tuned, to RF energy that has a frequency identical with the precession frequency (rate). This condition is known as resonance and is the basis for all MR procedures: NMR is the process in which a nucleus resonates, or "tunes in," when it is in a magnetic field.

Resonance is fundamental to the absorption and emission of energy by many objects and devices. Objects are most effective in exchanging energy at their resonant frequency. The resonance of an object or device is determined by certain physical characteristics. Let us consider two common examples. Radio receivers operate on the principle of resonant frequency. A receiver can select a specific broadcast station because each station transmits a different frequency. Tuning a radio is actually adjusting its resonant frequency. Its receiver is very sensitive to radio signals at its resonant frequency and insensitive to all other frequencies.

The strings of a musical instrument also have specific resonant frequencies. This is the frequency at which the string vibrates to produce a specific audio frequency, or note. The resonant frequency of a string depends on the amount of tension. It can be changed, or tuned, by changing the tension.

The resonant frequency of a nucleus is determined by a combination of nuclear characteristics and the strength of the magnetic field. The resonant frequency is also known as the Larmor frequency. The specific relationship between resonant frequency and field strength is an inherent characteristic of each nuclide and is generally designated the gyromagnetic ratio.

For all nuclides, the resonant frequency is proportional to the strength of the magnetic field. In a very general sense, increasing the magnetic field strength increases the tension on the nuclei (as with the strings of a musical instrument) and increases the resonant frequency. The Larmor frequencies for selected nuclides in a magnetic field of 1 T are:

- hydrogen-1, 42.58 MHz
- fluorine-19, 40.05 MHz
- phosphorus-31, 17.24 MHz
- sodium-23, 11.26 MHz.

The fact that different nuclides have different resonant frequencies means that most MR procedures can "look at" only one chemical element (nuclide) at a time. The fact that a specific nuclide can be tuned to different radio frequencies by varying the field strength (applying gradients) is used in the imaging process, as discussed later.

Excitation

If RF energy with a frequency corresponding to the nuclear resonant frequency is applied to the material, some of the energy will be absorbed by the individual nuclei. The absorption of energy by a nucleus shifts its alignment away from the direction of the magnetic field. This increased energy places the nucleus in an unnatural, or excited, state.

Relaxation

When a nucleus is in an excited state, it experiences an increased torque from the magnetic field, urging it to realign. The nucleus can return to a position of alignment by transferring its excess energy to other nuclei or to the general structure of the material. This process is known as relaxation.

Relaxation is not instantaneous following an excitation. It cannot occur until the nucleus is able to transfer its energy. How quickly the energy transfer takes place depends on the physical characteristics of the material. In fact, the nuclear relaxation rate (time) is, in many cases, the most significant factor in producing contrast among different types of tissue.

Figure 27-6 compares excitation and relaxation, which are the two fundamental interactions between RF energy and a resonant nucleus in a magnetic field.

MAGNETIZATION

We have considered the behavior of individual nuclei placed in a magnetic field. MRI depends on the collective, or net, magnetic effect of a large number of nuclei within a specific voxel of tissue. If a voxel of tissue contains more nuclei aligned in one direction than in other directions, the tissue will be temporarily magnetized in that particular direction. This process is illustrated in Figure 27-7.

In the absence of a magnetic field, the nuclei are randomly oriented and produce no net magnetic effect. This is the normal state of tissue before being placed into a magnetic field. When the tissue is placed in a field, and some of the nuclei align with the field, their combined effect is to magnetize the tissue in the direction of the field. An arrow, generally referred to as a *magnetization vector,* is used to indicate the amount and direction of the magnetization. When tissue is placed in a field, the maximum magnetization that can be produced depends on three factors: (1) the concentration (density) of magnetic nuclei in the tissue voxel, (2) the magnetic sensitivity of the nuclide, and (3) the strength of the magnetic field. Since an imaging magnetic field aligns a very small fraction of the magnetic nuclei, the tissues are never fully magnetized. The amount of tissue magnetization determines the strength of the RF signals emitted by the tissue during an imaging or analytical procedure. This, in turn, affects image quality and imaging time, as explained in the next chapter.

When tissue is placed in a magnetic field, it reaches its maximum magnetization within a few seconds and remains at that level unless it is disturbed by a change in the magnetic field or pulses of RF energy. The MRI procedure is a dynamic

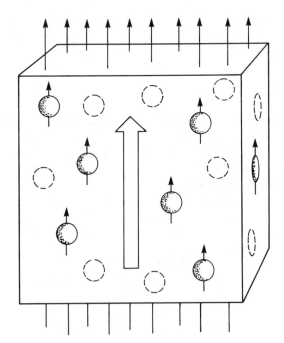

Figure 27-7 Magnetization of a Tissue Voxel Resulting from the Alignment of Individual Nuclei

process in which tissue is cycled through changes in its magnetization during each imaging cycle.

The direction of tissue magnetization is specified in reference to the direction of the applied magnetic field, as shown in Figure 27-8. With longitudinal magnetization, the tissue is magnetized in a direction parallel to the direction of the field. With transverse magnetization, the direction of tissue magnetization is at a 90° angle with respect to the direction of the magnetic field.

The actual direction of magnetization is not limited to longitudinal or transverse. It can exist in any direction. In principle, magnetization can have both longitudinal and transverse components. Since the two components have distinctly different characteristics, we consider them independently.

Longitudinal Magnetization and Relaxation

When tissue is placed in a magnetic field, it becomes magnetized in the longitudinal direction. It will remain in this state until the magnetic field is changed or the magnetization is redirected by the application of an RF pulse to the tissue. If the magnetization is temporarily redirected by an RF pulse, it will then, over a period of time, return to its original longitudinal position. The regrowth of

Tissue Magnetization

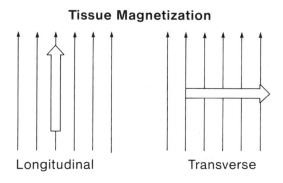

Longitudinal   Transverse

Figure 27-8 The Two Basic Directions of Tissue Magnetization

longitudinal magnetization is the relaxation process, which occurs after an excitation. The time required for the longitudinal magnetization to regrow, or relax, depends on characteristics of the material and the strength of the magnetic field.

Longitudinal magnetization does not grow at a constant rate but at an exponential rate, as shown in Figure 27-9. The factor that varies from one type of tissue to another, and can be used to produce image contrast, is the time required for the magnetization to regrow, or the relaxation time. Because of its exponential nature, it is difficult to determine exactly when the magnetization has reached its maximum. The convention is to specify the relaxation time in terms of the time

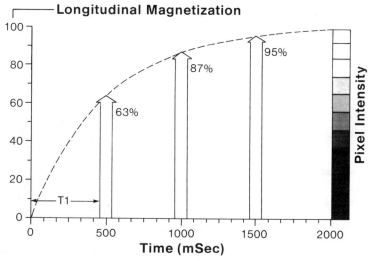

Figure 27-9 Growth of Longitudinal Magnetization During the Relaxation Process

required for the magnetization to reach 63% of its maximum. This time, ie, the longitudinal relaxation time, is designated T1. The 63% value is used because of mathematical, rather than clinical, considerations. Longitudinal magnetization continues to grow with time, and reaches 87% of its maximum after two T1 intervals, and 95% after three T1 intervals. For practical purposes, the magnetization can be considered fully recovered after approximately three times the T1 value of the specific tissue. We will see that this must be taken into consideration in setting up an imaging procedure.

At the beginning of each imaging cycle, the longitudinal magnetization is reduced to zero (or a negative value) by an RF pulse, and then allowed to regrow, or relax, during the cycle. The cycle terminates during the regrowth phase and the magnetization value is measured and displayed as a pixel intensity, or brightness.

The time required for a specific level of longitudinal magnetization regrowth varies from tissue to tissue. Figure 27-10 shows the regrowth curves for three tissues with different T1 values. The important thing to notice is that the tissue with the shortest T1 has the most magnetization at any particular time. The clinical significance of this is that tissues with short T1 values will be bright in T1-weighted images.

Typical T1 values for various tissues are listed in Table 27-1. Two materials establish the lower and upper values for the T1 range: Fat has a short T1, and fluid falls at the other extreme. Therefore, in T1-weighted images, fat is generally

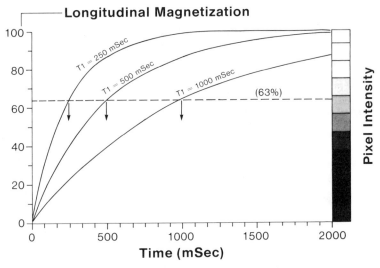

Figure 27-10 Comparison of Longitudinal Relaxation (Growth) for Tissues with Different T1 Values

Table 27-1 T2 and T1 Values for Various Tissues

Tissue	T2 (msec)	T1(0.5T) (msec)	T1(1.5T) (msec)
Adipose	80	210	260
Liver	42	350	500
Muscle	45	550	870
White Matter	90	500	780
Gray Matter	100	650	920
CSF	160	1800	2400

bright, and fluid (cerebrospinal fluid, cyst, etc.) is dark. Most other body tissues are within the range between fat and fluid.

In principle, at the beginning of each imaging cycle all tissues are dark. As the tissues regain longitudinal magnetization, they become brighter. The brightness, or intensity, with which they appear in the image depends on which moment during the regrowth process the cycle is terminated and "the picture is snapped." When a short TR is used, the regrowth of the longitudinal magnetization is interrupted before it reaches its maximum. This reduces signal intensity and tissue brightness within the image. Increasing TR increases signal intensity and brightness up to the point at which magnetization is fully recovered. For practical purposes, this occurs when the TR exceeds approximately three times the T1 value for the specific tissue. Although it takes many cycles to form a complete image, the longitudinal magnetization is always measured at the same time in each cycle.

T1 Contrast

Longitudinal relaxation time is one of the three basic tissue characteristics that can be translated into image contrast. The extent to which the T1 values of tissue contribute to image contrast is determined by the TR values. The TR also determines the moment during the regrowth of longitudinal magnetization at which "the picture is snapped." This is illustrated in Figure 27-11. In this illustration, we use two tissues, one with a T1 of 250 msec and the other with a T1 of 500 msec. T1 contrast is the difference between the two magnetization curves at any point in time. Notice that at the beginning of the cycle (time = 0), there is no contrast. As the two tissues regain magnetization, they do so at different rates. Therefore, a difference in magnetization (ie, T1 contrast) develops between the two tissues. As the tissues approach maximum magnetization, the difference between the two magnetization levels diminishes.

In order to produce a T1-weighted image, a value for TR must be selected to correspond with the time at which T1 contrast is significant between the two tissues. Several factors must be considered in selecting TR. T1 contrast is

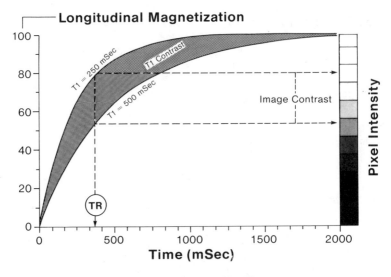

Figure 27-11 Development of T1 Contrast between Two Tissues

represented by the ratio of the tissue magnetization levels, and is at its maximum very early in the relaxation process. However, the low magnetization levels present at that time do not generally produce adequate RF signal levels for many clinical applications. The selection of a longer TR produces greater signal strength but less T1 contrast.

The selection of TR must be appropriate for the T1 values of the tissues being imaged. If a TR value is selected that is equal to the T1 value of a tissue, the picture will be snapped when the tissue has regained 63% of its magnetization. This generally represents a good compromise between T1 contrast and signal intensity.

In Figure 27-11 we show both tissues approaching the same level of maximum magnetization. This occurs only when both tissues have the same proton (nuclei) density and is usually not the case with tissues within the body.

Proton Density Contrast

The density, or concentration, of protons in each voxel determines the maximum level to which the magnetization will grow during the relaxation process. Differences in proton density among tissues can be used to produce image contrast, as illustrated in Figure 27-12. This illustration shows the regrowth of magnetization for two tissues with the same T1 values but different relative proton densities. The tissue with the lowest proton density (80) reaches a maximum magnetization level that is only 80% that of the other tissue. The difference in magnetization levels at any point in time is because of the difference in proton density and is therefore the source of proton density contrast.

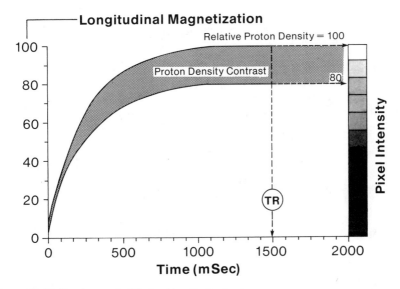

Figure 27-12 Development of Proton Density Contrast

Although there is some proton density contrast early in the cycle, it is generally quite small in comparison with the T1 contrast, which is not shown in this illustration. The basic difference between T1 contrast and proton density contrast is that T1 contrast is produced by the rate of growth, and proton density contrast is produced by the maximum level to which the magnetization grows. In general, T1 contrast predominates in the early part of the relaxation phase, and proton density contrast predominates in the later portion. In most situations, T1 contrast gradually gives way to proton density contrast as magnetization approaches the maximum value. A proton-density-weighted image is produced by selecting a TR value that falls in the later portion of the relaxation phase, where tissue magnetizations approach their maximum values. The TR values at which this occurs depend on the T1 values of the tissues being imaged. It was shown earlier that tissue reaches 95% of its magnetization in three T1s. Therefore, a TR value that is at least three times the T1 values for the tissues being imaged produces almost pure proton density contrast.

Most tissues encountered in MRI differ in both T1 and proton density. Therefore, both tissue characteristics can produce image contrast. Two possible situations are illustrated in Figure 27-13. In the first example, the tissue with the shorter T1 has the higher proton density. It will always appear brighter than the other tissue. Notice that the T1 contrast, which is present early in the relaxation phase, gradually gives way to the proton density contrast.

The second example is characteristic of the gray and white matter in the brain. White matter has the shorter T1 and the lower proton density. During the early

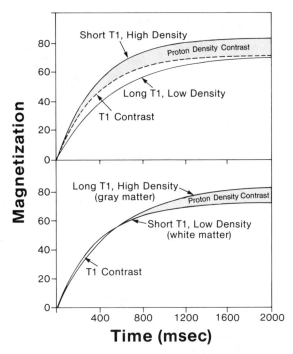

Figure 27-13 Comparison of T1 and Proton Density Contrast for Two Tissue Conditions

portion of the relaxation phase, the white matter magnetization exceeds that of the gray matter because it is growing at a faster rate (shorter T1). When a TR is selected to correspond to this general region, the white matter appears the brighter in the image. As the tissue magnetizations begin to approach their maximum values, the white matter brightness is below the gray. This is because of the difference in proton density. Notice there is a time where the two curves cross, indicating that both tissues have the same level of magnetization. If a TR is selected to correspond to this time, an image will be produced that shows no contrast between the gray and white matter. Late in the relaxation phase the proton density contrast predominates, and the gray matter is the brighter of the two.

Longitudinal magnetization does not produce an RF signal within the tissue. Therefore, when it becomes time to convert the magnetization into an RF signal to form an image, it is necessary to convert the longitudinal magnetization into transverse magnetization, which does produce RF signals.

Transverse Magnetization and Relaxation

Transverse magnetization is produced by applying a pulse of RF energy to the tissue. This is typically done with a 90° pulse, which converts longitudinal magnetization into transverse magnetization. Transverse magnetization is an unstable, or excited, condition and quickly decays after the termination of the excitation pulse. The decay of transverse magnetization is also a relaxation process, which can be characterized by specific relaxation times, or T2 values. Different types of tissue have different T2 values that can be used to discriminate among tissues and contribute to image contrast.

Transverse magnetization is used during the image formation process for two reasons: (1) to develop image contrast based on differences in T2 values and (2) to generate the RF signals emitted by the tissue.

The characteristics of transverse magnetization and relaxation are quite different from those for the longitudinal direction. A major difference is that the relaxation process results in the decay, or decrease, in magnetization, as shown in Figure 27-14. The T2 value is the time required for 63% of the initial magnetization to dissipate. After one T2, 37% of the initial magnetization is present. Transverse relaxation is generally much faster than longitudinal relaxation. In other words, T2 values are less than T1 values for most tissues. Typical T2 values for various types of tissue are listed in Table 27-1.

Figure 27-15 shows the decay of transverse magnetization for tissues with different T2 values. The tissue with the shortest T2 value loses its magnetization faster than the other tissues.

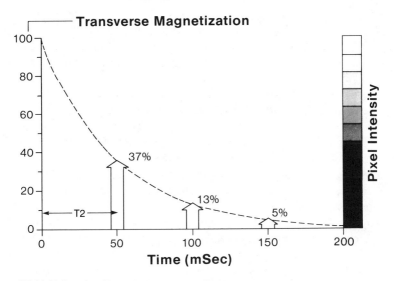

Figure 27-14 Relaxation (Decay) of Transverse Magnetization

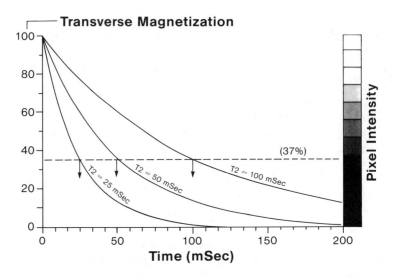

Figure 27-15 Comparison of Transverse Magnetization Decay for Tissues with Different T2 Values

---

T2 Contrast

Under certain imaging conditions, the difference in T2 values of tissue can be translated into image contrast, as illustrated in Figure 27-16. For the purpose of this illustration, we assume that the two tissues begin their transverse relaxation with the same level of magnetization (100%). The decay of the magnetization proceeds at different rates because of the different T2 values. The tissue with the longer T2 value (100 msec) maintains a higher level of magnetization than the other tissue. The ratio of the tissue magnetization at any point in time represents T2 contrast.

At the beginning of the cycle, there is no T2 contrast, but it develops and increases throughout the relaxation process. At some point in time, the magnetization levels are converted into RF signals and image pixel brightness; this is the TE (echo time) and is selected by the operator. Maximum T2 contrast is generally obtained by using a relatively long TE. However, when a very long TE value is used, the magnetization and RF signal are too low to form a useful image. In selecting TE values, a compromise must be made between T2 contrast and signal intensity.

In many clinical procedures, an imaging method that creates a series of images at different TE values is often used. This is known as multi-echo imaging.

The transverse magnetization characteristics of tissue (T2 values) are, in principle, added to the longitudinal characteristics (T1 and proton density) to form the

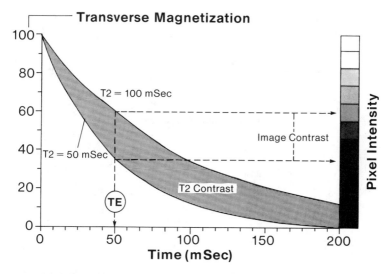

Figure 27-16 Development of T2 Contrast

MR image. We will see how this is achieved after considering additional characteristics of transverse magnetization.

The decay of transverse magnetization (ie, relaxation) occurs because of a dephasing among individual nuclei. Figure 27-17 is a much simplified model used to develop this concept.

Two basic conditions are required for transverse magnetization: The magnetic moments of the nuclei must be oriented in the transverse direction, or plane, and a majority of the moments must be in the same direction within the transverse plane. When a nucleus has a transverse orientation, it is actually spinning around an axis that is parallel to the magnetic field. In our example, we use four nuclei to represent the many nuclei involved in the process.

After the application of a 90° pulse, the nuclei have a transverse orientation and are rotating together, or in phase, around the magnetic field axis. This rotation is the normal precession discussed earlier. The precession rate, or resonant frequency, depends on the strength of the magnetic field where the nuclei are located. Nuclei located in fields with different strengths precess at different rates. Even within a very small volume of tissue, nuclei are in slightly different magnetic fields. As a result, some nuclei precess faster than others. After a short period of time, the nuclei are not precessing in phase. As the directions of the nuclei begin to spread, the magnetization of the tissue decreases. A short time later, the nuclei are randomly oriented in the transverse plane, and there is no transverse magnetization.

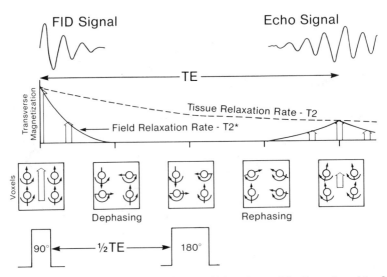

Figure 27-17 Events Contributing to Transverse Relaxation and the Formation of the Spin-Echo Signal

Two factors contribute to the dephasing of the nuclei and the resulting transverse relaxation. One is the exchange of energy among the spinning nuclei, which results in relatively slow dephasing and loss of magnetization. The rate at which this occurs is determined by characteristics of the tissue. It is this dephasing activity that is characterized by the T2 values. A second factor, which produces relatively rapid dephasing of the nuclei and loss of transverse magnetization, is the inherent inhomogeneity of the magnetic field. Even within a small volume of tissue, the field inhomogeneities are sufficient to produce rapid dephasing. This effect, which is unrelated to the characteristics of the tissue, tends to mask the true relaxation characteristics of the tissue. In other words, the actual transverse magnetization relaxes much faster than the tissue characteristics would indicate. This real relaxation time is designated as T2*. The value of T2* is always much less than the tissue T2 value.

SPIN ECHO

In most imaging procedures a special technique, called spin echo, is used to compensate for the dephasing and rapid relaxation caused by the field inhomogeneities. The sequence of events in the spin-echo process is illustrated in Figure 27-17.

Transverse magnetization is produced with a 90° RF pulse that rotates the longitudinal magnetization in the transverse plane. Immediately following the RF pulse, each voxel is magnetized in the transverse direction because protons are positioned in the transverse direction, and they are rotating in phase. However, because of the local magnetic field inhomogeneities within each voxel, the protons rotate at different rates and quickly slip out of phase.

If a 180° pulse is applied to the tissue, it rotates the spinning protons by 180° in the transverse plane and reverses their direction of rotation. This causes the fast protons to be located behind the slower ones. As the faster protons begin to catch up with the slower ones, they regain a common alignment, or come back into phase. This, in turn, causes the transverse magnetization to reappear. However, the magnetization does not grow to the initial value because the relaxation (dephasing) produced by the tissue is not reversible. The rephasing of the protons causes the magnetization to build up to a level determined by the T2 characteristics of the tissue. As soon as the magnetization reaches this maximum, the protons begin to move out of phase again, and the transverse magnetization dissipates. Another 180° pulse can be used to produce another rephasing. In fact, this is what is done in multi-echo imaging.

Transverse magnetization always produces an RF signal. The signal intensity is proportional to the amount of magnetization. The first signal is produced immediately following the 90° excitation pulse. It starts at its maximum value and rapidly decays, along with the transverse magnetization. This is designated a free induction decay (FID) signal. It is not used in most conventional imaging procedures. The second signal appears when the protons rephase, producing the recurrence of the transverse magnetization. This is known as the *echo signal*.

The intensity of the echo signal is proportional to the level of transverse magnetization as determined by the tissue relaxation rate, T2. In most imaging procedures, the intensity of the echo signal determines the brightness of the corresponding image pixel. The time between the initial excitation and the echo signal is TE. This is controlled by adjusting the time interval between the 90° and the 180° pulses.

IMAGE CONTRAST

The brightness of individual tissues and the contrast between different tissues is determined by the relationship between TR and TE and the basic tissue characteristics: proton density, T1, and T2. In most MR images, the contrast is not determined by a single tissue characteristic but by a combination of the three tissue factors. The weighting of image contrast with respect to a particular tissue characteristic is achieved by adjusting the TR and TE values. We now consider the sequence of events during an imaging cycle and how the various factors determine the final image contrast.

Figure 27-18 illustrates the development of contrast between two tissues, A and B. The process extends over a portion of two cycles. Although the same events occur in each cycle, the process is easier to visualize when it is separated as shown.

The first cycle begins with a 90° pulse that converts longitudinal magnetization into transverse magnetization. Therefore, the cycle begins with no longitudinal magnetization. The magnetization begins to grow (relax) at a rate determined by the T1 value for the specific tissue. If two tissues have different T1 values, a difference in magnetization, or contrast, will develop between the tissues. This is T1 contrast. As the tissues begin to approach their maximum magnetization, proton density becomes the major factor affecting magnetization level and contrast between the tissues. This cycle is terminated, and the next cycle begins by the application of another 90° pulse. The pulse interrupts the growth of the longitudinal magnetization and converts it to transverse magnetization. The transverse magnetization in each cycle is created from the longitudinal magnetization of the previous cycle.

At the beginning of the cycle, the two tissues have different levels of transverse magnetization (contrast) brought over from the previous cycle. This is a combination of T1 and proton density contrast. However, as the transverse magnetization begins to decay, it will do so at different rates if the two tissues have different T2 values. This leads to the development of T2 contrast. In general, the proton density and T1 contrast are gradually replaced by T2 contrast. In this example, we show the decay of the transverse magnetization as it relates to tissue characteristics,

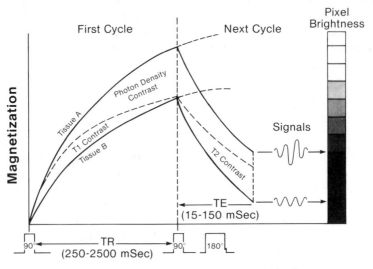

Figure 27-18 Sequence of Events and Factors that Determine Image Contrast

rather than the magnetic field effects as discussed previously. At the appropriate time, a 180° pulse is applied to produce an echo signal from the transverse magnetization. The intensity of the signal is proportional to the level of transverse magnetization. The signal intensity, in turn, determines the brightness of the tissue as it appears in the image. The two tissues will produce image contrast if their signal intensities are different.

To produce image contrast based on T1 differences between tissues, two factors must be considered. Since T1 contrast develops during the early growth phase of longitudinal magnetization, relatively short TR values must be used to capture the contrast. The second factor is to preserve the T1 contrast during the time of transverse relaxation. The basic problem is that if T2 contrast is allowed to develop, it generally counteracts T1 contrast. This is because tissues with short T1 values also have short T2 values. The problem arises because tissues with short T1s are generally bright, whereas tissues with short T2s have reduced brightness when T2 contrast is present. T2 develops during the TE time interval. Therefore, a short TE minimizes T2 contrast and the related loss of T1 contrast. A T1-weighted image is produced by using short TR and TE values.

Proton density contrast develops as the longitudinal magnetization approaches its maximum, which is determined by the proton density of each specific tissue. Therefore, relatively long TR values are required to produce a proton-density-weighted image. Short T2 values are generally used to reduce T2 contrast contamination and to maintain a relatively high signal intensity.

The first step in producing an image with significant T2 contrast is to select a relatively long TR value. This minimizes T1 contrast contamination and the transverse relaxation process begins at a relatively high level of magnetization. Long TE values are then used to allow T2 contrast time to develop.

CONTRAST OF FLOWING BLOOD

The movement, or flow, of blood usually alters signal intensity and produces contrast with respect to stationary tissue structures. Several flow-related mechanisms alter contrast. Under certain conditions, one mechanism causes flowing blood to emit a more intense signal. Under other conditions, mechanisms can cause the flowing blood to emit a signal with reduced intensity.

Flow-Related Enhancement

The process that causes flowing blood to show an increased intensity, or brightness, is illustrated in Figure 27-19. This occurs when the direction of flow is through the slice, as illustrated. The degree of enhancement is determined by the relationship of flow velocity to TR. Four conditions are illustrated. The arrow

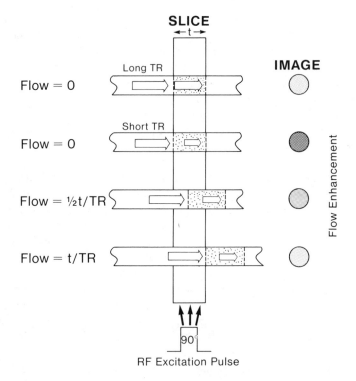

Figure 27-19 Conditions that Produce an Increase in Image Brightness with Flow

indicates the amount of longitudinal magnetization at the end of each imaging cycle. The RF pulses affect only the blood within the slice.

When a long TR is used in the absence of flow, the longitudinal magnetization regrows to a relatively high value during each cycle, as indicated at the top. This condition produces a relatively bright image. If a short TR value is used, each cycle will begin before the longitudinal magnetization has approached its maximum. This results in a relatively dark image.

The effect of flow is to replace some of the blood by fully magnetized blood from outside the slice. The increased magnetization at the end of each cycle increases image brightness. The enhancement increases with flow until the flow velocity becomes equal to the slice thickness divided by TR. This represents full replacement and maximum enhancement.

Intensity Reduction

Relatively high flow velocities through a slice reduce signal intensity and image brightness. In Figure 27-20, the arrow indicates the level of residual transverse

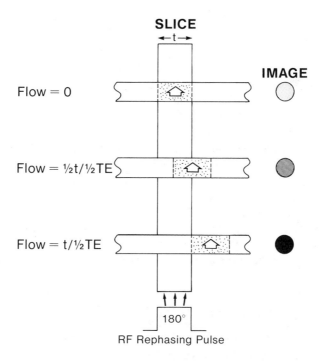

Figure 27-20 The Process of Flow-Related Reduction of Image Brightness

magnetization when the 180° pulse is applied to form the spin-echo signal. This is the transverse magnetization produced by the preceding 90° pulse. The time interval between the 90° and 180° pulses is one-half TE. If the blood is not moving, the blood that was magnetized (transversely) by the 90° pulse will be within the slice when the 180° pulse is applied. This results in maximum rephasing of the transverse protons and a relatively bright image.

If blood moves out of the slice between the 90° and 180° pulses, complete rephasing will not occur. This is because the 180° pulse can affect only the blood within the slice. The spin-echo signal is reduced, and the flowing blood appears darker than blood moving with a lower velocity. The intensity continues to drop as flow is increased until the flow velocity removes all magnetized blood from the slice during the interval between the two pulses (one-half TE).

Dephasing

Blood flowing within the slice plane is often imaged with reduced intensity. This is usually caused by a dephasing of the protons in the transverse plane. Dephasing of the protons reduces the transverse magnetization and the resulting RF signal. The dephasing is produced as the blood flows through a gradient (non-uniform) magnetic field. Gradient fields are present several times during each imaging cycle.

ALTERNATE IMAGING METHODS

The basic imaging method is determined by the sequence of RF pulses and magnetic field gradients applied during each imaging cycle. The conventional spin-echo method uses one 90° and one 180° pulse in each cycle. Some of the other imaging methods are, in principle, modifications of the spin-echo sequence.

Inversion Recovery

Inversion recovery is an imaging method used to produce greater T1 contrast. The inversion recovery pulse sequence is obtained by adding an additional 180° pulse to the conventional spin-echo sequence, as shown in Figure 27-21. The pulse is added at the beginning of each cycle. In inversion recovery, each cycle begins as the 180° pulse inverts the direction of the longitudinal magnetization. The regrowth (recovery) of the magnetization starts from a negative (inverted) value, rather than from zero, as in spin-echo. The increased relaxation time allows more T1 contrast to develop than in the conventional spin-echo technique.

The typical inversion recovery method uses a 90° pulse to produce transverse magnetization, and a final 180° pulse to produce a spin echo signal. An additional time interval is associated with the pulse sequence. The time between the initial 180° pulse and the 90° pulse is designated the inversion time, TI. It can be varied by the user and can be used as a contrast control.

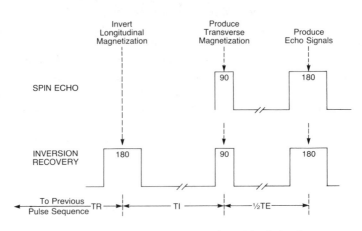

Figure 27-21 Comparison of Inversion Recovery and Spin-Echo Pulse Sequences

Fast Imaging Methods

The fast imaging methods differ from conventional spin echo in several respects and can be used to acquire an image much faster than with conventional spin echo.

The RF pulse used to convert longitudinal into transverse magnetization is less than 90°. Therefore, the longitudinal magnetization is not at zero at the beginning of each cycle. This permits a significant reduction in TR.

The second basic difference is that a magnetic field gradient is used to produce the spin-echo signal rather than a 180° pulse.

SPATIAL CHARACTERISTICS OF THE MR IMAGE

During the MRI procedure, the RF signal from each voxel must be isolated from RF signals from other voxels, and then converted into pixel brightness. This involves a number of steps during both the acquisition and reconstruction phases of an image procedure.

Two basic approaches are used to create the spatial characteristics of MR images. In most procedures, the individual slices are defined during the acquisition phase. This is usually described as two-dimensional (2D), or slice, imaging. When this method is used, multiple slices can be imaged at the same time. Three-dimensional (3D), or volume, imaging is an alternative method in which signals are acquired simultaneously from a large volume of tissue, and the slices are created during the reconstruction process.

Gradients

Individual tissue voxels are formed by creating a series of magnetic field gradients during each imaging cycle. A gradient is a gradual variation in magnetic-field strength along an axis passing through the magnetic field. Gradients are produced by energizing a set of coils within the bore of the magnet. The typical imaging system contains three sets of gradient coils that are positioned to produce gradients in three orthogonal directions.

During an imaging cycle, each gradient is turned on at a specific time to create a sequence of actions that ultimately form the individual voxels.

Slice Selection

The first gradient action in a cycle defines the location and thickness of the tissue slice to be imaged. We will illustrate the procedure for conventional transaxial slice orientation. Other orientations, such as sagittal and coronal, are created by interchanging the gradient directions.

Slice selection uses the principle of selective excitation, as illustrated in Figure 27-22. When a magnetic field gradient is oriented along the patient axis, each slice of tissue is tuned to a different resonant frequency. This is because the resonant frequency of protons is directly proportional to the strength of the magnetic field. The slice selection gradient is present whenever RF pulses are applied to the body. Since RF pulses contain frequencies within a limited range (bandwidth), they can excite tissue only in a specific slice. The location of the slice can be changed by using a slightly different RF pulse frequency. The thickness of the slice is determined by a combination of two factors: (1) the strength, or steepness, of the gradient and (2) the range of frequencies (bandwidth) in the RF pulse.

Phase Encoding

Phase encoding is the second function performed by a field gradient during each cycle and is also known as the *preparation* process. Phase encoding is used to define the voxels in one dimension of the slice.

The basic concept of phase encoding is illustrated in Figure 27-23. We use a vertical column of four voxels to illustrate the process. Immediately after the 90° excitation pulse, each voxel contains transverse magnetization that is rotating about the main field axis. If the four voxels are located in areas with the same field strength, the magnetization will continue to rotate at the same rate. Each voxel produces an RF signal with the same frequency and phase as signals from the other voxels. Since the signals are emitted simultaneously, they are indistinguishable.

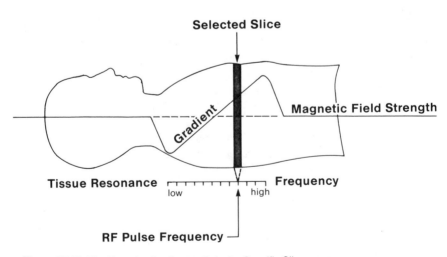

Figure 27-22 The Use of a Gradient to Select a Specific Slice

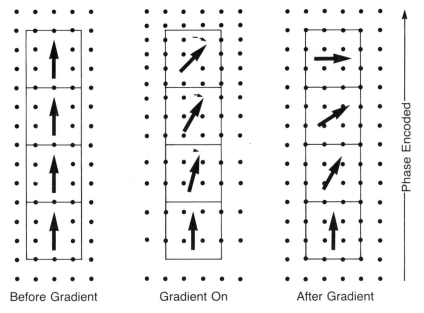

Before Gradient   Gradient On   After Gradient

Figure 27-23 The Concept of Phase Encoding

The next step is to turn on the gradient. Since the individual voxels are now located in areas of the magnetic field with different strengths, the voxel magnetizations rotate at different rates. This causes them to move out of phase. When the gradient is turned off, they resume the same rotation rate but the phase shift remains. The signals from each voxel are then emitted with a phase difference. This phase difference is used during the reconstruction process to sort individual signals.

During each pass through an imaging cycle, the phase-encoding gradient is set to a slightly different value. The different settings create the different "views" required to reconstruct the final image. The concept of a view in MRI is quite different from a view in CT. An MRI view is the composite signal obtained from all voxels during each imaging cycle. The difference from one view to another is that individual voxel signals have a different phase relationship within each composite signal.

To reconstruct an image by the conventional 2D Fourier transformation method, one composite signal, or view, must be collected for each voxel to be created in the phase-encoding direction. Therefore, the minimum number of cycles required to produce an image is determined by the size of the image matrix. A 128 × 128 matrix image can be created in 128 cycles. It takes 256 cycles to produce an image with a 256 × 256 matrix.

Frequency Encoding

Frequency encoding is used to define the individual voxels in the other dimension of the image. Frequency encoding of the signals is obtained by applying a gradient when the echo signals are actually created within the voxels. The basic principle is illustrated in Figure 27-24. We use a row of four voxels to illustrate the principle. When the gradient is applied, the voxels are located in areas with different field strengths. This causes the voxel magnetization to rotate at different rates and produce RF signals with different frequencies. During reconstruction, the frequency of the various signal components are used to determine voxel location in this direction.

The frequency-encoding gradient is on while the echo signals are produced within the tissue.

The Gradient Cycle

We have seen that various gradients are turned on and off at specific times within each imaging cycle. The relationship of each gradient to the other events during an imaging cycle is shown in Figure 27-25. The three gradient activities are the following:

1. The slice selection gradient is on when RF pulses are applied to the tissue. This limits magnetic excitation and echo formation to the tissue located within the specific slice.
2. The phase-encoding (preparation) gradient is turned on for a short period in each cycle to produce a phase difference in one dimension of the image. The strength of this gradient is changed slightly from one cycle to another to create the different "views" needed to form the image.
3. The frequency-encoding (measurement) gradient is turned on during the time when the signals are actually emitted by the tissue. This causes the different voxel columns to emit signals with different frequencies.

Because of the combined action of the three gradients, the individual voxels within each slice emit signals that are different in two respects, as shown in Figure 27-26. They have a phase difference in one direction and a frequency difference in the other. Although these signals are emitted at the same time, and picked up by the imaging system as one composite signal, the reconstruction process can sort the signals into the respective components.

Multi-Slice Imaging

In most clinical applications, it is desirable to have a series of images (slices) covering a specific anatomical region. By using the multi-slice mode, an entire set

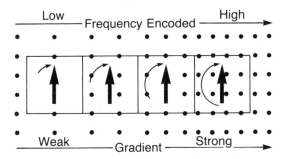

Figure 27-24 The Concept of Frequency Encoding

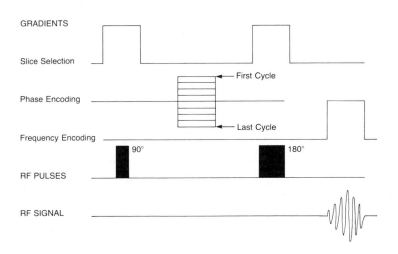

Figure 27-25 Sequence of Events During a Typical Imaging Cycle

of images can be acquired simultaneously. The basic principle is illustrated in Figure 27-27. The slices are separated by exciting and detecting the signals from the different slices in sequence during each imaging cycle.

When the slice selection gradient is turned on, each slice is tuned to a different resonant frequency. A specific slice can be selected for excitation by adjusting the RF pulse frequency to correspond to the resonant frequency of the slice. The process begins by applying an excitation pulse to one slice. Then, while that slice undergoes relaxation, the excitation pulse frequency is shifted to excite the next slice. This process is repeated to excite the entire set of slices at slightly different times within one TR interval.

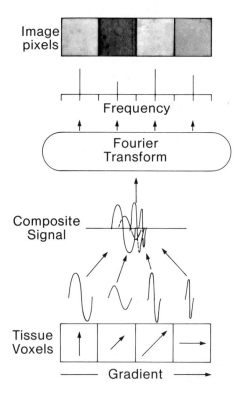

Figure 27-26 One-Dimensional Encoding and Image Reconstruction

Volume Imaging

Volume (3D) image acquisition has some advantages and disadvantages with respect to slice (2D) imaging. With this method, no gradient is present when the RF pulse is applied to the tissue. Since all tissue within an anatomical region, eg, the head, is tuned to the same resonant frequency, all tissue is excited simultaneously. The next step is to apply a phase-encoding gradient in the slice selection direction. In volume imaging, phase encoding is used to create the slices in addition to creating the voxel rows as in conventional slice imaging. The phase-encoding gradient used to define the slices must be indexed to different values corresponding to the number of slices to be created. At each gradient setting, a complete set of imaging cycles must be executed. Therefore, the total number of cycles required in one acquisition is multiplied by the number of slices to be produced. This has the disadvantage of increasing total acquisition time.

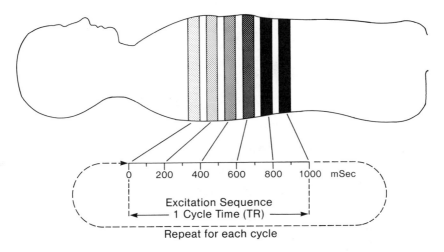

Figure 27-27 Multi-Slice Imaging

The primary advantage of volume imaging is that the phase-encoding process can generally produce thinner slices than the selected excitation process used in slice imaging.

IMAGE RECONSTRUCTION

The next major step in the creation of an MR image is the reconstruction process. Reconstruction is the mathematical process performed by the computer that converts the collected signals into an actual image. There are several reconstruction methods, but the one used for most clinical applications is the 2D Fourier transformation.

The basic concept of the Fourier transformation is illustrated in Figure 27-26. It is a mathematical procedure that can sort a composite signal into individual frequency components. Since each column of voxels emits a different signal frequency, the Fourier transformation can determine the location of each signal component and direct it to the corresponding column of pixels.

The sorting of the signals in the phase-encoded direction is also done by a Fourier transformation in a rather complex process.

The reconstruction process calculates a relative signal intensity value for each image pixel. The relationship between pixel value and pixel brightness is determined by the setting of the window controls.

Chapter 28

Nuclear Magnetic Resonance Image Characteristics

INTRODUCTION AND OVERVIEW

The ability of an MR image to show specific anatomical structures and pathologic conditions is dependent on the factors used during the imaging process. Essentially all aspects of image quality can be controlled by altering the imaging factors. However, MRI is like many other imaging methods in that compromises must be made among the various image quality characteristics. Image acquisition time must also be considered in selecting imaging factors.

The three image characteristics that must be considered in each imaging procedure are (1) contrast, (2) detail, and (3) noise. Figure 28-1 identifies the factors that must be selected for an imaging procedure and shows the image quality characteristics that are affected by each. Additional image quality characteristics, such as artifacts, uniformity, and distortion, are not so directly related to the imaging factors as are contrast, detail, and noise.

We now consider the various aspects of MR image quality and show how each is affected by the imaging process and the selection of imaging factors.

CONTRAST SENSITIVITY

High contrast sensitivity is one of the outstanding characteristics of MRI. The basic principles of contrast production were described in the last chapter. At this time we summarize the factors that contribute to image contrast and give special emphasis to the selection of factors to produce specific image types. The three basic image types are shown in Figure 28-2 along with the factors used to produce them.

In conventional MRI, the three tissue characteristics that contribute to image brightness and contrast are: (1) active proton density, (2) T1, and (3) T2. In general, an image can show contrast if the tissues differ in any one of the

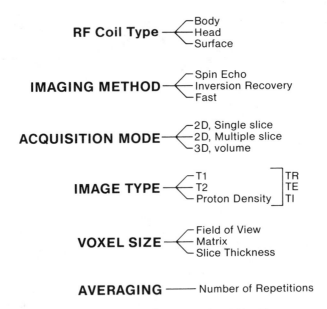

Figure 28-1 MRI Factors that Affect Image Quality and Acquisition Time

characteristics. In reality, there is usually a difference in all three characteristics between most tissues, but the difference is usually larger for one of the characteristics than for the others. In a conventional MR image, the contrast is usually affected to some extent by all three characteristics. However, the selection of the imaging variables determines which of the three factors is the predominant contributor to image contrast. Images are generally described as being weighted with respect to either proton density, T1, or T2.

The contrast of an MR image is controlled by the sequence of RF pulses used in the imaging process. The system operator first chooses the composition of the pulse sequence with respect to 90° and 180° pulses. The two most common pulse sequences are the spin echo (90-180) and the inversion recovery (180-90-180). The next step is to select the time intervals between the pulses. For the spin-echo pulse sequence, the two intervals are TR and TE. The inversion-recovery pulse sequence has an additional time interval, TI.

Since spin echo is the most prevalent pulse sequence, we will use it to illustrate the principles of weighting.

Although TR and TE are related to the time intervals between RF pulses, a more significant factor is that they represent the specific points in time at which the image is created during the magnetic relaxation process. There are two distinct phases to the relaxation process: (1) the regrowth of longitudinal magnetization, and (2) the decay of transverse magnetization. The image brightness of a specific

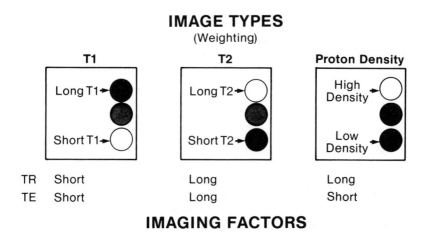

IMAGE TYPES
(Weighting)

T1	T2	Proton Density
Long T1 → ●	Long T2 → ○	High Density → ○
Short T1 → ○	Short T2 → ●	Low Density → ●

TR	Short	Long	Long
TE	Short	Long	Short

IMAGING FACTORS

Figure 28-2 Basic Image Types and Factors Associated with Their Production

---

tissue depends on the magnitude of the transverse magnetization at the time the image data are acquired during the relaxation process. The value of TR, which is selected by the operator, terminates the regrowth of the longitudinal magnetization by rotating it into the transverse orientation. In general, increasing the TR value allows the longitudinal magnetization to reach a larger value, ultimately resulting in a brighter image.

The value of TE determines when the image is acquired during the decay of transverse magnetization. In this case, increasing the TE value decreases image brightness. The important factor is that the contrast between tissues changes with TR and TE because of the differences in T1 and T2.

The general relationship between image types and the TR and TE values is shown in Figure 28-2. Let us now consider the different types in more detail.

Proton-Density-Weighted Images

A proton-density-weighted image is one in which the brightness of each tissue is determined by the density, or concentration, of active protons. Both fat and nonmoving fluids have relatively high proton concentrations. Gray matter has a higher proton concentration than white matter and therefore appears brighter in a proton-density-weighted image. Such an image is obtained by selecting TR and TE values that minimize the effects of tissue T1 and T2 on image brightness and contrast. A relatively long TR value allows all tissues to reach their maximum longitudinal magnetization, which is proportional to proton density. This condition is reached when TR is approximately three times longer than the T1 values of the tissue. This condition is usually not achieved with fluids, which have T1 values of approximately 2 seconds. Therefore, in a typical proton-density-weighted image, acquired with a reasonable TR value of approximately 2 seconds, the fluid appears less bright than its proton density would indicate. Proton density images also require a short TE. The short TE prevents the proton density contrast from becoming heavily "contaminated" by T2 contrast. The ideal value would be a TE of 0, but for most systems the minimum TE value is in the range of 15 to 30 milliseconds.

T1-Weighted Images

In a T1-weighted image, the contrast between tissues is determined by their T1 values. The tissues with the shorter T1 values appear brighter. This is because they regain their longitudinal magnetization faster than the tissues with the longer T1 values. Fat has a relatively short T1, which causes it to be bright in a T1-weighted image. The other extreme is represented by fluid, which typically has a long T1 value and is dark in an image of this type. White matter has a shorter T1 value than gray matter and therefore appears brighter in a T1-weighted image. However, in actual practice this can be observed only with very short TR values. As the TR value is increased, the influence of proton density, which makes gray matter brighter, begins to counteract the T1 contrast. In fact, there are TR values at which very little gray-white contrast is observed because of the combination of these two effects.

A T1-weighted image is obtained by selecting a relatively short TR value. T1 contrast is developed during the early regrowth of longitudinal magnetization. Therefore, a relatively short TR value is required in order to acquire the image when T1 contrast is high. Good T1 contrast is obtained when the TR is approximately equal to the T1 values of the tissue.

A short TE is used to minimize contributions from the T2 characteristics of the tissue.

T2-Weighted Images

Tissue brightness and contrast in a T2-weighted image are determined by the T2 values of the tissue. In this case, the tissue with the longer T2 values appears brighter. This is because these tissues maintain their transverse magnetization longer than the tissues with the shorter T2 values. It is important to recognize that this is essentially a reversal of the development of T1 contrast. In a T2-weighted image, fluids, which have long T2 values, are often the brightest. Fat is much less bright in this type of image because of its short T2 value; gray matter is brighter than white matter because it has a longer T2 value. In practice, this contrast is also enhanced by the higher proton density found in gray matter.

T2-weighted images are obtained by using a combination of long TR and TE values. The long TR value is used to minimize the effects of T1 dependence, and long TE values are used to allow T2 contrast adequate time to develop during the decay of the transverse magnetization.

The two primary variables, TR and TE, for spin-echo imaging can be adjusted to determine the specific tissue characteristic (proton density, T1, or T2) that will have the greatest effect on image contrast. It is not possible, with conventional imaging procedures, to produce an image with contrast limited to one tissue characteristic. There is always some contribution from at least one of the other factors. The general objective is to select TR and TE values that will minimize this contribution and produce maximum contrast for the tissues of interest.

IMAGE DETAIL

The ability of a magnetic resonance image to show detail is determined primarily by the size of the tissue voxels and corresponding image pixels. In principle, all structures within an individual voxel are blurred together and represented by a single signal intensity. The amount of image blurring is determined by the dimensions of the individual voxel.

Three basic imaging factors determine the dimensions of a tissue voxel, as illustrated in Figure 28-3. The dimension of a voxel in the plane of the image is determined by the ratio of the field of view (FOV) and the dimensions of the matrix. Both of these factors can be used, to some extent, to adjust image detail.

The selection of the FOV is determined primarily by the size of the body part being imaged. One problem that often occurs is the appearance of a foldover artifact when the FOV is smaller than the body section. The maximum FOV is usually limited by the dimensions and characteristics of the RF coil.

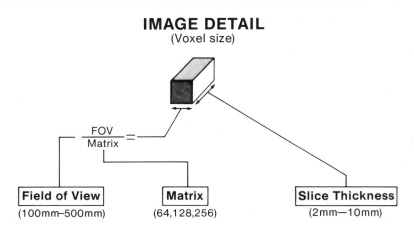

Figure 28-3 Factors that Affect Detail in MR Images

Matrix dimension refers to the number of voxels in the rows or columns of the matrix. The matrix dimension is selected by the operator before the imaging procedure. Typical dimensions are 64, 128, and 256.

There is a considerable range of voxel sizes (image detail) because of the possible choices of FOV and matrix dimension. The third dimension of a voxel is the thickness of the imaged slice of tissue. In most imaging procedures, this is the largest dimension of a voxel. The amount of blurring can be reduced and the visibility of detail improved by reducing voxel size. Unfortunately, there is a compromise. Signal strength is directly proportional to the volume of a voxel. Therefore, reducing voxel size to improve image detail reduces signal intensity. This becomes especially significant with respect to image noise.

IMAGE NOISE

MR image noise is produced primarily by random RF energy picked up along with the signals forming the image. The presence of image noise limits image quality both directly and indirectly and often requires extended acquisition times to partially compensate for its presence. If it were not for this form of noise, it would be possible to acquire images with greater contrast sensitivity, and more detail, and to acquire them in less time than is required for current image acquisition.

Noise Sources

Random RF energy can be generated by thermal activity within electrical conductors and circuit components. In principle, the patient's body is one of the components in the RF receiver circuit. Therefore, because of its mass, it becomes the most significant source of image noise in most imaging procedures. The specific noise source is the tissue contained within the sensitive FOV of the RF receiver coils. Some noise is generated within the receiver coils, but it is usually much less than from the patient.

Many devices in the environment produce RF noise or signals that can interfere with MRI. These include radio and TV transmitters, electrosurgery units, fluorescent lights, and computing equipment. All MR units are installed with an RF shield to reduce the interference from these external sources. External interference is not usually a problem with a properly shielded unit. When it does occur, it generally appears as an image artifact rather than the conventional random noise pattern.

Signal-to-Noise Considerations

Image quality is not dependent on the absolute intensity of the noise but rather the amount of noise in relationship to the image signal intensity. Image quality

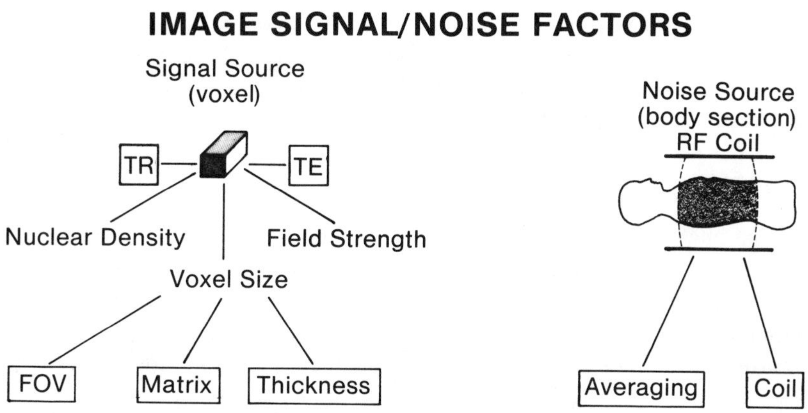

IMAGE SIGNAL/NOISE FACTORS

Figure 28-4 Factors that Affect Signal-to-Noise Ratios in MR Images

---

increases in proportion to the signal-to-noise ratio. When the intensity of the RF noise is low in proportion to the intensity of the image signal, the noise has a low visibility. In situations where the signal is relatively weak, the noise becomes much more visible. The principle is essentially the same as with conventional TV reception. When a strong signal is received, image noise (snow) is generally not visible; when one attempts to tune in to a weak signal from a distant station, the noise becomes significant.

In MRI, the interference from noise is reduced by either reducing the noise intensity or increasing the intensity of the signals that create the image, as illustrated in Figure 28-4. Let us now see how this can be achieved.

Voxel Size

One of the major factors that affects signal strength is the volume of the individual voxels. The signal intensity is proportional to the total number of protons contained within a voxel. Large voxels emit stronger signals and produce less image noise. Unfortunately, large voxels reduce image detail. Therefore, when the factors for an imaging procedure are being selected, this compromise between signal-to-noise and image detail must be considered. The major reason for imaging with relatively thick slices is to increase the voxel signal intensity.

Field Strength

The strength of the RF signal from an individual voxel generally increases in proportion to the square of the magnetic field strength. However, the amount of noise picked up from the patient's body often increases with field strength because of adjustments made to reduce artifacts at the higher fields. Because of differences in system design, no single precise relationship between signal-to-noise ratio and magnetic field strength applies to all systems. In general, MRI systems operating at relatively high field strengths produce images with higher signal-to-noise ratios than images produced at lower field strengths.

Tissue Characteristics

Signal intensity, and thus the signal-to-noise ratio, depends to some extent on the magnetic characteristics of the tissue being imaged. For a specific set of imaging factors, the tissue characteristics that enhance the signal-to-noise relationship are high magnetic nuclei (proton) concentration, short T1, and long T2. The primary limitation in imaging nuclei other than hydrogen (protons) is the low tissue concentration and the resulting low signal intensity.

TR and TE

TR (repetition time) and TE (echo time) are the factors used to control contrast in conventional spin-echo imaging. We have observed that these two factors also control signal intensity. This must be taken into consideration in selecting the factors for a specific imaging procedure.

When a short TR is used to obtain a T1-weighted image, the longitudinal magnetization does not have the opportunity to approach its maximum and produce high signal intensity. In this case, some signal strength must be sacrificed to gain a specific type of image contrast. Also, when TR is reduced to decrease image acquisition time, image noise often becomes a limiting factor.

When relatively long TE values are used to produce T2 contrast, noise often becomes a problem. The long TE values allow the transverse magnetization and the signal it produces to decay to very low values.

RF Coils

The most direct control over the amount of noise picked up from the patient's body is to select appropriate characteristics of the RF receiver coil. In principle, noise is reduced by reducing the amount of tissue within the sensitive region of the coil. Most imaging systems are equipped with interchangeable coils. These include a body coil, a head coil, and a set of surface coils. The body coil is the largest and usually contains a major part of the patient's tissue within its sensitive region. Therefore, body coils pick up the greatest amount of noise. Also, the distance between the coil and the tissue being imaged (voxels) is greater than in other types of coils. This reduces the intensity of the signals actually received from the individual voxels. Because of the combination of less signal intensity and higher noise pickup, body coils generally produce a poorer signal-to-noise ratio than the other coil types.

In comparison to body coils, head coils are both closer to the imaged tissue and generally contain a smaller total volume of tissue within their sensitive region. Because of the increased signal-to-noise characteristic of head coils, relatively small voxels can be used to obtain better image detail.

The surface coil provides the highest signal-to-noise ratio of the three coil types. Because of its small size, it has a limited sensitive region and picks up less noise from the tissue. When it is placed on or near the surface of the patient, it is usually quite close to the region of interest (ROI) and picks up a stronger signal than the other coil types. The compromise with surface coils is that their limited sensitive region restricts the useful field of view, and the sensitivity of the coil is not uniform within the imaged area. This non-uniformity results in very intense signals from tissue near the surface and a significant decrease in signal intensity with increasing depth. The relatively high signal-to-noise ratio obtained with surface coils can be traded for increased image detail by using smaller voxels.

Averaging

One of the most direct methods used to control the signal-to-noise characteristics of MR images is the process of averaging. In principle, each imaging cycle is repeated several times and the results are averaged to form the final image. The averaging process tends to reduce the noise level because of its statistical fluctuation nature from one cycle to another.

The disadvantage of averaging is that it increases the total image acquisition time in proportion to the number of cycle repetitions (2, 4, etc.).

PROCEDURE OPTIMIZATION

Maximum visibility of specific anatomical structures and tissue characteristics is obtained by selecting imaging factors that produce a proper balance among the image characteristics of contrast, detail, noise, and image acquisition time. The general relationships are summarized in Figure 28-5.

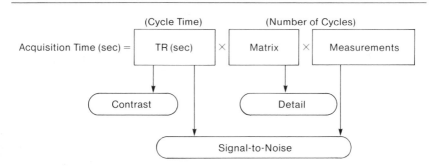

Figure 28-5 Factors that Must Be Considered in Optimizing an Imaging Procedure

Chapter 29

The Gamma Camera

INTRODUCTION AND OVERVIEW

Many nuclear medicine procedures require an image that shows the distribution of a radioactive substance within the patient's body. For many years nuclear images were obtained by using a rectilinear scanner. Today most imaging is done with the gamma camera. The gamma camera takes a picture of a gamma-emitting radioactive source much like a conventional camera takes a picture of an illuminated object. All gamma cameras in use today are not identical in design, but most have a number of common features. This chapter considers the general construction, function, and characteristics of a typical gamma camera.

The gamma camera consists of a number of components, as shown in Figure 29-1. Each component performs a specific function in converting the gamma image into a light image and transferring it to an appropriate viewing device or film. The first component, the collimator, projects the gamma image onto the surface of the crystal. The scintillation crystal absorbs the gamma image and converts it into a light image. The light image that appears on the rear surface of the scintillation crystal has a very low intensity (brightness) and cannot be viewed or photographed directly at this stage. The photomultiplier (PM) tube array, which is behind the crystal, performs two specific functions. It converts the light image into an image of electrical pulses, and it amplifies, or increases, the intensity of the image. The electrical pulses from the tube array go to an electronic circuit that creates three specific signals for each gamma photon detected by the camera. One signal is an electrical pulse whose size represents the energy of the gamma photon. The other two signals describe the location of the photon within the image area. Typically, the size of one pulse represents the horizontal position, and the size of the other pulse the vertical position.

The pulse representing the energy of the photon goes to the input of a pulse height analyzer (PHA). (The PHA function is discussed in detail later.) If the pulse

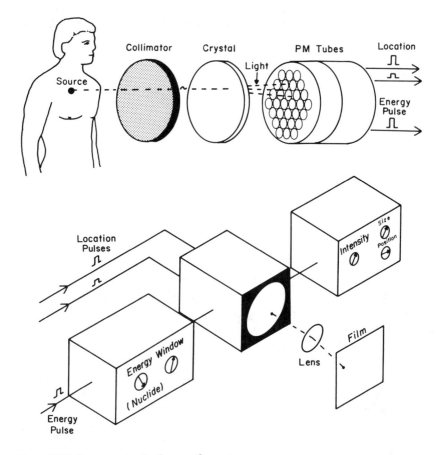

Figure 29-1 Components of a Gamma Camera

is within the selected window (energy) range, it will pass through the PHA onto either the viewing or storage unit. When the pulse from the PHA arrives at the viewing unit, a small dot of light is created on the screen. The location of the dot is determined by the horizontal and vertical position signals. Each gamma photon detected by the camera and accepted by the PHA creates one dot on the viewing screen. The location of the dot corresponds to the location of the gamma photon source within the patient's body. The image of the radioactive material is made up of dots that are images of the individual photons.

Most camera systems have at least two screens on which the image appears. One is used for viewing the image, and the other for photographing the image onto the film. In many camera systems, the data pulses go to a computer where they are stored for future processing, viewing, and analysis.

CAMERA CHARACTERISTICS

To use a gamma camera properly for various types of examinations, one must be familiar with its imaging characteristics. In some instances, it is desirable to alter the characteristics of the camera to fit the examination being conducted. After considering the significance of basic camera characteristics, we will see how they depend on the various components that make up the camera system.

Sensitivity

In a typical imaging situation, only a small fraction of the gamma photons emitted by the radioactive material contribute to the formation of the image. Consider the situation illustrated in Figure 29-2. The photons leave the small radioactive source equally distributed in all directions. The only photons that contribute to the image are the ones passing through the appropriate collimator hole and absorbed in the crystal. Photons from the source that are not absorbed in the crystal are, in effect, wasted and do not contribute to image formation. This characteristic of a gamma camera is generally referred to as the *sensitivity*. The sensitivity of a camera can be described in terms of the number of photons detected and used in the image for each unit (μCi) of radioactivity, as illustrated in Figure 29-2.

The sensitivity of a camera system is affected by several of its components; it is, for example, very dependent on the design of the collimator. Most camera systems have interchangeable collimators, and this is one factor that can be used to alter the sensitivity. The problem is that a collimator that yields maximum sensitivity

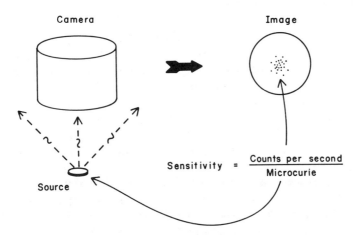

Figure 29-2 The Concept of Gamma Camera Sensitivity

usually produces maximum image blur. The compromise between these two factors is discussed in detail in a later chapter.

The thickness of a scintillation crystal has an effect on detector efficiency. Detector efficiency and camera sensitivity are reduced when photons pass through the crystal. Therefore, a thick crystal tends to yield higher sensitivity, especially for high-energy photons, but also produces more image blur.

Another factor that affects the sensitivity of a camera system is the setting of the PHA, which will be discussed later. The only photons that contribute to the image are the ones within the PHA window. A window that is very small or incorrectly positioned with respect to the photon energy spectrum can significantly reduce camera sensitivity.

Many cameras have a short dead time after each photon is detected during which an arriving photon is not counted. Dead time reduces sensitivity when the photon rate is high and the photons tend to overlap.

Camera sensitivities are generally in the range of 100 to 1,000 cps/μCi. Since 1 μCi typically yields 37,000 photons per second, this means that less than 3% of the emitted photons are used for image formation.

Field of View

The field of view (FOV) of a gamma camera is an important characteristic because it determines how much of a patient's body can be imaged at any one time. The FOV depends on the size of the crystal, the type of collimator, and, in some systems, the distance between the object being imaged and the camera crystal.

COLLIMATORS

The purpose of the collimator is to "project" an image of the radioactivity onto the surface of the camera crystal. The manner in which this is accomplished is illustrated in Figure 29-3. The collimator is constructed of a metal that is a good photon absorber, such as lead or tungsten. Holes are positioned in the collimator so that each point on the crystal's surface has a direct view of only one point on the surface of the body. In effect, each point of the crystal is able to see only the radiation originating from a corresponding point on the patient's body. Although the illustration shows only a few holes in the collimator, actual collimators contain hundreds of holes located very close together in order to see all points within the FOV. The one exception is the pin-hole collimator, which is discussed later.

Typically, a gamma camera is equipped with several interchangeable collimators. The differences among the collimators are the thickness, number, and size of the holes and the way they are arranged or oriented. This, in turn, has an effect on the camera sensitivity, FOV image magnification, and image blur. The

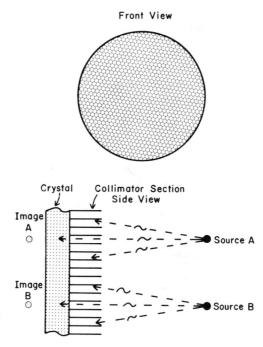

Front View

Crystal   Collimator Section
Side View

Figure 29-3 The Basic Function of a Collimator

user must be aware of these differences in order to select the best collimator for a given examination.

When selecting a collimator, it is necessary to consider the energy of the gamma photons. The ability of a photon to penetrate a given material generally increases with photon energy. In other words, it takes a thicker piece of material to absorb high-energy photons than it does to absorb low-energy photons. The purpose of the collimator septa (thin dividing walls) is to prevent photons from penetrating from one hole to another. This depends on the relationship of the photon energy to the thickness of the metal septa separating the holes. With low-energy photons, relatively thin septa are adequate. The advantage of thin septa is that more holes can be located in a given area, and this results in a higher sensitivity. However, thicker septa must be used with high-energy photons in order to prevent photons from crossing over from one hole to another.

Figure 29-4 compares sections of low-energy and high-energy collimators. If a low-energy collimator is used with high-energy photons, significant septal penetration will occur, and the image will be abnormally blurred. If a high-energy collimator is used with low-energy photons, an image of normal quality will be obtained, but the camera will be operating with less than optimum sensitivity. Collimator holes are oriented in different ways, which affects collimator function.

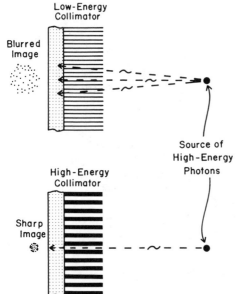

Figure 29-4 Comparison of Low-Energy and High-Energy Collimators

Parallel-Hole Collimators

A common arrangement is for the collimator holes to be parallel, as illustrated in Figure 29-5. The FOV is determined by the size (diameter) of the crystal and remains the same at all source-to-camera distances. The size of the image at the crystal is the same as the actual size of the radioactive source being imaged. This relationship does not change with distance. Therefore, the parallel-hole collimator does not produce either magnification or minification of the image. The photons that pass through the parallel-hole collimator are the ones moving in a direction parallel to the holes. Assuming there is no photon absorption between the source and collimator, the number of these parallel photons does not change significantly with the source-to-camera distance. Therefore, camera sensitivity with a parallel-hole collimator is generally not affected by changing the distance between the source and camera. Note that the inverse-square effect does not occur with a collimated system of this type.

Diverging Collimators

In the diverging collimator, the holes fan out from the surface of the crystal, as shown in Figure 29-6. With this arrangement of holes, the camera can image a source larger than the crystal. The FOV increases with distance from the face of the collimator. The major advantage of the diverging collimator is the increased

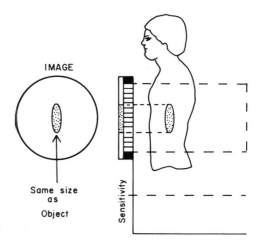

Figure 29-5 Parallel-Hole Collimator

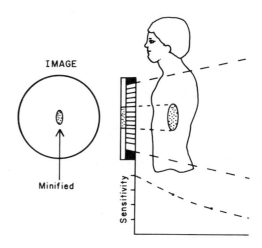

Figure 29-6 Diverging Collimator

FOV. The rate at which the FOV increases with distance depends on the angulation of the holes. For a typical diverging collimator, the FOV at a distance of 15 cm is approximately 1.6 times the FOV at the collimator surface.

With the diverging collimator, the image at the crystal surface is smaller than the actual size of the radioactive source. For a given collimator, the degree of minification increases with the distance between the source and collimator face. The change in minification with distance can produce distortion in the image, because objects close to the camera are minified less than objects located at a greater distance from the camera surface. For example, two identical lesions will appear to have different sizes if they are not located at the same distance from the camera.

The sensitivity of a camera equipped with a diverging collimator decreases with distance between the source and camera. As the radioactive source is moved away from the face of the collimator, it is in the FOV of a smaller number of holes. This reduces the number of photons that reach the crystal and decreases camera sensitivity.

Converging Collimators

The holes in the converging collimator are arranged so that they point to, or converge on, a point located in front of the collimator, as shown in Figure 29-7. This is, in effect, the reverse arrangement of the diverging collimator. In fact, some collimators are reversible so that they can be used as either a diverging or converging collimator. As might be expected, the FOV for a converging collimator decreases with increased distance from the collimator face. The converging collimator produces image magnification. The degree of magnification depends on the design of the collimator and the distance from the collimator surface. As a radioactive source is moved away from the collimator, it comes into the view of more collimator holes, and this produces an increase in sensitivity. The sensitivity increases approximately as the square of the distance from the collimator. Because of its magnification and sensitivity properties, the converging collimator is useful for imaging small organs, such as the thyroid gland, kidneys, and heart. However, converging collimators tend to produce distortion around the edges.

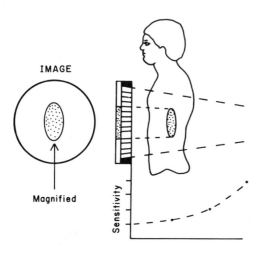

Figure 29-7 Converging Collimator

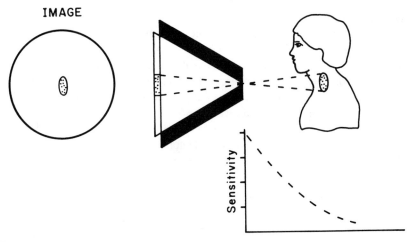

Figure 29-8 Pin-hole Collimator

Pin-Hole Collimators

The pin-hole collimator differs from other collimators in that it has a single small hole rather than several thousand holes. A typical pin-hole collimator is shown in Figure 29-8. The basic principle of this collimator is the same as that of the pin-hole camera from the early days of photography. The "lens" of the camera is a small hole (pin-hole) in an absorbing material. Radiation from each point within the body is limited to a corresponding point on the crystal as the radiation passes through the hole. This creates an image of the source on the crystal surface. With this type of collimator, the orientation of the image at the crystal is inverted with respect to the source. The FOV of a pin-hole collimator is very dependent on the distance between the source and the collimator. When the source is located as far in front of the collimator as the crystal is behind the collimator, the FOV is equal to the size of the crystal. If the source is located closer, the image will be magnified. The degree of magnification increases as the source approaches the collimator. Because it has only one hole, the sensitivity of the pin-hole collimator is obviously less than for typical multihole collimators. It also decreases as the distance between the source and pin-hole is increased. In many cameras, the pin-hole can be changed. A large hole gives more sensitivity, but also more blur.

CRYSTALS

As in any scintillation detector system, the crystal in the gamma camera has two basic functions: (1) to absorb the gamma photons and (2) to convert the gamma image into a light image. Crystals used for this purpose are typically in the form of disks. Both dimensions, diameter and thickness, have an effect on the characteristics of the camera. The diameter of the crystal establishes the basic FOV, which is then modified by the type of collimator used and the distance between the camera and the source being imaged. The thickness of the crystal affects sensitivity and image blur. Increasing crystal thickness generally decreases crystal penetration and improves sensitivity. However, increasing the thickness also increases image blur, which is discussed in the next chapter. Therefore, a crystal thickness is used that provides a reasonable compromise between sensitivity and image quality. Typical thicknesses are in the range of one-fourth to one-half inch.

PHOTOMULTIPLIER TUBE ARRAY

The photomultiplier (PM) tubes are generally arranged in a hexagonal array; the number that will completely fill a circular area depends on the relative diameters of the area and the PM tubes. Specific numbers of PM tubes uniformly fill a given circular area: 7, 19, 37, 61, 91, etc. The first gamma camera used seven PM tubes. Throughout the evolution of the camera, both the size of the array and the number of PM tubes have gradually increased.

In addition to converting the light from the crystal into electrical pulses and amplifying the pulses, the PM tube array also detects where each gamma photon is absorbed in the crystal. This information is necessary to transfer the image from the crystal to the viewing unit. The manner in which the location of a photon interaction is measured is illustrated in Figure 29-9. Assume that a gamma photon is absorbed in the crystal at the location shown. The light spreads throughout the crystal and light pipe and is viewed by a number of PM tubes. The brightness of the scintillation, as seen by a specific PM tube, depends on the distance between the PM tube and the scintillation. In the illustration, PM tube B is closest and sees the brightest scintillation and receives the most light from it. It responds by producing a relatively large electrical pulse. PM tube C receives less light and produces a correspondingly smaller electrical pulse. Because it is even farther away from the scintillation, PM tube A produces an even smaller electrical pulse. In other words, when one photon is absorbed by the crystal, a number of PM tubes around the specific point see the light and produce electrical pulses. The relative size of the pulses from the various PM tubes represents the location of the scintillation, or gamma photon, within the image area.

IMAGE FORMATION

The gamma camera must take the pulses from the PM tube array and use them to form an image. This function is performed by an electronic circuit. The first

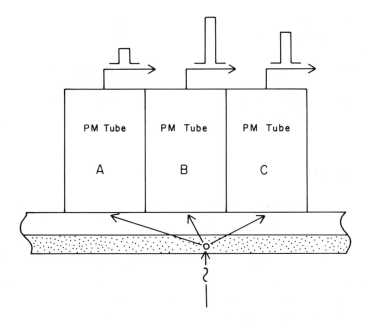

Figure 29-9 Three of the PM Tube Pulses Generated by the Capture of a Single Photon

function of this circuit is to take all of the electrical pulses created by a single photon interaction and use them to calculate, or determine, the location of the interaction within the image area. The circuit then produces two new pulses that describe the location of the photon. The amplitude of one pulse represents the location of the photon in the horizontal (H) direction, and the amplitude of the other pulse specifies the vertical (V) location.

A second function of the circuitry is to combine all of the PM tube pulses into one electrical pulse whose amplitude represents the energy of the photon. This pulse is passed on to a pulse height analyzer (PHA) in the viewing unit.

The function of the viewing unit is the formation of a visible image from electrical pulses. Most conventional viewing units create the image on the screen of a cathode ray tube (CRT), more commonly known as a picture tube, especially when found in television equipment. In a CRT the image is formed on the screen by a small electron beam striking the screen from the rear. The image is actually created by controlling the position of the electron beam. When the electron beam strikes the CRT screen, which is made of a fluorescent material, it creates a small spot of light. When the two position pulses arrive at the CRT, they are used to position the electron beam to the appropriate location on the CRT screen. If the energy pulse is within the appropriate range to pass through the PHA, it is also directed to the CRT. When this pulse arrives at the CRT, it turns on the electron beam, momentarily causing a small spot of light to be formed on the CRT screen. This spot of light is, in effect, the image of a single gamma photon coming from the patient's body. This process is repeated for each photon accepted by the gamma camera. Many CRTs can store or maintain each light spot while the total image is being formed.

A viewing unit generally has an intensity control that can be used to adjust the brightness of each spot. This control also adjusts the film exposure when the image is transferred from the CRT screen to film.

SPECTROMETRY

In many nuclear medicine procedures, it is desirable for the counting or imaging system to respond only to radiation from a specific primary source within the patient or sample. A problem arises because radiation from other sources might be present and enter the detector, as shown in Figure 29-10. Also, some of the radiation from the primary source undergoes Compton interactions with materials outside the source volume. This produces scattered radiation, which can enter the detector. If an imaging system responds to this scattered radiation, the resulting image will include areas around the primary source. This distorts the image and makes it impossible to determine the actual size, shape, and activity of the primary source organ or lesion. Radiation from other sources might also be present. Cosmic radiation, naturally occurring radioactive nuclides in building materials, and radioactive contamination of the environment produce what is generally

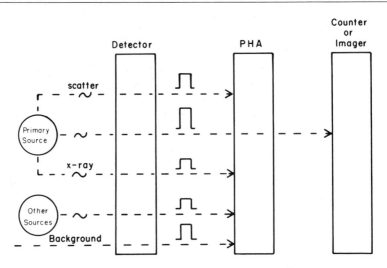

Figure 29-10 The Rejection of Unwanted Detector Pulses by the Spectrometer

referred to as background radiation. Background radiation can reduce contrast in images and introduce errors into the counting of radioactive samples. Occasionally, two radioactive materials are administered to a patient, and the system must selectively respond to each source at the appropriate time.

An imaging or counting system can be made selective by adding an energy spectrometer after the detector and amplifier, as shown in Figure 29-10. The spectrometer is actually a PHA that works with the electrical pulses produced by the detector. The purpose of the PHA is to allow pulses created by the desired (primary) source of radiation to pass on to the counting and imaging devices and to reject the pulses associated with other sources of radiation. The user must always adjust the controls of the PHA to ensure the proper selection of pulses.

The Gamma Spectrum

The pulses from a scintillation detector will not be the same size because most radioactive materials emit gamma photons of several energies. Variation in pulse size is also created by Compton interactions, energy escaping from the crystal, and statistical factors within the crystal and PM tube. We now consider some of these factors in detail and show how they relate to the proper use of a PHA.

For simplicity, we assume that the radioactive material emits all of its photons with the same energy. The spectrum of such a monoenergetic source and the pulses it would produce in an ideal detector system are shown in Figure 29-11. In an ideal detector system, monoenergetic photons would produce a series of pulses of the same size. The spectrum of these pulses would be a single line, as shown in Figure 29-11. Remember that pulse size height now represents photon energy. The

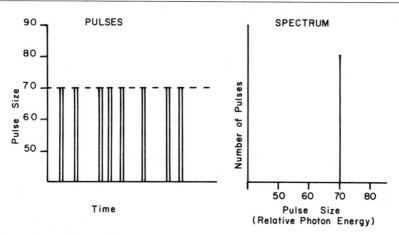

Figure 29-11 The Pulse Spectrum That Would Be Produced by a Monoenergetic Radiation Source and an Ideal Detector

spectrum shown here is the spectrum of a monoenergetic gamma emitter as seen "through the eyes of" an ideal detector system. Unfortunately, real detector systems do not produce a pulse size spectrum that precisely represents the photon energy spectrum. The various factors that affect the pulse size spectrum will now be considered.

Statistical Fluctuations

The various events taking place between the absorption of the gamma photon and the formation of the electrical pulse are illustrated in Figure 29-12. A gamma photon is absorbed in the crystal and creates a cluster of light photons. There is always variation in the number of light photons created by a specific gamma energy. Also, all of the light photons associated with one scintillation are not necessarily absorbed by the photocathode of the PM tube; some are absorbed within the crystal itself. The number absorbed within the crystal is influenced, to some extent, by the location of the scintillation within the crystal. The number of electrons emitted from the photocathode by a cluster of light photons is also subject to statistical fluctuation. The number of electrons also fluctuates at each of the dynodes. The cluster of electrons (electrical pulse) varies in size because of the combined effect of the various fluctuations. A series of typical pulses and the resulting spectrum are shown in Figure 29-13.

The variation in pulse size causes the pulse spectrum to assume the form of a broadened peak rather than a narrow line. An important characteristic of a detector system is the amount of variation in pulse size, or spreading, of the spectrum it produces. This characteristic is known as the energy resolution of the detector system and is generally expressed in terms of the full width at half maximum (FWHM). The FWHM is the full width of the spectrum peak measured at one-half of the maximum height of the peak. It is generally expressed as a percentage of the average pulse size (photon energy). In the example shown in Figure 29-13, the full width is 10 units and the average pulse size is 70 units. Therefore,

$$FWHM = 10/70 \times 100 = 14\%.$$

The FWHM might be considered as an expression of the "average" variation in pulse size. The ideal detector system would have an FWHM of 0. Actual scintillation detector systems generally have an energy resolution capability (FWHM) of approximately 10% to 15%. The energy resolution of a detector system generally depends on the overall quality of the crystal and PM tube and the stability of the pulse amplifier. Severe loss of energy resolution capability can result from conditions such as a fractured crystal or inadequate light transmission between the crystal and PM tube.

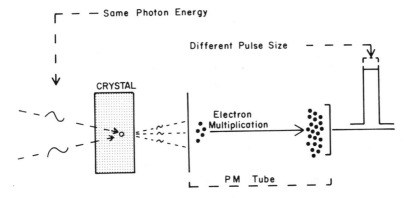

Figure 29-12 Factors That Produce a Variation in Detector Pulse Size

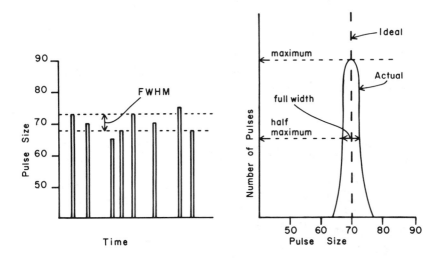

Figure 29-13 Pulse Spectrum Produced by a Monoenergetic Radiation Source and a Typical Detector

Poor energy resolution, or high FWHM values, means that the pulse size associated with the monoenergetic photons from the primary source varies considerably. This makes it difficult for the PHA to separate these pulses from the pulses arising from other radiation sources.

The peaked spectrum shown in Figure 29-13 results from the complete absorption of the gamma photons in the crystal by the photoelectric process. It is therefore often referred to as the photopeak portion of the spectrum. The following sections discuss other portions of the pulse spectrum created by other interactions.

Compton Scatter

When a gamma photon is engaged in a Compton interaction with a material, it both loses energy at the site of interaction and changes direction, as discussed in Chapter 10. Compton interactions can take place between the photon and the material containing the radioactive source, the detector crystal, or material located between the source and crystal.

In radionuclide imaging procedures, a significant number of Compton interactions usually occur in the tissue surrounding the radioactive material. If these scattered photons are included in the image, the image will not be a true representation of the distribution of radioactive material. It is therefore desirable to exclude the scattered photons from the imaging process. This can be achieved, to some extent, because their energy is different from the energy of the primary photons.

For a given primary energy, such as 140 keV, the energy of the scattered photon depends on the angle of scatter. Scatter that takes place within the body adds a component to the spectrum, as shown in Figure 29-14. Photons that scatter in the forward direction (directly toward the detector) lose very little energy in the scattering interaction and have energies very close to 140 keV. The statistical fluctuation within the detector causes some of these to appear to have energies greater than 140 keV. The fluctuations within the detector system cause the

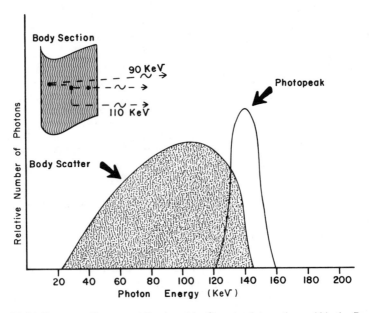

Figure 29-14 Spectrum Component Produced by Compton Interactions within the Body

overlap between the scatter component and the photopeak of the spectrum. Photons that scatter in the backward direction (180°) have the lowest energy. For 140-keV primary photons, complete backscatter produces 90-keV photons. This means that the scattered radiation produced by a 140-keV primary source has photon energies ranging from 90 keV to 140 keV. However, some photons may undergo two or more Compton interactions before leaving the body, and this creates some photons with energies well below 90 keV. The exact shape of the scatter portion of the spectrum and its amplitude relative to the photopeak depend on a number of factors, especially the thickness of tissue covering the radioactive material.

If Compton interactions take place within the detector crystal, a different spectrum component is created. The spectrum as seen "through the eyes of" the detector represents energy deposited within the detector. If a 140-keV photon undergoes a single Compton interaction in the crystal, the maximum energy it can deposit is 50 keV. This occurs when the photon is scattered back out of the crystal (180°) and carries an energy of 90 keV. The energy deposited in the crystal (50 keV) is the difference between the primary photon energy (140 keV) and the scattered photon energy (90 keV). Photons that scatter in a more forward direction have higher energies and therefore deposit less energy in the crystal. The high-energy side of this spectrum component is known as the Compton edge.

Characteristic X-Rays

When gamma photons interact with materials with relatively high atomic numbers, photoelectric interactions can occur. A photoelectric interaction removes an electron from an atom and creates a vacancy in one of the shell locations. When the vacancy is refilled, a characteristic x-ray photon is often produced. The energy of the characteristic photon is essentially the same as the binding energy of the K-shell electrons. This type of interaction and the resulting characteristic x-ray photons can produce distinct components in the spectrum.

If the interaction occurs in a material other than the crystal, the spectrum component corresponds to the energy of the characteristic x-ray. In many procedures, a lead collimator is located between the radioactive source and detector crystals. The predominant characteristic x-ray produced in lead has an energy of 77 keV, which gives rise to a lead x-ray peak centered at about this energy.

If the characteristic x-ray photon is created within the crystal, a different type of spectrum component is created, as shown in Figure 29-15. This particular component occurs only if the x-ray photon escapes from the crystal. The energy deposited in the crystal is the difference between the energy of the primary photon and the escaping characteristic x-ray photon. In a sodium iodide crystal, the predominant characteristic x-ray is the 28-keV iodine x-ray. When a 140-keV photon produces a 28-keV x-ray photon that escapes from the crystal, the energy deposited is the

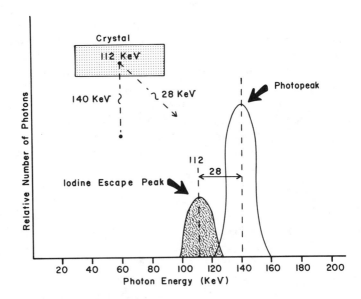

Figure 29-15 Spectrum Component (Escape Peak) Produced by X-Ray Photons Leaving the Crystal

difference between these two, or 112 keV. In other words, the detector sees only 112 keV rather than 140 keV. This gives rise to a spectrum component generally referred to as an iodine escape peak. The energy of an iodine escape peak is always 28 keV below the photopeak energy.

Background

No facility is completely free of background radiation. Sources of background radiation include cosmic radiation, naturally occurring radioactive nuclides in building materials, and environmental contamination. The photon energy spectrum for background radiation depends on the relative contribution from these sources. For simplicity, it is usually assumed to be evenly distributed throughout the energy range.

The Composite Spectrum

The photon energy spectrum as presented through a typical detector system consists of several components produced by the different types of interactions that have been discussed. The composite spectrum is the sum of all the components, as shown in Figure 29-16. The relative contribution of each component depends on

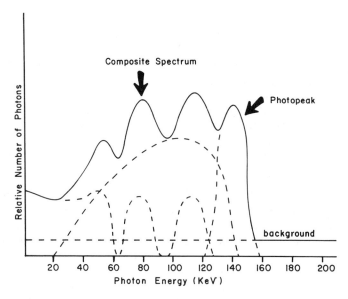

Figure 29-16 Composite Spectrum Produced by Adding the Different Spectral Components

many factors and varies considerably from one type of procedure to another. The spectrum shown in Figure 29-16 illustrates the concept, rather than presents its exact form. In most cases, the composite spectrum can be considered to be made up of "desirable" and "undesirable" components. The photopeak is usually considered a desirable component because it represents photons coming directly from the radioactive source. What constitutes an undesirable component depends, to some extent, on the nature of the procedure. For example, in most imaging procedures the body scatter component is undesirable. This subject is discussed in more detail later.

THE PULSE HEIGHT ANALYZER

A spectrometer is, in general, a device that allows the operator to select and use a specific portion of a spectrum. The type of spectrometer used in most nuclear medicine systems is a PHA. The PHA is located between the detector and the counting or imaging components of the system. The pulses from the detector must pass through the PHA in order to contribute to the image or counting data. The basic characteristic of a PHA is that it can be set to permit only pulses of a specific height to pass through.

Figure 29-17 illustrates the general function of a PHA. The pulse sizes that pass through the PHA are determined by the setting of two controls, the baseline and window.

Most PHAs operate on an arbitrary pulse height scale. The PHA shown in Figure 29-17 has a pulse height scale ranging from 0 to 100 units. By properly calibrating the detector and amplifier components, the PHA scale can be made to correspond to a specific photon energy range. For example, we will assume that the PHA scale of 0 to 100 is being used to represent a photon energy range of 0 to 200. This is achieved by adjusting the detector and amplifier gain so that a 200-keV photon produces a pulse with an amplitude of 100 units. Other photon energies and pulse amplitudes are related in the same manner.

The baseline control sets the minimum pulse amplitude that will pass through the PHA. The window control sets the range of pulse amplitudes that will pass through. Window controls are usually calibrated in either pulse height units, like the baseline control, or as a percentage of the pulse height scale. In the example shown in Figure 29-17, the baseline is set at 60 pulse height units and the window has a width of 20 units. The only pulses that can pass through the analyzer with this setting are those within the range of 60 units (120 keV) and 80 units (160 keV).

Let us now consider the action of the PHA with regard to the three pulses shown in Figure 29-17. The 50-unit pulse (100 keV) is below the baseline setting and is blocked by the analyzer. The 70-unit pulse (140 keV) is well within the range of acceptable pulse sizes established by the baseline and window and therefore passes through the analyzer. Since the 90-unit pulse (180 keV) is above the top of the window, it is also blocked by the analyzer.

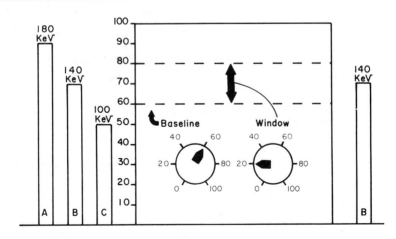

Figure 29-17 Basic Function of a Pulse Height Analyzer

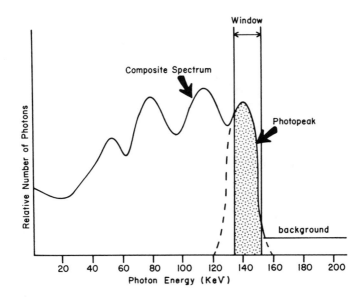

Figure 29-18 PHA Window Positioned to Select the Photopeak from the Other Components of the Spectrum

PHA settings should be considered in relation to the photon energy spectrum, as illustrated in Figure 29-18. In effect, the baseline and window settings determine the portion of the spectrum that will be used for imaging or data collection. The window is generally positioned over the desired portion of the spectrum, such as the photopeak. The area under the spectrum curve that falls within the window (shaded area) represents the relative number of photons that are being collected and used. A wide window setting, which encompasses more of the spectrum, produces an increase in the rate at which photons are counted. With a wide window, an image can be formed faster, or a certain number of counts can be collected in a shorter period. The problem with increasing window width is that it decreases the ability to discriminate between the desirable and undesirable portion of the spectrum.

In many situations, most of the undesirable portions of the spectrum are at energies below the desirable portion, or photopeak. Good data collection can be achieved by carefully positioning the baseline and opening the window to include all energies above the baseline setting. This is referred to as an integral counting.

Chapter 30

Radionuclide Image Quality

INTRODUCTION AND OVERVIEW

The radionuclide image produced by a gamma camera is distinctly different when compared with images from the other imaging methods. It is difficult to compare the contrast sensitivities because a gamma camera looks at a different tissue characteristic: the concentration of a specific radionuclide. The sensitivity generally depends on a specific tissue's ability to collect a specific pharmaceutical. There are a variety of pathologic conditions for which radionuclide imaging has a high contrast sensitivity.

The gamma camera image generally shows much less detail and a higher noise level than other medical images.

In this chapter we explore the factors that determine radionuclide image quality and how they can be used by the operator to optimize an imaging procedure.

CONTRAST

Contrast can exist when the radiation from an object is either more or less than the radiation from the background area. If the radiation from the object is greater than from the background, the object is commonly referred to as being "hot," and if it is less, it is referred to as being "cold" (eg, a nodule).

Figure 30-1 illustrates the three stages in the imaging process. The object within the patient has a certain amount of inherent contrast with respect to its surrounding background. The background can consist of radiation from a number of different sources, including

- radiation from the same radionuclide in the surrounding tissue
- scattered radiation

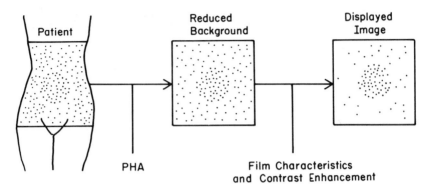

Figure 30-1 Contrast at Three Different Points in the Imaging Process

- radiation from other nuclides within the patient
- radiation from external sources.

The amount of inherent contrast generally depends on the amount of activity contained in the object of interest in comparison with the "activity" of the background area. Many factors affect the inherent contrast. A very significant factor is the physiologic function of the object (such as a tumor), which affects the radionuclide uptake.

One of the functions of the gamma camera is to increase the contrast between a radioactive object and the surrounding background. This is usually achieved by using the pulse height analyzer (PHA) to "separate" the object radiation from the background area radiation. Using the PHA usually creates an intermediate radiation image whose contrast is greater than the inherent contrast from the object being imaged.

Since the energy of scattered photons is less than the energy of the photons coming directly from the radioactive source, it is possible to produce some separation with a PHA. The difference between the energy of a scattered photon and the primary radiation depends on two factors: the angle of scatter and the initial energy of the primary radiation. For example, a 140-keV photon scattered at an angle of 90° has an energy of 116 keV. This is less than a 20% difference between the scattered and primary radiation. If we assume that one half of the scatter occurs at angles less than 90°, much of the scattered radiation is very close in energy to the primary radiation.

As discussed in Chapter 29, a scintillation detector system produces a certain amount of energy spreading, or loss of energy resolution. This spreading and the relatively small energy difference between scatter and primary radiations make it impossible in many cases to remove all of the scattered radiation from an image.

Figure 30-2 shows a typical photon energy spectrum for both the direct and the scattered radiation. By carefully positioning the PHA window, it is usually possible to exclude a significant amount of the scattered radiation from the image. Figure 30-3 compares two images of a radioactive object. In the one on the left, the amount of scattered radiation was reduced by using a PHA.

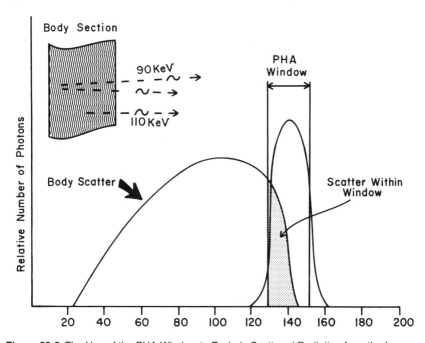

Figure 30-2 The Use of the PHA Window to Exclude Scattered Radiation from the Image

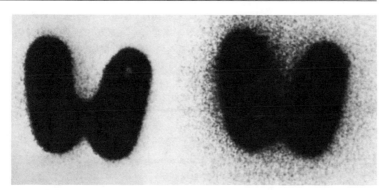

Figure 30-3 Radioactive Object Imaged without and with Scattered Radiation Present

Scattered radiation is generally more of a problem in imaging a "cold" lesion, which is surrounded by activity, than a "hot" lesion.

In some cases it is desirable to image one radionuclide when another radioactive substance is present in the same area. The ability to separate the two radiations depends very heavily on their relative energies. The problem can be appreciated by considering the photon energy spectra of the two nuclides shown in Figure 30-4. If there is a sufficient energy difference between the two photon peaks, it will be possible to set the PHA window to image nuclide B. The problem arises when we attempt to image nuclide A. Because the photopeak energy of nuclide A is less than that of nuclide B, it might coincide with a significant amount of scattered radiation from nuclide B.

BLUR AND VISIBILITY OF DETAIL

The method commonly used in nuclear medicine to assign a value to blur is illustrated in Figure 30-5. The blurred image of an object point is generally not a circle of uniform intensity or film density. Typically the image is most intense at the center with a gradual decrease toward the periphery, best illustrated by means of a profile, as shown. Since the blur is not uniform in intensity, the question arises

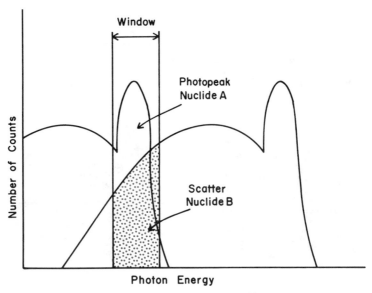

Figure 30-4 Overlapping of the Energy Spectra of Two Nuclides

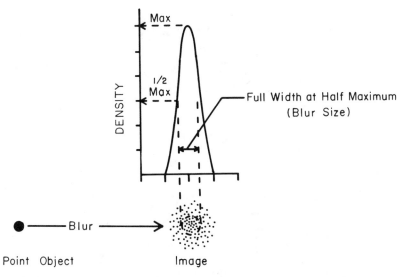

Figure 30-5 Profile of the Blurred Image of a Small Object (Radioactive Source)

as to which dimension should be used to express the size of the blur pattern. The common practice is to use the diameter of a circle located at one half of the maximum intensity. With respect to the profile, this corresponds to the full width of the profile at one half of its maximum height. This blur value is generally expressed in millimeters and is the FWHM. This is also the name of the parameter used to express radiation detector energy resolution, but the two entirely different applications of the term FWHM should not be confused.

The image profile of a point object, such as in Figure 30-5, is generally designated as a point spread function (PSF). It is usually easier to measure the image spread, or blur, of a source that is in the form of a thin line, ie, a small tube filled with radioactive material. The profile obtained in this manner is known as a line spread function (LSF). In either case, the blur width is expressed in terms of the FWHM.

Because blur tends to spread image points, it can make it difficult to resolve, or separate, small objects or features that are located close together. Because of this, the term *resolution* is often used to describe the blur characteristics of an imaging system. This results from the common practice of using resolution test objects to measure blur. An image of a typical test object used for this purpose is illustrated in Figure 30-6. The object consists of a series of lead strips that are placed over a large uniform source of radiation. In the four sections of the test object, the width and separation distance between the lead strips varies from section to section. Each section is characterized by the number of line pairs (one lead strip and one space) per centimeter. The blur is measured by imaging the test object and determining

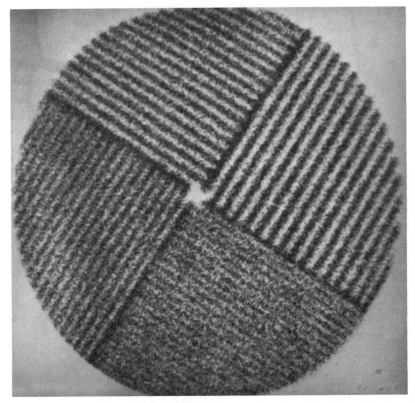

Figure 30-6 Image of a Test Object Used to Measure the Resolving Ability (Amount of Blur) of a Gamma Camera

the closest strips that can be resolved. The approximate relationship between resolution and blur is

$$\text{Resolution (lp/cm)} = 1/\text{FWHM (cm)}.$$

The two quantities are inversely related: As blur increases, resolution decreases.

There are several sources of image blur in a nuclear imaging procedure. The equipment user should be familiar with them so that blur can be minimized as much as possible.

Motion

Motion of the patient during the imaging procedure is an obvious source of blur. The amount of blur is equal to the distance that each point within the object moves during the time the image is actually being formed.

Gamma Camera Blur

Two kinds of blur are introduced by the gamma camera itself: intrinsic blur and collimator blur. The distinction between them can be made by referring to Figure 30-7.

Intrinsic Blur

Consider an image point that has been formed within the camera crystal. (For the moment we are assuming that the gamma photons from a point source have all been absorbed in the crystal at this point.) The light spreads as it moves from the image point to the surface of the crystal. This spreading, or diffusion, of light within the crystal causes the image at the crystal surface to be blurred. The amount of blurring introduced by the crystal is more or less proportional to crystal thickness. This is similar to what happens in intensifying screens. The selection of a crystal thickness involves a compromise between blur and camera sensitivity (detector efficiency). A thick crystal captures more photons, and therefore increases camera sensitivity, but it also increases the amount of intrinsic blur. Thin crystals, which reduce image blur, can be effectively used with radionuclides that emit relatively low energy photons.

The light image from the crystal is transferred electronically to the viewing device. The inability of the electronic circuitry to position precisely each image point on the viewing screen can be an additional source of intrinsic blur.

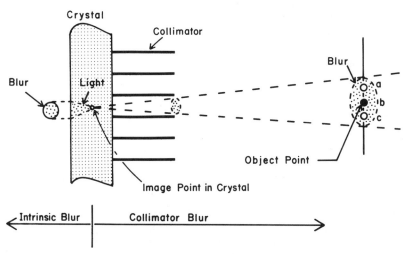

Figure 30-7 The Two Basic Components of Gamma Camera Blur: Intrinsic Blur and Collimator Blur

At the present time, gamma cameras have intrinsic blur values in the approximate range of 3 mm to 6 mm when measured at the crystal surface. The amount of intrinsic blur in gamma cameras has been reduced over the years, with improvements in both the crystals and electronic circuits.

When considering the blur value for a specific camera application, one must consider the location of the object being imaged. The degree of image quality usually depends on the relationship of the amount of blur to the size of the object. Therefore, the amount of blur must be considered not only at the crystal surface but at the location of the object. If a parallel-hole collimator is used, the value of the intrinsic blur will be the same for an object located at any distance from the camera. If either a diverging, converging, or pin-hole collimator is used, the amount of intrinsic blur projected to the object location will depend on the distance between the object and the camera surface. This is illustrated in Figure 30-8.

If a diverging collimator is used, the amount of intrinsic blur, expressed at the object location, increases with an increase in the distance between the object and the camera. This occurs because a diverging collimator minifies the image and minification increases with distance between the object and camera. Therefore, as the object is moved away from the camera surface, the image becomes smaller, and the ratio of intrinsic blur to apparent object size increases. For reasons discussed later, this effect is represented as an increase in blur with respect to object size.

If a converging collimator, which produces image magnification, is used, the intrinsic blur with respect to object size decreases as the object is moved away from the camera surface.

In summary, the amount of intrinsic blur with respect to object size depends on whether the image is magnified or minified by the collimator. Minification increases the effective blur, whereas magnification reduces it.

Collimator Blur

The purpose of the collimator is to "focus" the radiation from each point of the object to a corresponding point on the crystal. Because of the finite size of the collimator holes, each image point in the crystal cannot correspond to a single object point, as shown in Figure 30-7. This causes the gamma photon image that is focused onto the crystal by the collimator to be blurred. This effect is generally designated *collimator blur*.

It is best to analyze collimator blur by starting from an image point within the crystal, as shown in Figure 30-7. In the ideal, no-blur, imaging system, the field of view (FOV) from the image point would be limited to a corresponding object point of equal size. However, with an actual collimator, the FOV from a single image point is much larger than the corresponding object point. From the standpoint of an image point within the crystal, this causes each object point to look larger than it really is, or, in other words, to be blurred. If an object point (small source) is

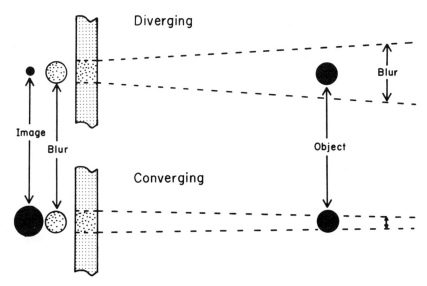

Figure 30-8 Illustration of How Collimator Characteristics Affect the Relationship of Intrinsic Blur to Object Size

located at the face of the collimator, it appears to be the same size as the collimator hole; if the object point is moved away from the face of the collimator, as shown in Figure 30-7, it appears to become even larger, or more blurred. This effect should not be confused with the minification and magnification produced by converging and diverging collimators. Here we are considering the characteristics of an individual collimator hole. The amount of blur is, in effect, the FOV from a point within the crystal through an individual collimator hole.

Because of the increased FOV of an individual hole, the camera cannot resolve, or separate, small sources located near each other. For example, in Figure 30-7, three small sources located at points a, b, and c would be blurred together and appear as one.

The amount of collimator blur is primarily dependent on three factors:

1. size of the collimator hole
2. length of the collimator hole (collimator thickness)
3. distance between the camera and the object being imaged.

The three factors determine the FOV from a point on the crystal through a single collimator hole. To the camera, a small point source appears to be the size of the FOV through a single hole. Figure 30-9 compares the blur produced by collimators with different hole sizes. As the collimator thickness is increased, the single-hole FOV or blur, is decreased. Figure 30-9 also shows that a reduction in collimator hole size (diameter) reduces blur at a specific object location.

When selecting a collimator for a specific application, consideration must be given to the compromise between blur and sensitivity. Design factors that decrease blur, such as decreased hole diameter and increased hole length (collimator thickness), also reduce detector efficiency and camera sensitivity. This rela-

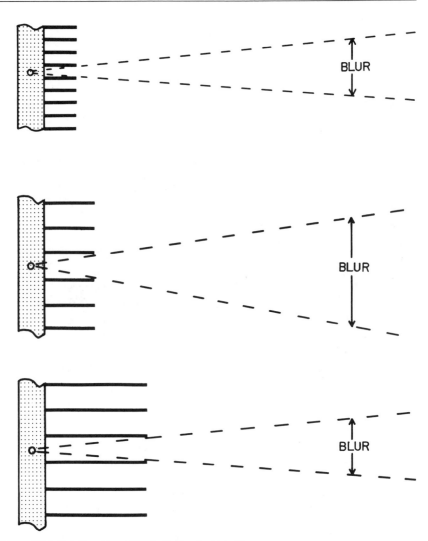

Figure 30-9 Relationship of Blur to Collimator Hole Size

tionship is shown in Figure 30-10 for some typical collimators. Collimators are often placed into general categories by virtue of their blur/sensitivity characteristics. Names for the various categories are usually chosen that emphasize the positive aspects of a particular collimator. These general categories are indicated in Figure 30-10.

With all collimators, blur increases with distance from the collimator face, as shown in Figures 30-7 and 30-9. This is a rather significant factor when the object being imaged is not in direct contact with the collimator face. Figure 30-11 shows the general relationship between collimator blur and the distance between the collimator face and the object being imaged. The blur value at a distance of 0 (at the collimator surface) represents the intrinsic blur of the camera plus the minimum value of collimator blur. As the object is moved away from the collimator surface, the collimator blur increases and adds to the intrinsic blur.

IMAGE NOISE

In nuclear imaging, the major source of noise is the random distribution of photons over the surface of the image. A gamma camera image typically contains much more noise than a conventional x-ray image. This is because nuclear images are generally formed with fewer photons than x-ray images. The amount of noise,

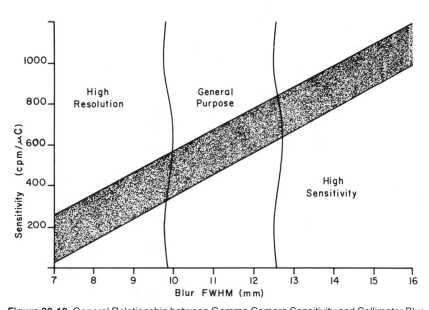

Figure 30-10 General Relationship between Gamma Camera Sensitivity and Collimator Blur

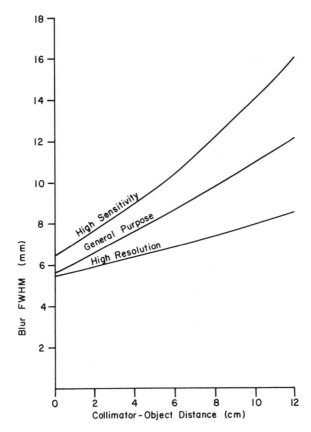

Figure 30-11 Relationship of Gamma Camera Blur to the Distance between the Radioactive Object and the Collimator

---

or variation in photon concentration, is inversely related to the number of photons used to form the image. The noise in an image can be reduced by increasing the number of photons used in the imaging procedure.

The relationship between image noise and photon concentration, or count density, is illustrated in Figure 30-12. A series of circular areas are drawn across the surface of an image. The size of the area that should be used to analyze image noise is approximately equal to the camera blur size (FWHM). For the purpose of this discussion, an area size of 1 cm^2 is used. A camera with a large blur value tends to produce an image with less noise because the blur, in effect, averages or blends the photons together over a larger area. The image section shown in Figure 30-12 was (theoretically) produced by a uniformly distributed radioactive source. That is, there is no variation in activity, as there would be from the

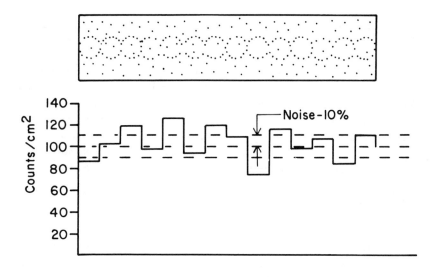

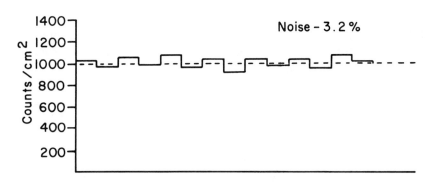

Figure 30-12 Area-to-Area Variation in Photon Concentration for Two Average Count Densities

presence of a lesion, that would provide useful information. Any variation in count density is produced by the natural random distribution of photons. The variation in the number of photons, or counts, from area to area is an indication of the image noise level.

The upper count-density profile in Figure 30-12 shows the variation in count density when the average is 100 counts per cm². The standard deviation of the count densities can be used to assign a numerical value to the noise. In our earlier discussion of image noise (Chapter 21), we showed that an average of 100 counts (photons) had a standard deviation of 10 counts, or 10%. Therefore, when the count density is 100 counts per area, the standard deviation noise level is 10%.

The lower profile shows the area-to-area variation when the average count density is 1,000 counts per cm^2. In this case, the standard deviation (the square root of 1,000) is 32 counts, or 3.2%. This demonstrates that as the number of photons used to form an image (count density) is increased, the area-to-area variation in photon concentration, or noise, is decreased. The noise level is inversely proportional to the square root of the average count density.

Lesion Visibility

Image noise degrades the overall quality of an image and makes it difficult to detect certain lesions. Let us consider the situation shown in Figure 30-13. Assume we have a lesion that has sufficient radioactive uptake to produce 20% contrast. If an imaging system that is completely noise-free is used, the lesion will be readily visible against a smooth background, illustrated by the upper graph. If, on the other hand, the image is produced with a gamma camera that collects, on the average, 100 counts per area, the situation changes rather dramatically. The ratio of the lesion contrast to the noise level will be only 2:1. It is generally considered that a lesion contrast-to-noise ratio of at least 4:1 is necessary in nuclear medicine to ensure reliable lesion detection. In this case, detectability can be improved simply by collecting more counts to form the image, so that it has a lower noise level.

UNIFORMITY

In order to produce an image that accurately shows the distribution of radioactive material, a gamma camera should have an equal sensitivity over the entire image area. A non-uniform sensitivity generally occurs when the various PM tube outputs are not properly balanced. Most modern gamma cameras use special circuits, usually containing microprocessors, to correct for the inherent non-uniformity in the detector array.

A gamma camera should be checked periodically to determine if it has a uniform sensitivity response. This procedure requires a source of radiation that will cover the entire crystal area with a uniform intensity. This can be achieved in two ways, as illustrated in Figure 30-14.

One method is to use a large flat radioactive source at least as large as the crystal, generally referred to as a *flood source*. To test for uniformity, the flood source is mounted on the face of the camera, usually with a collimator in place. Another

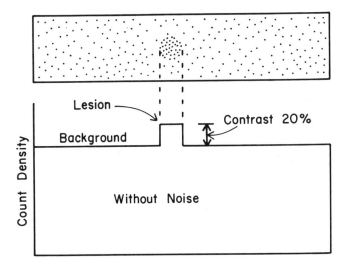

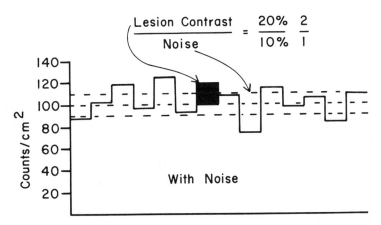

Figure 30-13 Relationship of Lesion Contrast to Background, Both with and without Noise

method is to use a small radioactive source located at least 1.5 m from the face of the camera. With this method, the collimator must be removed in order to produce a uniform exposure to the crystal surface.

SPATIAL DISTORTION

Because of the manner in which the image is transferred from the crystal to the viewing screen, a gamma camera may introduce spatial distortion. Distortion

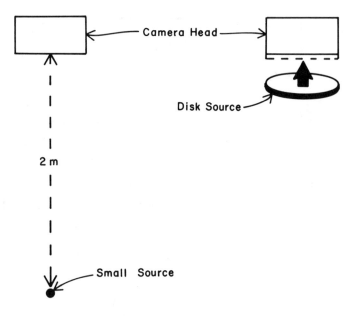

Figure 30-14 Radioactive Sources Used to Test a Gamma Camera for Uniformity Over the Image Area

occurs when various points within an image are moved with respect to each other in the transfer process. This distorts the size and shape of objects within the image.

A gamma camera can be checked for spatial distortion by using one of several types of test objects, or phantoms. For this test, the test object must have a series of lines or holes that are spaced uniformly within the image area. The test is performed by imaging the test object and then determining if the uniform spacing is maintained in the image.

Chapter 31

Statistics

INTRODUCTION AND OVERVIEW

Photons are emitted from a radioactive source in a random manner with respect to both time and location. The random emission of photons with respect to time makes it somewhat difficult to get a precise indication of source activity. This is because the random emission produces a fluctuation in the number of photons emitted from one time interval to another. If the photons from the sample are counted for several consecutive time intervals, the number of counts recorded will be different for each, as illustrated in Figure 31-1. This natural variation introduces an error in the measurement of activity that is generally referred to as the *statistical counting error*.

The random emission of photons with respect to location, or area, produces image noise. The presence of this spatial noise within an image decreases the ability to see and detect small objects, especially when their contrast is low.

In this chapter we first consider the nature of the random variation, or fluctuation, in photons from a radioactive source, and then show how this knowledge can be used to increase the precision of activity measurements (counting) and the quality of nuclear images.

We must first know something about the extent of the fluctuation, and if it is related to a factor over which we have control. One approach is to imagine we are conducting an experiment for the purpose of studying the random nature of photon emissions. Let us assume we have a source of radiation in a scintillation well counter that is being counted again and again for 1-minute intervals. We quickly notice that the number of counts, or photons, varies from one interval to another. Some of the values we observe might be 87, 102, 118, 96, 124, 92, 108, 73, 115, 97, 105, and 82. Although these data show that there is a fluctuation, they do not readily show the range of fluctuations. The amount of fluctuation will become more apparent if we arrange our data in the form of a graph, as shown in

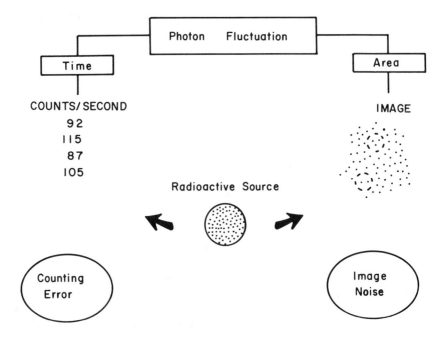

Figure 31-1 Statistical Photon Fluctuation as a Source of Counting Error and Image Noise

Figure 31-2. In this graph, we plotted the number of times we measured a specific number of counts versus the actual number of counts observed. Obviously, we would have to count the number of photons from our source many many times to obtain the data to plot this type of graph.

When the data are presented in this manner, it is apparent that some count values occurred more frequently than others. In our experiment we observed 100 counts more frequently than any other value. Also, most of the count values fell within the range of 70 to 130 counts. Within this range, the number of times we observed specific count values is distributed in the Gaussian, or normal, distribution pattern. (This is actually a special type of Gaussian distribution known as the Poisson distribution, and is discussed later.)

At this point we need to raise a very significant question: Of all of these values, which one is the "true" count rate that best represents the activity of our sample? In our example, the average, or mean, of all of the values is 100 counts. This is considered to be the value that best represents the true activity of the sample.

COUNTING ERROR

In our experiment, we took one sample of radioactive material and counted it many times to determine the fluctuation in the number of counts, or photons, from

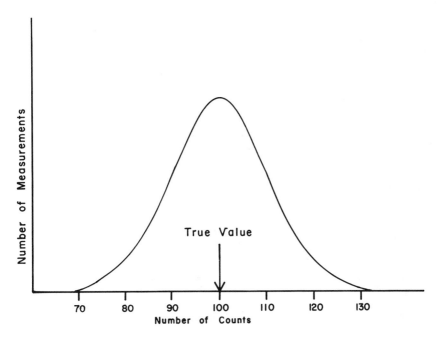

Figure 31-2 Graph Showing the Relative Number of Times Different Count Values (Number of Counts) Are Obtained When a Specific Radioactive Sample Is Counted Again and Again

the sample. However, in the clinical laboratory we normally count a sample only one time. Any time we make a single count on a source we are faced with a question: How close is our measured count value to the true count value for that particular sample? As illustrated in Figure 31-3, the difference between these two values is the error in our observed count value. At this point we have a problem: Since we do not know what the true count value is, we have no way of knowing what the error associated with a single measurement is.

Error Ranges

From our earlier experiment, we know that the value of any individual count falls within a certain range around the true count value. In our experiment, we observed that all counts fell within 30 counts (plus or minus) of the true value (100 counts). Based on this observation, we could predict the maximum error that could occur when we make a single count. In our case, the maximum error would be $\pm$ 30 counts ($\pm$ 30%). We also observed that very few count values approached the maximum error. In fact, a large proportion of the count values are clustered relatively close to the true value. In other words, the error associated with many individual counts is obviously much less than the maximum error. To assume that

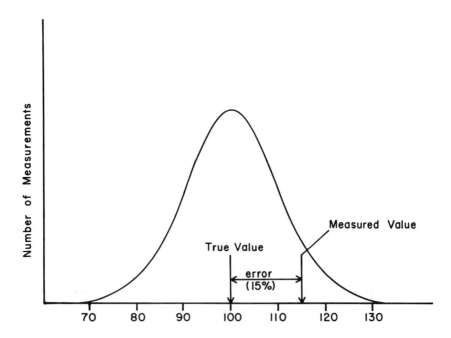

Figure 31-3 The Amount of Error Is the Difference between the Measured and True Count Values

the error in a single count is always the maximum possible error is overstating the problem. Although it is necessary to recognize that a certain maximum error is possible, we must be more realistic in assigning values to the error itself because it is usually much less than the maximum possible error.

If, at this point, we were to go back to the data from our earlier experiment and analyze it from the standpoint of how the individual count values are clustered around the true value (mean), we would get results similar to those illustrated in Figure 31-4. For the purpose of this analysis, we established three error ranges around the true value. In our particular case, the error ranges are in ten-count increments. The first range is ± 10 counts (10% error), the second range is ± 20 counts (20% error), and the largest range is ± 30 counts (30% error). At this point we are interested in how often the value of a single measurement fell within the various error ranges. Upon careful analysis of our data, we find that 68% of the time the count values are within the first error range (± 10%), 95% of all count values are within the next error range (± 20%), and essentially all values (theoretically 99.7%) are within the largest error range (± 30%).

With this information as background, let us now see what we can say about the error of an individual measurement. Note that in the case of a single measurement,

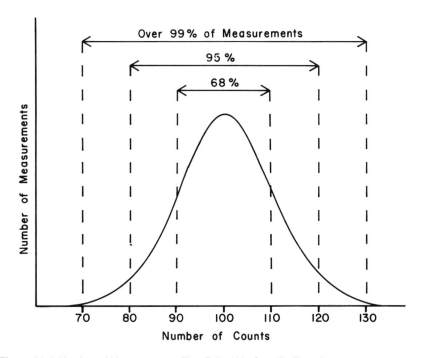

Figure 31-4 Number of Measurements That Fall within Specific Error Ranges

there is no way to determine the actual error because the true value is unknown. Therefore, we must think in terms of the probability of being within certain error ranges. With this in mind, we can now make several statements concerning the error of an individual measurement in our earlier experiment:

- There is a 68% probability (chance) that the error is within ± 10%.
- There is a 95% probability that the error is within ± 20%.
- There is a 99.7% probability that the error is within ± 30%.

While we are still not able to predict what the actual error is, we can make a statement as to the probability that the error is within certain stated limits.

It might appear that the error ranges used above were chosen because they were in simple increments of ten counts. Actually, they were chosen because they represent "standard" error ranges used for values distributed in a Gaussian manner. Error ranges can be expressed in units, or increments, of standard deviations (σ). In our example, one standard deviation (σ) is equivalent to ten counts. However, one standard deviation is not always equivalent to ten counts.

The general situation is illustrated in Figure 31-5. For values distributed in a Gaussian manner, the relationship between the probability of a value falling within a specific error range remains constant when the error range is expressed in terms of standard deviations. For the general case, we have the following relationship between error limits and the probability of a value falling within the specific limits.

Error Limits	Probability
± 1 σ	68.0%
± 2 σ	95.0%
± 3 σ	99.7%

It might be helpful to draw an analogy between the error limits and a bull's-eye target, as shown in Figure 31-6. The small bull's-eye in the center represents the true count value for a specific sample. If we make one measurement, we can expect the count value to "hit" somewhere within the overall target area. Although there is no way to predict where the value of a single measurement will fall, we do know something about the probability, or chance, of it falling within certain areas. For example, there is a 68% chance that our count value will fall within the smallest circle, which represents an error range of one standard deviation. There is a 95% probability that the value will fall within the next largest circle, which represents an error range of two standard deviations. Essentially all of the values (99.7%) will fall within the largest circle, which represents an error range of three standard deviations.

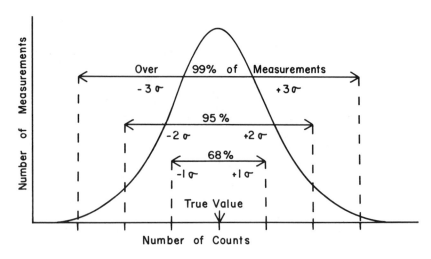

Figure 31-5 Relationship between the Number of Measurements within Error Limits When the Limits Are Expressed in Terms of Standard Deviations

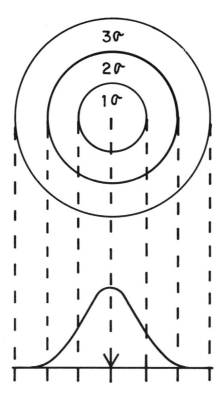

Figure 31-6 An Analogy between Counting Error and a Bull's-Eye Target

Measuring the relative activity of a radioactive sample is like shooting at a bull's-eye. We do not expect to get the true count value (hit the bull's-eye) each time. The problem is that after making a measurement (taking a shot) we do not know what our actual error is (by how far we missed the bull's-eye). This is because we do not know what the true value is, only the value of our single measurement. We must, therefore, describe our performance in terms of error ranges and the confidence we have of falling within the various ranges. We can express a level of confidence of falling within a certain error range if we know the probability of a single value falling within that range. For Gaussian distributed count values, 68% will fall within one standard deviation of the true, or mean, value. Based on this we could make the statement that we are 68% confident that the value of a single measurement will fall within the one standard deviation error range. A more complete description of our performance could be summarized as follows:

Error Range	Confidence Level
± 1 σ	68.0%
± 2 σ	95.0%
± 3 σ	99.7%

A clear distinction between an error range and a confidence level is necessary. Error range describes how far a single measurement value might deviate, or miss, the true count value of a sample. Confidence level expresses the probability, or chance, that a single measurement will fall within a specific error range. Notice that as we increase the size of our error range our confidence level also increases. In terms of our target, this simply means we are more confident that our shot will hit within a larger circle than within a smaller circle.

The relationship between confidence level and error range expressed in standard deviations does not change for measurement values distributed in a Gaussian manner. What does change, however, is the relationship between an error range expressed in standard deviations and an error range expressed in actual number of counts or percentages. In our earlier example, one standard deviation was equal to ten counts, or 10%. We will now find that for other measurements one standard deviation can be a different number of counts.

Radiation events (such as count values), unlike the value of many other nonradiation variables, are distributed in a very special way. The value of the standard deviation, expressed in number of counts, is related to the actual number of photons counted during the measurement. Theoretically, the value of the standard deviation is the square root of the mean of a large number of measurements. In actual practice, we never know what the true count value of a sample is. In most cases, our measurement value will be sufficiently close to the true value so that we can use it to estimate the value of the standard deviation as follows:

$$\text{Standard deviation} = \sqrt{\text{Measured value.}}$$

For example, if we make a measurement in which 100 counts will be recorded, the value of the standard deviation will be

$$\sigma = \sqrt{100} = 10 \text{ counts.}$$

This will be recognized as the count value in our earlier example, where it was stated that the value of one standard deviation was 10 counts, or 10%. Now let us examine the values of one standard deviation for other recorded count values shown in Table 31-1. Examination of this table shows that as the number of counts recorded during a single measurement increases, the value of the standard deviation, in number of counts, also increases; but it decreases when expressed as a percentage of the total number of counts. We can use this last fact to improve the precision of radiation measurements.

Table 31-1 Standard Deviation Expressed in Number of Counts and Percentage of Count Value

Number of Counts	Standard Deviation	
	Counts	Percent
100	10	10
1,000	32	3.2
10,000	100	1
100,000	316	0.32
1,000,000	1,000	0.1

Table 31-2 Error Limits for Different Count Values and Levels of Confidence

Number of Counts	Confidence Level		
	68%	95%	99.7%
100	10	20	30
1,000	3.2	6.3	9.5
10,000	1	2	3
100,000	0.32	0.63	0.95

The error range, expressed as a percentage of the measured value, decreases as the number of counts in an individual measurement is increased. The real significance of this is that the precision of a radiation measurement is determined by the actual number of counts recorded during the measurement. The error limits for different count values and levels of confidence are shown in Table 31-2.

We can use the information in Table 31-2 to plan a radiation measurement that has a specific precision. For example, if we want our measurement to be within a 2% error range at the 95% confidence level, it will be necessary to record at least 10,000 counts. Most radiation counters can be set to record counts either for a specific time interval or until a specific number of counts are accumulated. In either case, the count rate of the sample (relative activity) is determined by dividing the number of counts recorded by the amount of time. Presetting the number of counts and then measuring the time required for that number of counts to accumulate allows the user to obtain a specific precision in the measurement.

Combined Errors

In some applications, it is necessary to add or subtract counts in order to obtain a desired parameter. An example is the subtraction of background from a sample measurement. The first step is to count the sample. (Counts from background radiation are included in this measurement.) The next step is to remove the radioactive sample from the counting system, and then measure only the background radiation. The background count rate is then subtracted from the sample-plus-background count rate to obtain a measurement of the relative sample activity. The question now arises: What is the error in the sample count rate that was obtained by subtracting one count value from another?

Let us use the example shown in Figure 31-7 to investigate the error in the difference between two count values. Assume that we have two radiation sources. For the same counting time, one has a true value of 3,600 counts and the other a true value of 6,400 counts. The *true difference* between the two is 2,800 counts. If we now measure the two samples, we expect the *measured values* to fall somewhere within the error ranges indicated in Figure 31-7. With respect to the *measured difference* we now have two errors to contend with, one for each of the sample measurements. The question is now: What will be the error range for the difference between the two measured values? In some instances, the error in the measurement of one sample might be in a direction that compensates for the error in the measurement of the other sample, and the net error in the difference would be relatively small. There is also the possibility that the two errors are in opposite directions, in which case the error in the difference would be relatively large. When making measurements on two samples, we have no way of knowing either the amount or direction of the individual errors. Therefore, we must consider the range of errors possible in the difference between the two measured count values. Because of the possibility of errors compounding (by being in opposite directions), it should be obvious that the error range for the difference (σ_d) will be larger than the error range associated with the individual measurement (σ_1 and σ_2). When the error ranges are expressed in terms of standard deviations, the relationship becomes

$$\sigma_d = \sqrt{\sigma_1^2 + \sigma_2^2}.$$

Let us now examine the actual values in Figure 31-7 and see what the error range will be for the difference between the two count values. The first sample measurement has a true value of 3,600 counts. By taking the square root of this number, we find that the standard deviation is 60 counts, or 1.67%. The second sample has a count total of 6,400 counts with a standard deviation of 80 counts, or 1.25%. If we now determine the standard deviation for the difference by using the relationship given above, we see that

$$\sigma_d = \sqrt{(60)^2 + (80)^2} = 100.$$

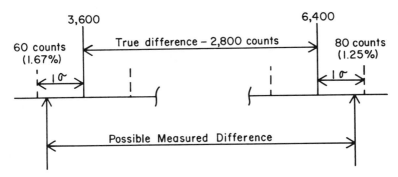

Figure 31-7 Errors Associated with the Difference between Two Count Values

A standard deviation of 100 counts is 3.6% of the difference between the two count values, 2,800 counts.

Any time we add or subtract count values, the error range (standard deviation) of the sum or difference will be larger than the error range of the individual measurements. When two count values are added, the standard deviation of the sum (σ_s) is related to the standard deviation of the individual measurements (σ_1 and σ_2) by

$$\sigma_s = \sqrt{\sigma_1^2 + \sigma_2^2}.$$

Notice that this is the same relationship as that for the difference between two count values. A common mistake is to assume that the sign between the two standard deviation values is different for addition and subtraction. It does not change; it is positive in both cases.

Let us now determine the error range of the sum of the two count values in Figure 31-7. As we have just seen, the standard deviation for the sum is the same as the standard deviation for the difference. That is, in this case, 100 counts, but since the sum of the two count values is 10,000 counts this now represents an error range of only 1%. This is the same error range as we would find on a single measurement of 10,000 counts.

When expressed as a percentage, the error range increases when we take the difference between two measurements, but it decreases when we add the results of the two measurements.

Chapter 32

Patient Exposure and Protection

INTRODUCTION AND OVERVIEW

All medical imaging methods deposit some form of energy in the patient's body. Although the quantity of energy is relatively low, it is a factor that should be given attention when conducting diagnostic examinations. In general, there is more concern for the energy deposited by the ionizing radiations, x-ray and gamma, than for ultrasound energy or radio frequency (RF) energy deposited in magnetic resonance imaging (MRI) examinations. Therefore, this chapter gives major emphasis to the issues relating to the exposure of patients to ionizing radiation.

Patients undergoing either x-ray or radionuclide examinations are subject to a wide range of exposure levels. One of our objectives is to explore the factors that affect patient exposure. This is followed by an explanation of methods that can be used to determine patient exposure values in the clinical setting.

Figure 32-1 identifies the major factors that affect patient exposure during a radiographic procedure. Some factors, such as thickness and density, are determined by the patient. Most of the others are determined by the medical staff. Many of the factors that affect patient exposure also affect image quality. In most instances when exposure can be decreased by changing a specific factor, image quality is also decreased. Therefore, the objective in setting up most x-ray procedures is to select factors that provide an appropriate compromise between patient exposure and image quality.

X-RAY EXPOSURE PATTERNS

In any x-ray examination, there is considerable variation in exposure from point to point within the patient's body. This must be considered when expressing values for patient exposure. In fact, when exposure values are given, the specific

477

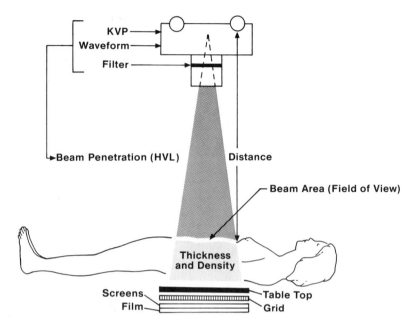

Figure 32-1 Factors That Affect Patient Exposure in a Radiographic Procedure

anatomical location of the value should also be stated. Some exposure patterns are characteristic of the different x-ray imaging methods. A review of these patterns will give us some background for considering factors that affect exposure and applying methods to determine actual exposure values.

Radiography

In the typical radiographic examination, the x-ray beam is projected through the patient's body, as shown in Figure 32-1. The point that receives maximum exposure is the entrance surface near the center of the beam. There are two reasons for this. The primary x-ray beam has not been attenuated by the tissue at this point, and the area is exposed by some of the scattered radiation from the body. The amount of surface exposure produced by the backscatter depends on the spectrum of the primary beam and the size of the exposed area. For typical radiographic situations, scattered radiation can add at least 20% to the surface exposure produced by the primary beam.

As the x-ray beam progresses through the body, it undergoes attenuation. The rate of attenuation (or penetration) is determined by the photon-energy spectrum (KV and filtration) and the type of tissue (fat, muscle, bone) through which the beam passes. For the purpose of this discussion, we assume a body consisting of homogeneous muscle tissue. In Figure 32-2, lines are drawn to divide the body into HVLs. The exposure is reduced by a factor of one half each time it passes through 1 HVL. The thickness of 1 HVL depends on the photon-energy spectrum. However, for the immediate discussion, we assume that 1 HVL is equivalent to 4 cm of tissue. A 20-cm thick body section consists of 5 HVLs. Therefore, the exposure decreases by one half as it passes through each 4 cm of tissue. At the exit surface, the exposure is a small fraction of the entrance surface exposure.

The exposure to a specific organ or point of interest within the direct x-ray beam depends on its proximity to the entrance surface.

Tissue located outside the primary beam receives some exposure from the scattered radiation produced within the beam area. The scatter exposure to the surrounding tissue is relatively low in comparison to the exposure levels within the primary beam.

Fluoroscopy

The fluoroscopic beam projected through the body will produce a pattern similar to a radiographic beam if the beam remains fixed in one position. If the beam is moved during the procedure, the radiation will be distributed over a large volume of tissue rather than being concentrated in one area. For a specific exposure time,

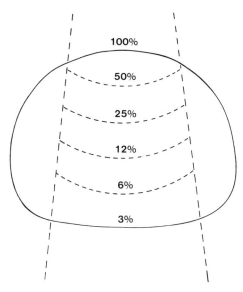

Figure 32-2 Typical Exposure Pattern (Depth Dose Curves) for an X-Ray Beam Passing through a Patient's Body

tissue exposure values (roentgens) are reduced by moving the beam, but the total radiation ($R - cm^2$) into the body is not changed. This was illustrated in Figure 3-5 (Chapter 3).

Computed Tomography

In computed tomography (CT) two factors are associated with exposure distribution and must be considered: (1) the distribution within an individual slice and (2) the effect of imaging multiple slices.

The rotation of the x-ray beam around the body produces a much more uniform distribution of radiation exposure than a stationary radiographic beam. A typical CT exposure pattern is shown in Figure 32-3. A relatively uniform distribution throughout the slice is obtained if a 360° scan is performed. However, if other scan angles that are not multiples of 360° are used, the exposure distribution will become less uniform.

When multiple slices are imaged, the exposure (roentgens) does not increase in proportion to the number of slices because the radiation is distributed over a larger volume of tissue. This point was also illustrated in Chapter 3. However, when slices are located close together, radiation from one slice can produce additional exposure in adjacent slices because slice edges are not sharply defined (as described in Chapter 23) and because of scattered radiation.

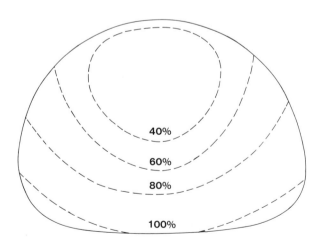

Figure 32-3 Typical Exposure (Dose) Pattern Produced with Computed Tomography

RADIATION AND IMAGE QUALITY

One of the major compromises that must be made in imaging procedures using ionizing radiation is between patient exposure and image quality. Within certain limits, increasing image quality requires an increase in patient exposure. It is usually the specific image quality requirements that determine the quantity of radiation that must be used in the imaging process. The three basic image quality factors (contrast sensitivity, detail, and noise) are each related to patient exposure. This holds true for both x-ray and nuclear radiation imaging procedures. The variables of an imaging procedure should be selected to produce adequate image quality with the lowest possible radiation exposure.

We now consider each factor that affects patient exposure and show how it relates to image quality.

FACTORS AFFECTING EXPOSURE

The exposure, or dose, to a specific point within a patient's body is determined by a combination of factors. One of the most significant is whether the point in question is in or out of the primary beam. Points not located in the direct beam can receive exposure from scattered radiation, but this is generally much less than the exposure to points within the beam area. The factors that determine exposure levels to points within the body will be discussed in reference to the situation illustrated in Figure 32-4.

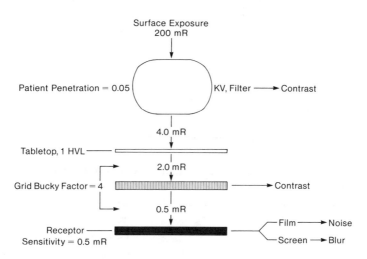

Figure 32-4 Factors That Determine Exposure Values in Radiography

Receptor Sensitivity

One of the most significant factors is the amount of radiation that must be delivered to the receptor to form a useful image. This is determined by the sensitivity of the receptor. It was shown in Chapter 14 that there is a rather wide range of sensitivity values encountered in radiography. It is generally desirable to use the most sensitive receptor that will give adequate image quality. The exposure to points within the patient's body will be a multiple of the receptor exposure.

The sensitivity of a radiographic receptor is determined both by characteristics of the intensifying screen (Chapter 14) and the film (Chapter 15). To produce a net film density of one, radiographic receptors require exposures ranging from 0.16 mR, for 800 speed systems, to more than 10 mR, for some mammographic receptors. We will illustrate our immediate discussion using a receptor that requires a 0.5-mR exposure, as shown in Figure 32-4.

Intensifying Screens

The selection of intensifying screens for a specific procedure involves a compromise between exposure and image blur or detail. The screens that require the least exposure generally produce more image blur, as discussed in Chapter 14.

Films

Films with different sensitivity (speed) values are available for radiographic procedures. The primary disadvantage in using high sensitivity film is that quantum noise is increased, as described in Chapter 21. In fact, it is possible to manufacture film that would require much less exposure than the film generally used. However, the image noise level would be unacceptable.

Grid

It was shown in Chapter 13 that the penetration of grids is generally in the range of 0.17 to 0.4. This corresponds to a Bucky factor ranging from 6.0 to 2.5. The exposure to the exit surface of the patient is the product of the receptor exposure and the grid Bucky factor. This is assuming that the receptor surface is not separated from the surface of the patient by a significant distance. The use of a high-ratio grid, which generally has a relatively low penetration, or high Bucky factor, tends to increase the ratio of patient-to-receptor exposure. Low-ratio grids reduce patient exposure by allowing more scattered radiation to contribute to the film exposure. In selecting grids, the user should be aware of the general compromise between patient exposure and image contrast.

Tabletop

In many x-ray examinations, the receptor is located below the table surface that supports the patient's body. The attenuation of radiation by the tabletop increases the ratio of patient-to-receptor exposure. It is generally recommended that the tabletop have a penetration of at least 0.5 (not more than 1 HVL). The patient exposure with a tabletop that has a penetration of 0.5 will be double the exposure if no tabletop is located between the patient and receptor.

Distance

Because of the diverging nature of an x-ray beam, the concentration of x-ray photons, or exposure, decreases with distance from the focal spot. This is the inverse-square effect. This effect increases the ratio of patient-to-receptor exposure.

Consider a point located 20% of the way between the receptor surface and the focal spot. The geometric magnification is 1.25. The exposure at this point is 1.56 times the receptor exposure because of the inverse-square effect. The distance between the surface, or point of interest, and receptor is generally fixed by the size of the patient. Therefore, the only factor that can be changed is the distance between the focal spot and point of interest.

Patient exposure is reduced by using the greatest distance possible between the focal spot and body. The effect of decreasing this distance on patient exposure is illustrated in Figure 32-5; two body sections are shown with x-ray beams that cover the same receptor area. The x-ray beam with the shorter focal-to-patient distance covers a smaller area at the entrance surface. Because the same radiation is concentrated into the smaller area, the exposure to the entrance surface and points within the patient is higher than for the x-ray beam with the greater focal-patient distance.

It is generally recommended that the distance between focal spot and patient surface should be at least 38 cm (15 in) in radiographic examinations. Fluoroscopic tables should be designed so that the focal spot is at least 38 cm below the tabletop.

The inverse-square effect increases the concentration of radiation (exposure and dose) in the patient's body. However, the total amount of radiation (surface integral exposure) is not significantly increased by decreasing the tube-to-patient distance. The same radiation energy, or number of photons, is concentrated in a smaller area.

In procedures in which the body section is separated from the receptor surface to achieve magnification, exposure can significantly increase because of the inverse-square effect. An air gap is also introduced, which reduces the amount of scattered radiation reaching the receptor. To compensate for this and to achieve the same

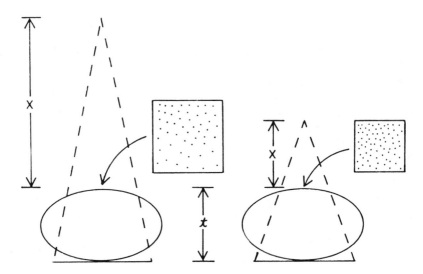

Figure 32-5 Decreasing the Distance between the X-Ray Tube Patient Surface Increases the Concentration of Radiation or Surface Exposure

film exposure, it is generally necessary to increase the x-ray machine output, which also increases exposure to the patient.

Tissue Penetration

If the point of interest, or organ, is not located at the exit surface of the body, the attenuation in the tissue layer between the organ and exit surface will further increase the exposure. The ratio of the organ-to-exit surface exposure is determined by the penetration of the tissue.

The penetration of the tissue between the point of interest and the exit surface is determined by the distance between the two points, the type of tissue (lung, soft tissue, bone, etc.), and the effective energy of the x-ray beam. For a given patient, the only factor that can be varied to alter penetration is the effective energy. This, in turn, depends on waveform, KV, and filtration. Generally speaking, three-phase, or constant potential, waveforms produce more penetrating radiation, which reduces patient exposure. It was shown earlier that adding filters to an x-ray beam selectively removes the low-energy, low-penetrating photons. This produces an x-ray beam with a greater penetrating ability. Filtration of an x-ray beam is especially significant in reducing the exposure to points near the entrance surface. Patient exposure is generally reduced by increasing KV. The problem is that the higher KV values give lower image contrast because of object penetration and more scattered radiation.

Exposure Values

The entrance surface exposure for a radiographic procedure covers a considerable range because of variations in the factors discussed above. Table 32-1 gives some typical values for a variety of procedures.

Beam Limiting

Changing the x-ray beam area (or field of view, FOV) has relatively little effect on the entrance surface exposure but has a significant effect on the total amount of radiation delivered to the patient. The surface integral exposure is directly proportional to the beam area. A large beam will deliver more radiation to the body than a small beam if all other factors are equal.

Limiting the FOV to the smallest area that fulfills the clinical requirements is an effective method for reducing unnecessary patient exposure. Under no circumstances should an x-ray beam cover an area that is larger than the receptor.

EXPOSURE DETERMINATION

The previous section identified the significant factors that affect the exposure, or dose, to a patient undergoing an x-ray examination. It is often desirable to determine the dose received by a patient in a specific examination. The relationships discussed above are generally not useful for this purpose because many of the factors, such as receptor sensitivity, scatter factor, etc., are not precisely known. It is usually easier to determine patient exposure and dose by starting with the technical factors, KV_p and MAS.

Table 32–1 Typical Patient Exposure Values for Various X-Ray Procedures

Procedure	Exposure
Skull (L)	40 – 60 mR
Chest (L)	50 – 100 mR
Chest (PA)	10 – 30 mR
Breast	500 – 2,000 mR
Abdomen	100 – 400 mR
Lumbar Spine (L)	500 – 1,500 mR
Pelvis	250 – 500 mR
Fluoroscopy (1 min)	2,000 – 5,000 mR
Computed Tomography	1,000 – 4,000 mR

The exposure (X) delivered to a point located 1 m from the focal spot is given by

$$X(mR) = E_x \times MAS$$

where E_x is the efficacy of the x-ray tube. In most facilities, x-ray machines are calibrated periodically, and the efficacy value can be obtained from the calibration reports. In the absence of a measured efficacy value for a specific machine, it might be necessary to use typical values such as are found in Figure 7-8. The efficacy values depend on KV_p, waveform, filtration, and the general condition of the x-ray tube anode. The exposure to points at other distances from the focal spot can be determined by adding an inverse-square correction to the above relationship. This gives

$$X(mR) = \frac{X}{d^2} = \frac{E_x \times MAS}{d^2}$$

where d is the distance between the focal spot and the point of interest. This relationship will apply if there is no attenuation of the x-ray beam by materials such as tissue.

When the point of interest is within the body, two additional factors must be considered: (1) the attenuation of the radiation as it passes through the overlying tissue and (2) the contribution of scattered radiation to the exposure. This can be done by multiplying the exposure value in air by the appropriate tissue-air ratio (TAR), as illustrated in Figure 32-6. Some typical TAR values for diagnostic x-ray examinations are given in Table 32-2. TAR values depend on the depth of

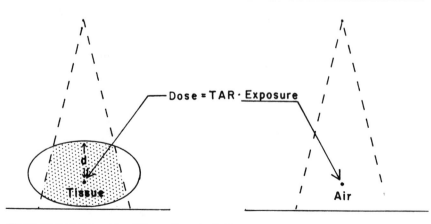

Figure 32-6 Relationship of Tissue Dose to Air Exposure

Table 32-2 TAR Values for a 40 cm × 40 cm Field and 2.5 mm
Aluminum Filtration

Tissue depth (cm)	kVp				
	70	80	90	100	120
0	1.07	1.10	1.12	1.14	1.15
2	1.06	1.09	1.11	1.15	1.20
4	0.791	0.845	0.904	0.955	1.09
6	0.566	0.625	0.679	0.726	0.813
8	0.406	0.461	0.510	0.552	0.630
10	0.291	0.340	0.383	0.420	0.489
12	0.208	0.250	0.288	0.320	0.379
14	0.149	0.185	0.217	0.243	0.294
16	0.107	0.136	0.163	0.185	0.228
18	0.077	0.100	0.122	0.141	0.177
20	0.055	0.074	0.092	0.107	0.137

[a]Data provided by R. J. Schulz.

the point of interest within the body, the penetrating ability of the x-ray beam (KV, filtration, waveform) and the size of the x-ray beam field that affects the amount of scattered radiation produced.

The relationships discussed above can be combined to give

$$\text{Dose (mrad)} = X \times \text{TAR} = \frac{E_x \times \text{MAS} \times \text{TAR}}{d^2}.$$

The fact that both x-ray tube efficacy, E, and TAR increase with KV does not mean that patients receive more radiation when the KV is increased in an examination. An increase in KV must be compensated for by decreasing MAS to obtain the same film exposure. This results in less radiation to the patient because of better penetration.

RADIONUCLIDE DOSIMETRY

One of the problems with using radioactive materials for diagnostic purposes is that a significant portion of the radiation energy is deposited in the human body. In this section we consider the characteristics of the radioactive material and the human body that determine the amount of energy that will be deposited.

Total Energy (Integral Dose)

The determination of the integral dose, or total energy deposited, is rather straightforward. As illustrated in Figure 32-7, the two factors that determine integral dose are (1) the total number of radioactive transitions that occur within the body and (2) the average energy emitted by each transition. The product of these two quantities is the total energy emitted by the radionuclide, excluding the energy carried away by the neutrino. If the radionuclide is located within the body, it can generally be assumed that most of the emitted energy will be absorbed by the body. This, however, depends on the penetrating characteristic of the radiation. If the emitted radiation is in the form of high-energy photons, some of the energy will escape from the body, but this will usually be a relatively small fraction of the total amount.

The relationship among total energy (integral dose), the average energy per transition, and the number of transitions expressed in terms of the cumulated activity is shown in Figure 32-7.

Cumulated Activity

Cumulated activity, $\bar{A}$, is a convenient way of expressing the number of transitions that occur. The units used for this quantity are microcurie-hours. Recall that 1 μCi-hr is equivalent to 1.33×10^8 radioactive transitions.

The first step in determining the amount of radiation energy deposited in a body is to determine the cumulated activity. The cumulated activity depends on two

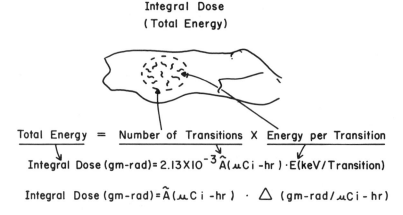

Integral Dose
(Total Energy)

Total Energy = Number of Transitions X Energy per Transition

Integral Dose (gm-rad) = $2.13 \times 10^{-3} \bar{A}(\mu Ci\text{-}hr) \cdot E(keV/Transition)$

Integral Dose (gm-rad) = $\bar{A}(\mu Ci\text{-}hr) \cdot \triangle (gm\text{-}rad/\mu Ci\text{-}hr)$

Figure 32-7 Factors That Determine the Total Amount of Radiation Energy (Integral Dose) Imparted to the Patient's Body

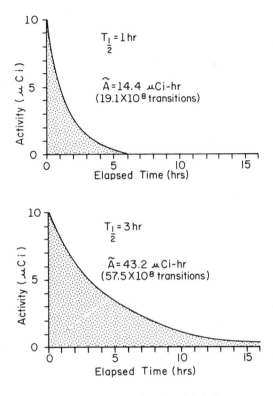

Figure 32-8 Effect of Radioactive Lifetime on Cumulated Activity

factors: (1) the amount of activity administered to the patient (A_o) and (2) the lifetime of the radioactive material within the body or organ of interest. The relationship between cumulated activity and these two quantities is

$$\tilde{A} = 1.44\, A_o\, T_e.$$

The half-life that determines cumulative activity is always the effective half-life, T_e. The relationship shown above applies only if the radioactive material is administered to or taken up by the body or organ of interest very quickly. This is usually the situation after administering a radiopharmaceutical in a single dose.

It is important to recognize the dependence of the number of transitions (cumulated activity) on the lifetime of the radionuclide. This is illustrated in Figure 32-8 for two nuclides with different half-lives. In both cases the administered activity is the same, ie, 10 μCi. The illustrations show the relationship between activity remaining in the body and elapsed time. The cumulated activity, or number of transitions, is represented by the shaded area under the curve. The point to be made is simply this: For a given amount of administered activity, the number of transitions that occur within the body (cumulated activity) is directly proportional to the half-life of the radionuclide.

In many cases when a radionuclide is administered to the patient, there is some delay in the build-up of activity in a specific organ, as illustrated in Figure 32-9. In determining the cumulated activity for the organ, it is necessary to take this delay into account. If the build-up of activity in the organ has an exponential relationship with time, the rate of uptake can be expressed in terms of an uptake "half-life." When there is a delay in organ uptake, and the uptake half-life, T_u, is significant with respect to the effective removal half-life, T_e, the relationship for finding cumulated activity becomes

$$\tilde{A} = 1.44 \, A_o \, (T_e - T_u).$$

Cumulated activity is related to the characteristics of both the radionuclide and the patient. In other words, both physical and biological factors affect cumulated activity. The physical factors, ie, administered activity and physical half-life of the nuclide, are always known. The problem in determining cumulated activity is

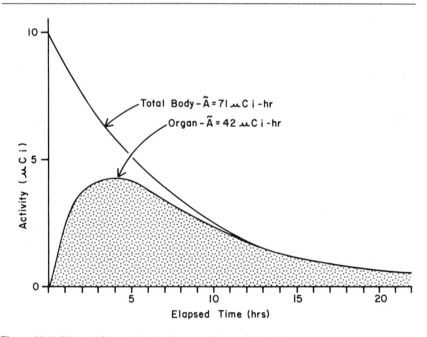

Figure 32-9 Effect of Organ Uptake Rate on Cumulated Activity

in assessing the rate of uptake and elimination. The uptake of a radionuclide in a specific organ often depends on the condition of the organ and can vary from patient to patient for the same radionuclide.

Transition Energy

Most radionuclides emit a mixture of radiations, as discussed in Chapter 5. The radiation can consist of both electrons and photons. Although the total transition energy is the same for all nuclei of a specific nuclide, the radiation energy might vary from nuclei to nuclei because of energy carried away by neutrinos and the fact that all nuclei do not go through exactly the same transition steps. The transition diagram and radiation spectrum for a hypothetical nuclide are shown in Figure 32-10. The total transition energy of 290 keV is shared by the beta electrons, neutrinos, and gamma photons.

This particular nuclide has two possible transition routes. Twenty percent of the nuclei emit a beta and neutrino followed by a 190-keV gamma photon (gamma 1). Eighty percent of the nuclei emit more energy in the form of beta and neutrino radiation and a 160-keV gamma photon (gamma 2). It is assumed in this example

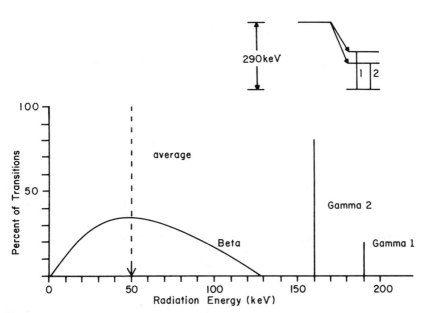

Figure 32-10 Components of a Radiation Spectrum That Must Be Considered when Determining Patient Exposure

that the average energy of all beta electrons is 50 keV. The average beta and gamma energy emitted per transition is

$$
\begin{aligned}
\text{Gamma 1: } 0.2 \times 190 &= 38 \\
\text{Gamma 2: } 0.8 \times 160 &= 128 \\
\text{Beta: } &= \underline{50} \\
&\ 216 \text{ keV.}
\end{aligned}
$$

Notice that the average radiation energy per transition (216 keV) is less than the total transition energy (290 keV) because we exclude the energy carried away from the body by the neutrinos.

The average transition energy is usually expressed in the units of gram-rad per microcurie-hour, which is designated the equilibrium dose constant, Δ. The equilibrium dose constant is the amount of radiation energy emitted by 1.33×10^8 transitions (1 μCi-hr). This is a useful quantity because the integral dose can be found by multiplying two quantities, the equilibrium dose constant and the cumulated activity, as shown in Figure 32-7. Since

$$1 \ \mu\text{Ci-hr} = 1.33 \times 10^8 \text{ transitions}$$

and

$$1 \ \text{g-rad} = 6.24 \times 10^{10} \text{ keV}$$

the relationship between the equilibrium dose constant, Δ, and the average energy per transition, E, is

$$\Delta \ (\text{g-rad}/\mu\text{Ci-hr}) = 2.13 \times 10^{-3} \ E \ (\text{keV/transition}).$$

ABSORBED DOSE

Absorbed dose is the concentration of absorbed radiation energy at a specific point. It is especially important to recognize that an absorbed dose value applies to a specific point within the body. Since radiation is usually not uniformly distributed throughout the body, there will be many absorbed dose values for the various points throughout the body or organ of interest.

Electron Radiation

If the radioactive material emits electron or particle radiation such as beta, internal conversion, Auger, or positron, the energy will be absorbed in the close vicinity of the radioactive material. Recall that a 300-keV electron can penetrate less than 1 mm of soft tissue. Most of the electron radiations encountered in nuclear medicine have energies much less than this and shorter ranges.

From the standpoint of dose estimation, the simplest situation is an organ that contains an electron emitter that is uniformly distributed throughout the organ, as illustrated in Figure 32-11. In this case, the absorbed dose is essentially the same throughout the organ and is simply the total emitted energy divided by the mass of the organ. The factors that determine the total emitted energy (integral dose) were discussed above. The absorbed dose is inversely related to organ mass. If the same amount of radiation energy is deposited in two organs that differ in size, the absorbed dose will be greater in the smaller organ.

Photon Radiation

Photon radiation, such as gamma, characteristic x-ray, and annihilation radiation, can penetrate a significant thickness of tissue and deposit energy a considerable distance from the radioactive material. This causes the absorbed dose from photon radiation to differ from that of electron radiation in two major respects: (1) Organs or parts of the body that do not contain a radioactive material can be exposed to radiation energy, and (2) the range of dose values throughout the body is generally wider.

In considering dosage factors associated with photon radiation, it is desirable to identify two organs, as shown in Figure 32-12. The organ that contains the radioactive material is designated the source organ. The organ in which the dosage is being considered is designated the target organ. With photon radiation, several target organs must usually be considered. Obviously, the source organ is also a target organ and is generally the organ that receives the greater dose.

In most cases, only a fraction of the emitted radiation energy is absorbed in a specific target organ. The fraction absorbed depends on

- the distance between the source and target organs
- the composition of the tissue between the source and target organs
- the penetrating ability (individual photon energy) of the radiation.

It was shown above that in the case of electron radiation, where the source and target organ are the same, the absorbed dose is inversely proportional to the mass of the organ. In the case of photon radiation and a target organ that is different from the source organ, the absorbed dose generally does not depend on the mass of the target organ. If the point of interest in each of two organs is located the same distance from the source organ, the points will receive the same absorbed dose regardless of the size of the target organ. The size of the target organ affects the

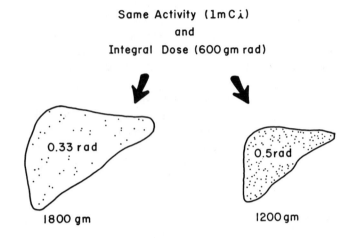

Figure 32-11 Effect of Organ Size on Absorbed Dose

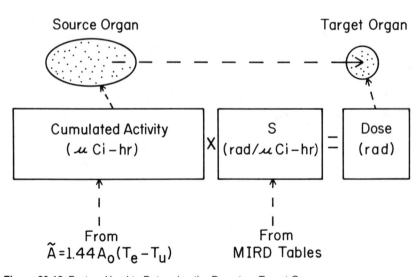

Figure 32-12 Factors Used to Determine the Dose to a Target Organ

total amount of energy absorbed by the organ, but has relatively little effect on the concentration or absorbed dose. The reason that changing target organ size might not significantly affect absorbed dose is that dose is the amount of absorbed energy per unit mass of tissue. A larger organ might absorb more energy, but because of its greater mass the energy per unit mass is essentially the same.

ESTIMATION OF DOSAGE VALUES

We have considered the factors that affect dose to a patient produced by an internal radioactive source. Some of the factors relate to the physical characteristics of the radioactive material, such as its half-life, initial activity, type of radiation, and radiation energy. Other factors relate to the anatomy and physiology of the patient's body. These include the size and location of the organs and the rates at which the body and specific organs concentrate and eliminate the radioactive material. The knowledge of these factors is helpful in understanding the variation in dose among different radionuclides and different patients. However, it is a rather difficult procedure to attempt to determine dosage values by starting from these basic factors.

The computation of estimated dosage values is greatly simplified by combining all of the physical, anatomical, and physiological factors into two composite factors, which can be multiplied together to obtain a dose estimate. One of these factors is cumulated activity, $\tilde{A}$. The other quantity is the absorbed dose per unit of cumulated activity, S (rad per microcurie-hour or rad per curie-hour). Values for S have been tabulated and published by the Medical Internal Radiation Dose (MIRD) Committee of the Society of Nuclear Medicine. A typical tabulation for a specific radionuclide is shown in Table 32-3. The MIRD tables contain the values of S for different combinations of source and target organs. The tabulated values of S are for one particular body size selected to represent a range of body sizes encountered in actual practice.

After values of $\tilde{A}$ and S are obtained for a particular radionuclide and patient, an estimation of the dose is obtained by multiplying the two factors:

$$\text{Dose (rad)} = \tilde{A} \ (\mu\text{Ci-hr}) \times S \ (\text{rad}/\mu\text{Ci-hr})$$

or

$$\text{Dose (rad)} = 10^{-6} \ A \ (\mu\text{Ci-hr}) \times S \ (\text{rad/Ci-hr})$$

when S is in the units of rad per curie-hour.

Table 32-3 Values of S, Absorbed Dose per Unit of Cumulated Activity (rad/Ci-hr), for Technetium-99m.

Target Organs	Source Organs			Intestinal Tract						
	Adrenals	Bladder Contents	Stomach Contents	SI Contents	ULI Contents	LLI Contents	Kidneys	Liver	Lungs	Other Tissue (Muscle)
Adrenals	3100.0	0.15	2.7	1.0	0.91	0.36	11.0	4.5	2.7	1.4
Bladder Wall	0.13	160.0	0.27	2.6	2.2	6.9	0.28	0.16	0.036	1.8
Bone (Total)	2.0	0.92	0.9	1.3	1.1	1.6	1.4	1.1	1.5	0.98
GI (Stomach wall)	2.9	0.27	130.0	3.7	3.8	1.8	3.6	1.9	1.8	1.3
GI (SI)	0.83	3.0	2.7	78.0	17.0	9.4	2.9	1.6	0.19	1.5
GI (ULI wall)	0.93	2.2	3.5	24.0	130.0	4.2	2.9	2.5	0.22	1.6
GI (LLI wall)	0.22	7.4	1.2	7.3	3.2	190.0	0.72	0.23	0.071	1.7
Kidneys	11.0	0.26	3.5	3.2	2.8	0.86	190.0	3.9	0.84	1.3
Liver	4.9	0.17	2.0	1.8	2.6	0.25	3.9	46.0	2.5	1.1
Lungs	2.4	0.024	1.7	0.22	0.26	0.079	0.85	2.5	52.0	1.3
Marrow (Red)	3.6	2.2	1.6	4.3	3.7	5.1	3.8	1.6	1.9	2.0
Other Tissue (Muscle)	1.4	1.8	1.4	1.5	1.5	1.7	1.3	1.1	1.3	2.7
Ovaries	0.61	7.3	0.5	11.0	12.0	18.0	1.1	0.45	0.094	2.0
Pancreas	9.0	0.23	18.0	2.1	2.3	0.74	6.6	4.2	2.6	1.8
Skin	0.51	0.55	0.44	0.41	0.41	0.48	0.53	0.49	0.53	0.72
Spleen	6.3	0.66	10.0	1.5	1.4	0.8	8.6	0.92	2.3	1.4
Testes	0.032	4.7	0.051	0.31	0.27	1.8	0.088	0.062	0.0079	1.1
Thyroid	0.13	0.0021	0.087	0.015	0.016	0.0054	0.048	0.15	0.92	1.3
Uterus (Nongravid)	1.1	16.0	0.77	0.6	5.4	7.1	0.94	0.39	0.082	2.3
Total Body	2.2	1.9	1.9	2.4	2.2	2.3	2.2	2.2	2.0	1.9

Source: Data from MIRD Pamphlet No. 11, Snyder, W.S., et al.

Chapter 33

Personnel Exposure and Protection

INTRODUCTION AND OVERVIEW

Personnel in the immediate vicinity of x-ray equipment or radioactive materials can be exposed to ionizing radiation. Therefore, certain actions must be taken to minimize their exposure and maintain it within acceptable levels.

This chapter covers the general concepts of radiation protection that apply to non-patient personnel in a medical imaging facility.

EXPOSURE LIMITS

Since it is not practical to eliminate human exposure, certain exposure limits have been established as part of the radiation protection guidelines. The exposure limits established by the National Council on Radiation Protection (NCRP) are generally adopted by other agencies involved in radiation protection. The established exposure limits do not represent levels that ensure absolute safety but rather exposure levels that carry acceptable risk to the persons involved. The recommendations of the NCRP are in the form of maximum permissible dose equivalent (MPD) values. The limits are used in designing radiation facilities and in monitoring the effectiveness of safety practices.

The recommended MPDs vary with the occupational status of the individual and the parts of the body, as shown in Figure 33-1. The exposure limits are not for exposure received as a patient undergoing an x-ray examination.

Occupational Exposure

One set of exposure limits applies to persons receiving radiation exposure because of their work. The MPD is 5 rem per year for all parts of the body that are

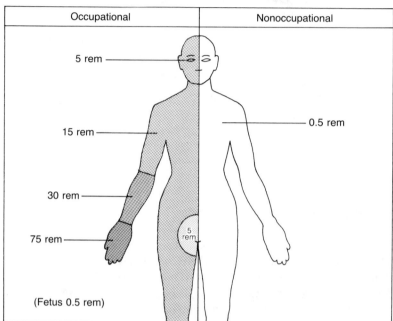

Figure 33-1 Maximum Permissible Dose Equivalent (MPD) Values

not permitted higher limits. The accumulative lifetime exposure should not exceed 5 rem per year for each year past the age of 18.

The limbs and the skin have higher MPD values than the other parts of the body. The higher limit for skin is of little practical significance for x-radiation because it is virtually impossible to expose the skin without exposing the underlying tissue.

Non-Occupationally Exposed Persons

Persons who enter a facility as patients, visitors, or persons who do not routinely work in the facility might be exposed to radiation. The MPD for the non-occupationally exposed person is one-tenth of the limit for occupationally exposed personnel.

Fetus

The MPD for a fetus is 0.5 rem for the total gestational period.

Area Exposure Limits

Areas adjacent to rooms containing radiation sources can receive significant exposure from radiation that penetrates through the walls. Wall penetration is reduced by adding a shielding or barrier material, such as lead, at the time of construction. The amount of lead added to the wall depends on the quantity of radiation produced within the room containing the equipment and the permissible levels of exposure in the adjacent areas. The permissible exposure into an area depends on two factors: (1) the MPD of the personnel occupying the areas and (2) the occupancy rate by specific individuals.

For purposes of evaluating shielding requirements, the occupancy rate of an area is assigned an occupancy factor (T). The occupancy factor represents the fraction of time the area is occupied by any one individual. Most work areas (offices, laboratories, etc.) have occupancy factor values of 1 because they are typically occupied by the same persons on a full-time basis. Areas such as stairways, toilets, etc., have relatively low occupancy factor values because the same persons are not present in these areas for any extended period of time. These areas are typically assigned minimum occupancy factor values of 1/16. Other areas, such as hallways, have occupancy factor values between these two extremes.

The maximum permissible exposure into any area is equal to the MPD for the personnel occupying the area divided by the appropriate occupancy factor, T. Areas with relatively low occupancy factors have greater area exposure limits than the MPD for the personnel in the area.

EXPOSURE SOURCES

The amount of radiation directed toward the walls of an x-ray room and producing exposure in the adjacent areas depends on several factors that must be evaluated to determine the amount of wall shielding required.

Workload

The workload, W, represents how much a specific x-ray machine is used during a typical week. It is expressed in the units of milliampere-minutes and is the sum of the MAS values for all exposures during 1 week divided by 60. For example, if we have a room that produces 250 exposures per week with an average MAS of 20 mAs per exposure, the workload would be calculated as follows:

Workload = 250 exposures $\times$ 20 mAs/exposure/60 sec/min $\cong$ 83 mA-min.

The total exposure produced each week is the product of 60 times the workload, W, and the factor K, which represents the average exposure (roentgens) at a distance of 1 from the focal spot for each 1 mAs of tube charge. The actual exposure produced by an x-ray tube depends on factors such as KV_p, waveform, and filtration, as discussed in Chapter 7. Values of K corresponding to the maximum x-ray machine KV_p are used to calculate exposure. A K value of 20 mR/mAs is a typical value for a three-phase x-ray machine operating at 120 kV_p, taken from Figure 7-10 (Chapter 7). The weekly exposure produced at this K value is

Exposure $= 60(\text{sec/min}) \times 83 \ (\text{mA/min}) \times 20(\text{mR/mAs}) \cong 100,000 \ \text{mR/wk.}$

Utilization Factor

The direction of the x-ray beam must also be considered. For the purposes of exposure analysis, x-ray beam direction is expressed in terms of a utilization factor, U, for each of the walls, ceiling, and floor of the room containing the x-ray equipment. Each surface (wall) has a utilization factor value that represents the fraction of time the x-ray beam is directed toward it. If an x-ray beam is fixed in one direction, that particular wall will have a utilization factor value of 1.

The exposure to each wall also depends on the distance, d, between the x-ray source and the wall. The exposure decreases inversely with the square of the distance. These two factors are used in conjunction with the machine exposure to determine the exposure to a specific wall.

We now carry our example one more step and determine the x-ray beam exposure to a wall located 3 m from the x-ray tube that has a utilization factor value of 0.5.

Exposure $= 100,000 \ \text{mR/wk} \times 0.5/3^2 = 5,555 \ \text{mR/wk.}$

Scattered Radiation

We have considered the possibility of a primary x-ray beam projecting exposure onto walls and into adjacent areas. Calculations of the type illustrated here generally produce a conservative overestimate of all exposure because the primary x-ray beam is always attenuated by the patient's body and the image receptor.

In most facilities, the most significant source of area exposure is the scattered radiation produced by the patient's body. The relationship used to calculate primary beam exposure is modified in the following manner to produce an estimate of exposure produced by scattered radiation.

It is generally assumed for this type of analysis that the scatter exposure at a distance of 1 m from a patient's body is 0.001 of the primary beam exposure entering the body; or, in other words, each roentgen of primary beam exposure produces 1 mR of scattered radiation. Since scattered radiation goes in virtually all directions, utilization factor values of 1 are assigned to all walls, ceilings, and floors. The distance between the irradiated portion of the patient's body and the wall is also used in the calculation.

If we assume that the wall of interest in our example is also 3 m from the patient's body, the scattered radiation exposure to the wall is

$$\text{Scatter Exposure} = 100,000 \ (\text{mR/wk}) \times 0.001 \ (\text{Scatter Factor})/3^2 \cong 11 \ \text{mR/wk}.$$

AREA SHIELDING

If the exposure to a wall exceeds the exposure limit for the adjacent area, a barrier or shield is required. A specific barrier or shield is characterized by its penetration value. The maximum permissible wall penetration is the ratio of the area exposure limit to the calculated wall exposure. As an example, if the wall of an area that has an exposure limit of 100 mR per week receives an exposure of 5,555 mR per week, the maximum barrier penetration will be:

$$\text{Wall Penetration} = 100 \ (\text{mR/wk})/5,555 (\text{mR/wk}) = 0.018.$$

Several materials are used to shield areas within an x-ray facility. Many building materials provide significant shielding. Where the building material shielding is inadequate, sheets of lead are added to the walls to reduce the total penetration to an acceptable level.

PERSONNEL SHIELDING

Shielding is usually required for personnel located in the same area as a patient undergoing an x-ray examination. Although the scattered exposure produced by a single procedure is relatively small, significant exposures can result from working with patients on a regular basis. The greatest potential for personnel exposure usually comes from fluoroscopic procedures. If we assume a side scatter value of 0.001 (1 mR/R), a 10-minute fluoroscopic procedure with a patient exposure rate of 3 R/min will produce a scatter exposure of 30 mR at a distance of 1 m from the patient. This is approximately one-third the MPD for 1 week. At a distance of 0.5 m from the patient, the exposure from this one procedure could easily exceed the MPD for 1 week.

Exposure to personnel can be reduced to acceptable levels by using lead aprons, drapes, and other shielding devices.

EXPOSURE FROM RADIOACTIVE SOURCES

It is occasionally necessary to consider the exposure produced by a radiation source external to the body. This is primarily a problem with photon radiation. Since electron radiation has a short penetrating range and is easily contained or shielded, it generally does not present an exposure problem when the source is not within the body. We therefore limit this discussion to exposure produced by photon radiation.

Several factors affect the exposure produced by an external radioactive source, as illustrated in Figure 33-2. At this point, we need to distinguish between exposure (milliroentgens) and exposure rate (milliroentgens per hour). The exposure produced by a radioactive source is related to the cumulated activity (microcurie-hours), whereas exposure rate is related to the activity, A (microcuries), at a particular time.

The number of photons per transition and photon energy have characteristic values for each radionuclide. When these factors are known, it is possible to determine the exposure rate at a standard distance, such as 1 m from a radioactive source. This exposure value is generally designated the gamma constant (Γ). The value of the gamma constant is the exposure rate (mR/hr) at a distance of 1 m from a 1-mCi source. It also is the exposure (mR) produced by a cumulated activity of 1 mCi-hr. The gamma constant can therefore be expressed in the units of milliroentgens per millicurie-hour or milliroentgens per hour per millicurie.

The gamma constants for three selected nuclides are

Nuclide	Gamma Constant (mR/mCi-hr)
Technetium-99m	0.072
Iodine-131	0.22
Cobalt-57	0.093

Values for other nuclides are tabulated in various nuclear medicine reference books. The precise calculation of the gamma constant value for a specific nuclide requires a knowledge of the attenuation coefficient of air at each photon energy. However, over the range of photon energies normally encountered in nuclear medicine, the approximate gamma constant can be calculated from

$$\Gamma \ (\text{mR/mCi-hr}) \cong 0.0005n \times E(\text{keV})$$

where n is the fraction of transitions that produce a specific energy photon (yield) and E is the energy of the photons. If a radionuclide produces photons of more than one energy, the gamma constant value for the nuclide will be the sum of the values for each photon energy.

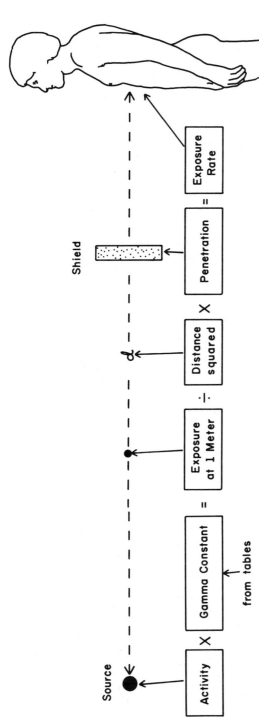

Figure 33-2 Factors That Determine Human Exposure from an External Gamma-Emitting Radioactive Source

Since the gamma constant value represents the exposure (or exposure rate) for 1 unit of cumulated activity (or activity), it is necessary to multiply the gamma constant value by the actual activity value. This product is the exposure at a distance of 1 m from the source. The exposure at any other distance is determined by dividing the exposure at 1 m by the square of the distance (d^2) because of the inverse-square effect. If the radiation passes through a material that has significant absorption characteristics, such as a shield, the exposure value must be multiplied by the penetration value of the material (P).

The relationship of these factors can be summarized as follows:

$$\text{Exposure Rate (mR/hr)} = [A(mCi)\ \Gamma\ (mR/hr/mCi)\ P]/d^2(m^2)$$

$$\text{Exposure (mR)} = [\tilde{A}(mCi\text{-}hr)\ \Gamma\ (mR/mCi\text{-}hr)\ P]/d^2(m^2).$$

In many instances the exposure time (t) to an external source is relatively short in comparison with the lifetime (half-life) of the radionuclide. If there is no significant radioactive decay during the exposure interval, then the cumulative activity ($\tilde{A}$) will be the product of the activity (A) and the exposure time (t). In this case, the expression for exposure is

$$\text{Exposure (mR)} = [A(mCi) \times t(hr) \times \Gamma(mR/mCi\text{-}hr) \times P]/d^2(m^2).$$

Chapter 34

Radiation Measurement

INTRODUCTION AND OVERVIEW

There are many occasions when it is necessary to measure the radiation used in diagnostic procedures. Several instruments are used for this purpose. The selection of a specific measuring device depends on several factors including the relative intensity of the radiation and the required measurement accuracy.

The most general radiation measurement activities and the devices used to measure each are

Measurement	Device
X-ray beam exposure	Ionization chambers
Environment exposure	Survey meters
Personnel exposure	Film badges
	Thermoluminescence dosimeters
Radioactivity	Scintillation detectors
	Activity calibrators

IONIZATION CHAMBERS

Exposure is defined in terms of the amount of ionization produced by the radiation. Therefore, the most direct way to measure exposure is to collect and measure the ions produced by the radiation in air. This can be done by using an ionization chamber. All chambers consist of a volume of air located between two electrical conductors, or electrodes, mounted on insulating material. The electrodes collect the ions formed within the air volume. Ionization chambers are generally used in two modes of operation: (1) to measure exposure rates and (2) to measure total accumulated exposure over a period of time.

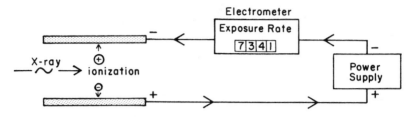

Figure 34-1 Ionization Chamber System for Measuring Exposure Rate

Exposure Rate Measurements

The basic system for measuring exposure rate with an ionization chamber is shown in Figure 34-1. In addition to the ionization chamber, a power supply and a device that will measure small electrical currents are required. The device normally used to measure the currents is the electrometer.

The three components are connected in a circuit, as shown. The power supply applies a voltage to the chamber, which causes one electrode to be negative and the other positive. If the air between the electrodes is not ionized, it is an insulator, and no electrical current can flow between the electrodes and through the circuit. However, when the air is exposed to x-radiation, it becomes ionized and electrically conductive. Ionization is a process that either adds or removes electrons from an atom. This causes the atom to take on an electrical charge.

Figure 34-1 shows how conduction takes place when an electron is removed from an atom by the radiation. The electron is attracted to the positive electrode, where it is collected and pumped through the circuit by the power supply. The arrows indicate the direction of electron flow. The positive ion is attracted to the negative electrode. When it reaches the electrode, it picks up an electron and becomes neutral. The electron that was absorbed from the negative electrode is replaced by an electron from the circuit. Because electrons enter the ionization chamber at the negative terminal and leave from the positive terminal, the ionization chamber becomes, in effect, a conductor. For a given ionization chamber, the amount of conduction, or current, is proportional to the exposure rate. When the system is calibrated, the electrometer indicates the exposure rate in units, such as roentgens per minute or milliroentgens per hour.

Exposure Measurements

Ionization chambers can also be used to measure accumulated exposure. One method is a three-step process, as illustrated in Figure 34-2.

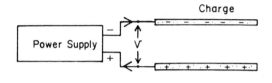

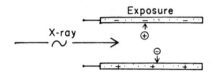

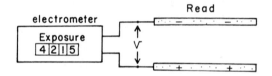

Figure 34-2 Ionization Chamber System for Measuring Accumulated Exposure

The first step is to "charge" the ionization chamber by connecting it to a power supply. This is done before the chamber is exposed to the radiation. Since an ionization chamber consists of two conductors separated by an insulator (non-ionized air), it forms an electrical capacitor. The power supply pumps some of the electrons from the positive electrode to the negative. The quantity of electrons moved depends on the size of the chamber and the voltage applied by the power supply. The movement of electrons is what is generally referred to as charging the chamber. If the ionization chamber is disconnected from the power supply, the charge will remain until a conductive path is formed between the two electrodes. Voltage is present between the two electrodes even after the power supply is removed. For a given ionization chamber, the voltage is proportional to the charge, or number, of displaced electrons.

In the second step, the charged chamber is exposed to ionizing radiation, and the air becomes conductive and discharges the chamber. This happens in the following way. The positively charged ions are attracted to the negative electrode, where they pick up some of the excess electrons. The electrons formed in the air by the ionization are attracted to and collected by the positive electrode. The number of electrons that are returned to their normal locations is proportional to the exposure to the air within the chamber.

The third step is to determine the exposure value by reading the voltage that remains across the chamber after it is exposed to radiation. The voltage is usually read with an electrometer. By using appropriate calibration factors, the drop in chamber voltage produced by the ionization can be converted into appropriate exposure units, such as roentgens or milliroentgens.

In practice, exposure measurements should be made over relatively short time intervals to avoid error from chamber leakage. Leakage is the discharge of the chamber from sources other than radiation, such as moisture on the insulating materials.

Errors in Exposure Measurement

Several factors must be considered when using ionization chambers to make exposure measurements. Most ionization chambers are not absolute devices and must be calibrated against a standard. A "free air ionization chamber" is used as the standard in most calibration laboratories. The device is a specially designed instrument in which the sensitive air volume is not in direct contact with the electrodes but is surrounded by a buffer region of air. This prevents x-ray interactions with the electrodes from influencing the amount of ionization within the sensitive air volume. In the free air ionization chamber, the ions are collected from a precisely determined volume of air. When the amount of ionization is measured with a properly calibrated electrometer, an accurate exposure determination can be made. Free air ionization chambers are not used for routine exposure measurements but as a standard for calibrating other types of ionization chambers.

The response of an ionization chamber in terms of the number of ions produced and collected per unit of exposure can change with exposure conditions. Because of this, it is often necessary to use various correction factors to get precise exposure measurements.

Photon Energy Dependence

In most ionization chambers the amount of ionization produced per exposure unit varies with photon energy. This is usually related to the interaction of the x-ray beam with the walls of the chamber. A significant portion of the x-ray photons that contribute to the ionization are absorbed in the chamber walls. Some of the energetic electrons created by photoelectric and Compton interactions within the walls enter the air volume and produce ionization. For a given energy, there is a specific wall thickness that allows maximum ionization. This is known as the equilibrium thickness and is approximately proportional to the photon energy. At low photon energies, a thick chamber wall attenuates the x-ray beam and reduces the chamber response. At high photon energies, a thin chamber wall does not provide adequate material to interact with the x-ray beam and produce maximum ionization.

An ionization chamber should be selected for the particular type of radiation to be measured. For example, most chambers designed for high-energy therapy radiation are generally not well suited to the measurement of diagnostic radiation. Even when a chamber is designed for a specific photon energy range or beam quality, it is often necessary to use correction factors for the different beam quality (KV) values.

Saturation

There are conditions in which all ions formed by the radiation are not collected and measured. The electrons and positive ions that result from the ionization process are known as ion pairs. Unless they are quickly separated, there is a good chance they will recombine because of their opposite electrical charges. The ion pairs that recombine do not contribute to the exposure measurement. Therefore, in order to get an accurate indication of the amount of ionization produced, it is necessary to separate the ion pairs before recombination can occur. This is achieved by applying a sufficient voltage between the electrodes. As the voltage across the chamber is increased, the force on the ions is also increased, and they are separated more quickly. When the voltage applied to the chamber is enough to prevent any recombination, the chamber is said to be saturated. The voltage required to produce saturation depends on the size and shape of the chamber and the rate at which ionization is being produced. Large chambers require a higher voltage to produce saturation than small chambers. For a given chamber, the voltage required to produce saturation depends on the exposure rate. When some chambers are used to make measurements at high exposure rates, saturation is not achieved, and it is necessary to apply a saturation correction factor to obtain the correct exposure value.

SURVEY METERS

Laboratories that use radioactive materials are usually required to have an instrument that can be used to measure exposure to personnel and to locate and measure the relative activity of sources, such as a spilled radionuclide. From time to time, it is also necessary to measure the environmental exposure produced by scattered radiation during an x-ray procedure. An instrument that can be used for these purposes is generally referred to as a survey meter. Survey meters can be constructed using several radiation detectors. The most common detectors used for this purpose are Geiger-Mueller (GM) tubes and ionization chambers. Scintillation detectors are not widely used for this purpose because they are generally larger, more complex, and more expensive than the other types of detectors.

Geiger-Mueller Detector

The major components of a GM survey meter are shown in Figure 34-3. The detector (GM or Geiger tube) is a cylindrical tube that contains a specially formulated gas mixture and two electrodes. One electrode is a small wire running along the axis of the cylinder. The other electrode is the wall of the cylinder, which is electrically conductive. The tube is connected to a power supply that applies a relatively high voltage (500 to 1,000 V) between the two electrodes. The other two components are a count-rate meter and a device, such as a small speaker or earphones, that produces an audible signal.

When a radiation photon or electron enters the tube and interacts, it produces ionization within the gas. Generally, each ionization produces an ion pair consisting of an electron and an atom with a positive charge. Because the electrons and ions have electrical charges, they are attracted to the electrodes that have the opposite electrical polarity. For example, the negative electrons produced in the initial ionization process are pulled toward the positive electrode located at the

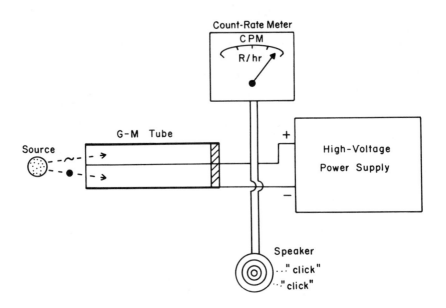

Figure 34-3 Geiger-Mueller (GM) Survey Meter

center of the tube. Because of the relatively high voltage applied between the electrodes, the electrons are accelerated as they move along. After moving a short distance, the electrons gain sufficient kinetic energy so that they, in turn, collide with and ionize other gas atoms and molecules. This process produces a second generation of electrons that is larger in number than the first generation produced by the radiation. The second-generation electrons are also accelerated until they can produce additional ionizations and an even larger third generation of electrons. This electron multiplying process is repeated until the ionization spreads throughout the tube. Because of this avalanche effect, the number of electrons that eventually reach the central electrode is many times larger than the number of electrons produced by the radiation photon or particle. When the electrons reach the electrode, they are collected and conducted out of the tube in the form of an electrical pulse. An important characteristic of a GM tube is that the pulse is relatively large and requires very little, if any, additional amplification. The avalanche effect is a form of amplification that occurs within the tube.

The number of pulses produced by a GM tube is proportional to the number of photons or radiation electrons interacting with the detector. The efficiency of a GM detector, compared with a scintillation detector, for gamma photons is relatively low. This is because many photons can penetrate the tube without interacting. Recall that radiation must interact with and be absorbed in a detector before a signal can be created. Even so, a GM survey meter can detect low levels of radiation because it can respond to individual photons.

The basic problem in measuring beta radiation is getting the electrons into the tube. Most beta electrons cannot penetrate the glass walls of the tube. This problem is overcome by constructing tubes with a thin window in the end that can be penetrated by radiation particles, such as beta electrons. A GM tube cannot generally distinguish between a photon and a beta electron.

The pulses from the GM tube can be counted in two ways. Many instruments are equipped with a speaker or earphone in which each pulse is heard as a sharp "click." This type of output is useful when searching for a source, such as spilled radioactive material. When listening to the pulses, it is relatively easy to detect small changes in the radiation level.

A more precise indication of radiation level can be obtained by electronically counting the pulses and displaying the count rate on a meter. On most survey meters, the count-rate meter has two scales. One scale indicates the count rate in counts per minute (cpm), and the other scale indicates exposure rate, typically in the units of milliroentgens per hour (mR/hr). GM survey meters usually do not produce precise measurements of exposure rate. This is because the response of GM tubes is often photon-energy dependent. In other words, an exposure of 1 mR of 100-keV photons might produce a different number of counts than a 1-mR exposure of 300-keV photons. Survey meters are usually calibrated at one specific photon energy. If the instrument is to be used to measure exposure rates, it is necessary to have some knowledge of its energy dependence.

The major advantage of a GM survey meter is that it is relatively simple and can detect low levels of radiation.

Ionization Chambers

Another type of survey meter uses an ionization chamber detector. The chambers designed for survey meters generally use the cylinder wall as one electrode and a wire along the cylinder axis for the other. The ionization chamber differs from the GM tube in several respects. It is generally much larger. Rather than a special gas mixture, the ionization chamber contains air at atmospheric pressure. The survey meter contains a power supply that applies a voltage between the two chamber electrodes. However, the voltage used to operate an ionization chamber is much less than that required to operate a GM tube.

When radiation enters the ionization chamber, it interacts with the air and produces ionization. The ions and electrons are attracted to the electrodes. Because a lower voltage is used, the electrons in the ionization chamber are not accelerated enough to produce additional ionization, as in the GM tube. The only electrons and ions collected by the electrodes are the ones produced directly by the radiation. Because no electron multiplication (amplification) occurs in the ionization chamber, the output signal is relatively small. The signal is in the form of a very weak current that is proportional to the radiation exposure rate. The current is amplified, and its value displayed on a meter calibrated to indicate exposure rate (mR/hr).

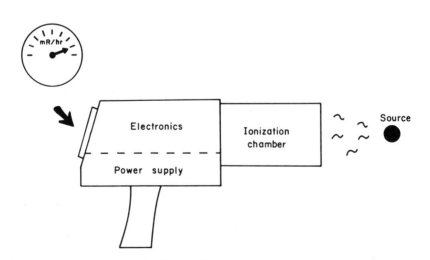

Figure 34-4 Ionization Chamber Survey Meter

In comparing an ionization chamber survey meter to a GM-tube type, the ionization chamber is generally less sensitive and does not detect low radiation levels. It is, however, a more precise instrument for measuring exposure levels.

A common configuration for this type of survey meter is one in which the chamber, electronics, and meter are mounted on a pistol-grip handle, as shown in Figure 34-4. This type of instrument is often referred to as a "cutie-pie."

Film Badges

Film can be used to measure exposure. The most common application of film is to measure personnel exposure within the clinical facility. This is normally done by placing a small piece of film in a badge that is then worn on the body. Film badges can be used to monitor personnel exposure over extended periods of time, such as 1 month or longer. Film badges generally cannot measure exposure with the same accuracy as most other devices.

Thermoluminescence Dosimetry

Thermoluminescence is a process in which materials emit light when they are heated. Certain thermoluminescent materials can be used as dosimeters because the amount of light emitted is proportional to the amount of radiation absorbed by the material before heating. Two materials used in thermoluminescence dosimetry (TLD) are lithium fluoride and calcium fluoride. These materials consist of small crystals that can be used in a powdered form or molded into various shapes.

TLD is a two-step procedure, as illustrated in Figure 34-5. The first step is to expose the TLD material to the radiation. A portion of the absorbed radiation

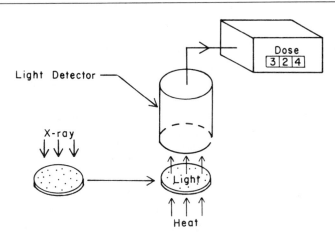

Figure 34-5 The Two Steps in Radiation Measurement Using a Thermoluminescence Dosimeter

energy is used to raise electrons to higher energy levels. A characteristic of TLD material is that some of the electrons are trapped in the higher energy locations. The number of electrons that remain in the elevated energy positions is proportional to the amount of radiation energy absorbed, or the absorbed dose. The second step is to place the irradiated TLD material in a special reader unit. This unit heats the TLD material and measures the amount of light emitted during the heating process. Heating frees the trapped electrons and allows them to drop to their normal low energy positions. The energy difference between the two electron locations is given off in the form of light. By calibrating the system, the light output is converted into absorbed dose values.

TLD dosimeters have several advantages over ionization chambers. A TLD can measure a much greater range of dose (or exposure) values than a single ionization chamber. They are also dose-rate independent and do not have the saturation problems common to ionization chambers. Another useful property is the ability of a TLD to collect radiation over a much longer period of time than is possible with ionization chambers. This makes them very useful for monitoring personnel and area exposures.

A TLD actually measures absorbed dose in the thermoluminescent material. Since most materials used as thermoluminescent dosimeters have approximately the same effective atomic number as soft tissue and air, the TLD reading will be proportional to both tissue absorbed dose and exposure in air. Some TLD materials have a response that changes more with photon energy than others. Therefore, it is desirable to calibrate a TLD system for the type of radiation (photon energy) to be measured.

ACTIVITY MEASUREMENT

In nuclear medicine procedures, diagnostic information is obtained by either measuring the relative activity in a specific organ or sample, or by forming an image that shows the spatial distribution of the radioactive material. In many situations, it is also desirable to measure the quantity of radioactive material (activity) before it is administered to a patient.

Most systems used for these purposes use a scintillation detector. The major components of such a system are shown in Figure 34-6. Systems used to measure relative activity do so by counting photons or radiation particles over a period of time, and are therefore generally referred to as scintillation counters.

All systems contain a detector that absorbs the photons and produces electrical pulses. The size of the pulses is generally proportional to the energy of the photons. The pulses then pass through a linear amplifier, which increases the size of each pulse. From the amplifier the pulses enter a pulse height analyzer (PHA). If the pulse size (height) is within a certain range (set by the operator), it will pass through the PHA. If the pulse size is not within the selected range, it will be blocked by the PHA. Since pulse size is proportional to photon energy, the PHA passes pulses that correspond to a specific range of photon energies. The main purpose of the PHA is to eliminate pulses created by scattered radiation, background radiation, or other radioactive materials in or near the patient. In order to measure relative activity, the pulses go to a counter circuit.

The Scintillation Detector

A scintillation, or scintilla, is a flash of light. In the scintillation detector, the radiation, typically a gamma photon, is absorbed by a crystal that converts some of the absorbed energy into a flash of light, or a scintillation. The light from the crystal enters a PM tube in which it is converted into an electrical pulse. The relationship of the crystal to the PM tube is shown in Figure 34-7.

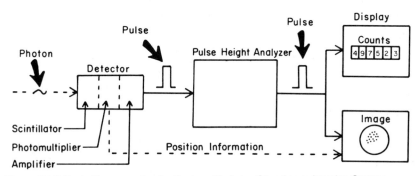

Figure 34-6 Basic Components of a Nuclear Medicine Counting or Imaging System

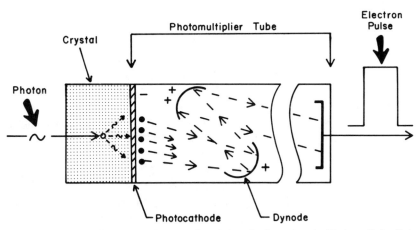

Figure 34-7 Typical Scintillation Detector Consisting of a Crystal and a Photomultiplier Tube

Crystals

The crystals in scintillation detectors perform two major functions: (1) to absorb the gamma photons and (2) to convert the energy into light. A number of materials will do this, but the most commonly used is sodium iodide (NaI). The presence of the iodine in the crystal enhances photon absorption. When the crystal is impregnated with an appropriate activator, such as thallium, NaI(Tl), it becomes an efficient scintillator.

An important characteristic of a detector crystal is its ability to capture the photons emitted by the radioactive material and produce a pulse. This is generally referred to as the efficiency of the detector. To a large extent, the efficiency is related to the size of the crystal. Photons from a radioactive source are emitted uniformly in all directions. Therefore, if the detector crystal is located at some distance from the source, only a small fraction of the emitted photons will enter the crystal. More photons can be captured by either increasing the size (surface area) of the crystal or by reducing the distance between the crystal and the radioactive source.

All photons intercepted by the crystal are not necessarily absorbed. A photon can penetrate the crystal without interacting and producing a scintillation. For a given crystal material, the chance of a photon penetrating the crystal is determined by photon energy and crystal thickness. The penetration through a specific crystal increases with photon energy, except when a K edge is encountered. The point to be made is simply this: The crystal thickness determines the absorption efficiency for the various photon energies. In general, thick crystals must be used with high energy photons to obtain good absorption efficiencies.

The size of the crystal does not affect the amount of light produced by a given photon energy. Its only significant effect is on the number of photons absorbed.

Photomultiplier Tubes

The scintillations produced in the crystal or liquid scintillators by the absorbed radiation is detected and converted into an electrical pulse by the PM tube. The basic construction of a PM tube is illustrated in Figure 34-7. The electrical components are contained in a glass cylinder approximately 15 cm long with a diameter between 2.5 cm and 5 cm. One end of the tube is a flat transparent window through which the light from the scintillator enters. Inside the window is a thin layer of material that forms a photocathode. When light photons strike the front surface of the photocathode, they undergo a photoelectric interaction, and electrons are emitted from the rear surface. The number of electrons emitted is proportional to the number of light photons, which, in turn, is proportional to the brightness of the scintillation. The number of electrons produced by a single scintillation is relatively small and would be a very weak electrical pulse. In order to have a pulse that can be counted or used to form an image, it is necessary to increase the size, or strength, of the pulse. This is the second function performed by the PM tube.

The PM tube contains a series of cup-shaped metal electrodes, commonly referred to as dynodes, positioned as shown in Figure 34-7. An electrical voltage from an external power supply is applied to the dynodes through wires that enter the rear end of the tube. The voltage is divided among the dynodes and applied so that each succeeding dynode is more positive than the one before it. The first dynode is positive with respect to the photocathode. The electrons emitted from the photocathode are therefore attracted to the first dynode. As they travel from the photocathode to the dynode, they are accelerated and gain kinetic energy. When one of the energetic electrons strikes the dynode, it has sufficient energy to knock out several electrons. This process increases the number of electrons in the group associated with a single scintillation. The group of electrons from the first dynode is accelerated toward the second dynode where they strike the surface and emit additional electrons. This process is repeated throughout the series of dynodes. The electron group reaching the last electrode is collected and conducted out of the tube in the form of an electrical pulse. The size of the pulse is determined by the number of electrons. The number of electrons reaching the last electrode is approximately 1 million times the number of electrons emitted from the cathode.

The output from the PM tube is an electrical pulse whose size is proportional to the brightness of the scintillation, which should be proportional to the energy of the radiation photon or particle. For a given scintillation brightness (photon energy), the size of the pulse depends on the electron multiplication, or gain, that occurs within the PM tube. This is influenced, to some extent, by the amount of voltage applied between the tube dynodes. As this voltage is increased, the electrons gain more energy in moving from one dynode to another. This causes each electron to produce a greater number of electrons when it strikes the next dynode. In some detector systems, the voltage applied to the PM tube is adjustable and can be used as a gain control to change the pulse size (and to calibrate a scintillation detector with respect to radiation energy).

Amplifier

Even though the pulse from the PM tube is increased in size approximately 1 million times, it is still too small to be processed by the counting or imaging components. The sizes of the pulse can be increased by passing it through an electronic amplifier, as shown in Figure 34-8. It is important that all pulses be amplified by the same factor so that a proportionality between pulse size and photon energy is maintained. An amplifier with this characteristic is generally known as a linear amplifier. In many systems, the gain, or amount of amplification, is adjustable. This can also be used to calibrate the system with respect to photon energy.

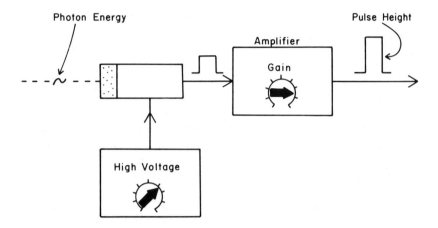

Figure 34-8 Two Factors, Amplifier Gain and PM Tube High Voltage, Used to Adjust the Size of the Pulse from a Scintillation Detector

Scintillation Probes

In a number of procedures it is necessary to measure the radiation coming from specific organs or areas of the body. While this can be done with a gamma camera, it may be more practical in some situations to perform the measurements with a collimated scintillation detector or probe. This type of detector consists of a single scintillation crystal mounted in a shield or collimator. The shield is usually constructed of lead and performs two basic functions: It shields the detector crystal from environmental radiation and produces a known field of view (FOV) for the crystal. The efficiency of the detector is determined by the size of the crystal and its distance from the radiation source.

Well Counters

When the radiation source is small and can be placed in a vial, maximum counting efficiency is obtained by inserting the source into a hole or well in the crystal, as shown in Figure 34-9. This configuration virtually surrounds the source with the crystal and gives a very high geometric efficiency. Maximum efficiency is obtained with small sources confined to the bottom portion of the well. If the source material fills the well, more of the radiation will escape out of the top, and the efficiency will be reduced.

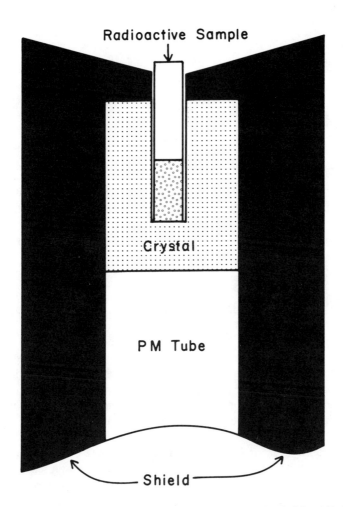

Figure 34-9 Scintillation Well Counter Used to Measure the Relative Activity of Radioactive Samples

Liquid Scintillator Counters

Solid scintillation materials are quite adequate for radiation that can penetrate into the scintillator, such as photon radiation. Beta radiation has a very short range and is normally absorbed within 1 mm of the point of origination. Liquid scintillators overcome this problem by allowing the radioactive material to be mixed into the scintillator itself, as shown in Figure 34-10. The scintillation liquid usually consists of three components: (1) a solvent, (2) a primary scintillator, and

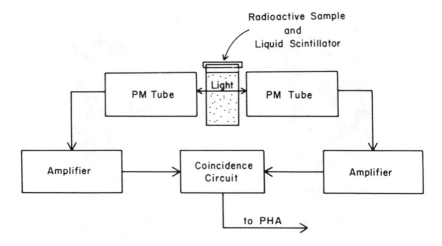

Figure 34-10 Liquid Scintillation Counter Used to Measure the Activity of Beta-Emitting Radionuclides

(3) a secondary scintillator. The scintillators are chemical compounds with fluorescent properties. The function of the primary scintillator is to convert some of the beta particle energy into light. A portion of the light from many primary scintillators is in the ultraviolet region of the spectrum and is not readily detectable by the PM tubes. The purpose of the secondary scintillator is to absorb the ultraviolet light and emit light of a color (wavelength) more readily detectable by the PM tubes.

The radioactive material must be properly prepared so that it does not significantly decrease the transparency of the liquid. Also, the presence of certain chemical substances reduces the energy transfer to the primary scintillator and thereby reduces light output. The reduction in light output produced by the presence of unwanted chemical substances is referred to as *quenching*.

Activity Calibrators

It is usually desirable to measure the activity of a radionuclide before it is administered to a patient. In most facilities, this is done with an instrument known as an activity or dose calibrator. The basic components of a typical calibrator are shown in Figure 34-11.

The detector used in most calibrators is an ionization chamber. The ionization chamber is generally filled with an inert gas, such as argon, to a pressure of several atmospheres. The radioactive material to be calibrated is placed into a well surrounded by the gas. Some of the photons from the radioactive material interact with the gas and produce ionization. Within limits, the rate at which ions are produced is proportional to the activity of the sample being calibrated. The activity of the sample can therefore be determined by measuring the amount of ionization produced in a known period of time. Two additional components are required to collect and measure the ionization. One is a high-voltage power supply and the other is an electrometer. These are connected to the ionization chamber, as shown in Figure 34-11. In addition to the gas, the ionization chamber has two electrodes, or conductors. When the power supply is energized, it causes one of the electrodes to assume a positive and the other a negative voltage. The ions formed in the gas are attracted to the electrode with a polarity opposite to the charge on the ion. Positive ions attracted to the negative electrode, and negative ions, or freed electrons, are attracted to the positive electrode. The ionization, in effect, makes the chamber electrically conductive. While ionization is taking place, electrons are collected by the positive electrode, and a current flows through the circuit as indicated. The current is proportional to the rate at which ions are being produced, which, in turn, is related to the activity. The current is measured by the electrometer. The system is calibrated so that the current value is displayed in units of activity, millicuries or microcuries.

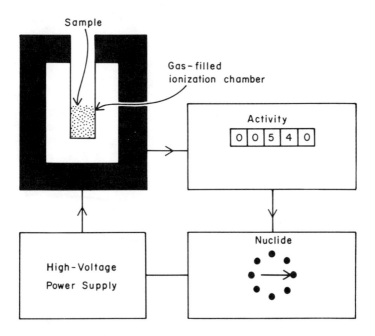

Figure 34-11 Basic Components of an Activity Calibrator

The relationship between ionization rate and sample activity is not the same for all radionuclides for several reasons. All nuclides do not emit exactly one photon per transition. (This was discussed in Chapter 5.) Some nuclei go through a transition process that creates only one photon, whereas others undergo transitions that create two or more photons. The various nuclides also produce photons with different energies. Both the percentage of photons that will interact with a gas and the number of ions produced by each photon depend on the photon energy. Because of this, it is necessary to use a different calibration factor to relate activity to ionization for each radionuclide. Most systems have a switch that can be used to set the correct calibration factor for a variety of radionuclides.

Index